Molecular Diagnosis of Cancer

METHODS IN MOLECULAR MEDICINE™

John M. Walker, Series Editor

102. Autoimmunity: *Methods and Protocols,* edited by *Andras Perl, 2004*

101. Cartilage and Osteoarthritis: *Volume 2, Structure and In Vivo Analysis,* edited by *Frederic De Ceuninck, Massimo Sabatini, and Philippe Pastoureau, 2004*

100. Cartilage and Osteoarthritis: *Volume 1, Cellular and Molecular Tools,* edited by *Massimo Sabatini, Philippe Pastoureau, and Frederic De Ceuninck, 2004*

99. Pain Research: *Methods and Protocols,* edited by *David Z. Luo, 2004*

98. Tumor Necrosis Factor: *Methods and Protocols,* edited by *Angelo Corti and Pietro Ghezzi, 2004*

97. Molecular Diagnosis of Cancer: *Methods and Protocols, Second Edition,* edited by *Joseph E. Roulston and John M. S. Bartlett, 2004*

96. Hepatitis B and D Protocols: *Volume 2, Immunology, Model Systems, and Clinical Studies,* edited by *Robert K. Hamatake and Johnson Y. N. Lau, 2004*

95. Hepatitis B and D Protocols: *Volume 1, Detection, Genotypes, and Characterization,* edited by *Robert K. Hamatake and Johnson Y. N. Lau, 2004*

94. Molecular Diagnosis of Infectious Diseases, *Second Edition,* edited by *Jochen Decker and Udo Reischl, 2004*

93. Anticoagulants, Antiplatelets, and Thrombolytics, edited by *Shaker A. Mousa, 2004*

92. Molecular Diagnosis of Genetic Diseases, *Second Edition,* edited by *Rob Elles and Roger Mountford, 2004*

91. Pediatric Hematology: *Methods and Protocols,* edited by *Nicholas J. Goulden and Colin G. Steward, 2003*

90. Suicide Gene Therapy: *Methods and Reviews,* edited by *Caroline J. Springer, 2004*

89. The Blood–Brain Barrier: *Biology and Research Protocols,* edited by *Sukriti Nag, 2003*

88. Cancer Cell Culture: *Methods and Protocols,* edited by *Simon P. Langdon, 2003*

87. Vaccine Protocols, *Second Edition,* edited by *Andrew Robinson, Michael J. Hudson, and Martin P. Cranage, 2003*

86. Renal Disease: *Techniques and Protocols,* edited by *Michael S. Goligorsky, 2003*

85. Novel Anticancer Drug Protocols, edited by *John K. Buolamwini and Alex A. Adjei, 2003*

84. Opioid Research: *Methods and Protocols,* edited by *Zhizhong Z. Pan, 2003*

83. Diabetes Mellitus: *Methods and Protocols,* edited by *Sabire Özcan, 2003*

82. Hemoglobin Disorders: *Molecular Methods and Protocols,* edited by *Ronald L. Nagel, 2003*

81. Prostate Cancer Methods and Protocols, edited by *Pamela J. Russell, Paul Jackson, and Elizabeth A. Kingsley, 2003*

80. Bone Research Protocols, edited by *Miep H. Helfrich and Stuart H. Ralston, 2003*

79. Drugs of Abuse: *Neurological Reviews and Protocols,* edited by *John Q. Wang, 2003*

78. Wound Healing: *Methods and Protocols,* edited by *Luisa A. DiPietro and Aime L. Burns, 2003*

77. Psychiatric Genetics: *Methods and Reviews,* edited by *Marion Leboyer and Frank Bellivier, 2003*

76. Viral Vectors for Gene Therapy: *Methods and Protocols,* edited by *Curtis A. Machida, 2003*

75. Lung Cancer: *Volume 2, Diagnostic and Therapeutic Methods and Reviews,* edited by *Barbara Driscoll, 2003*

74. Lung Cancer: *Volume 1, Molecular Pathology Methods and Reviews,* edited by *Barbara Driscoll, 2003*

73. *E. coli*: *Shiga Toxin Methods and Protocols,* edited by *Dana Philpott and Frank Ebel, 2003*

72. Malaria Methods and Protocols, edited by *Denise L. Doolan,* 2002

71. *Haemophilus influenzae* Protocols, edited by *Mark A. Herbert, Derek Hood, and E. Richard Moxon,* 2002

70. Cystic Fibrosis Methods and Protocols, edited by *William R. Skach,* 2002

69. Gene Therapy Protocols, *Second Edition,* edited by *Jeffrey R. Morgan,* 2002

68. Molecular Analysis of Cancer, edited by *Jacqueline Boultwood and Carrie Fidler,* 2002

METHODS IN MOLECULAR MEDICINE™

Molecular Diagnosis of Cancer

Methods and Protocols

Second Edition

Edited by

Joseph E. Roulston

Division of Reproductive and Developmental Sciences, The University of Edinburgh, The Royal Infirmary, Edinburgh, Scotland, UK

and

John M. S. Bartlett

Division of Cancer and Molecular Pathology, University Department of Surgery, Glasgow Royal Infirmary, Glasgow, Scotland, UK

HUMANA PRESS TOTOWA, NEW JERSEY

999 Riverview Drive, Suite 208
Totowa, New Jersey 07512

www.humanapress.com

This publication is printed on acid-free paper. ∞
ANSI Z39.48-1984 (American Standards Institute) Permanence of Paper for Printed Library Materials.

Production Editor: Wendy S. Kopf.
Cover design by Patricia F. Cleary.

Cover illustration: Courtesy of John M. S. Bartlett and Amanda Forsyth.

Printed in the United States of America. 10 9 8 7 6 5 4 3 2 1
ISBN: 978-1-61737-396-1 e-ISBN: 978-1-59259-760-4
Library of Congress Cataloging in Publication Data

Molecular diagnosis of cancer : methods and protocols / edited by Joseph
E. Roulston, John M. S. Bartlett.-- 2nd ed.
p. ; cm. -- (Methods in molecular medicine ; 97)
Includes bibliographical references and index.

ISSN: 1543-1894
1. Cancer--Molecular diagnosis.
[DNLM: 1. Neoplasms--diagnosis. 2. Neoplasms--genetics. 3.
Polymerase Chain Reaction--methods. QZ 241 M7173 2004] I. Roulston, J.
E. II. Bartlett, John M. S. III. Series.
RC270.M64 2004
616.99'40756--dc22

2003020791

Preface

We are currently experiencing a fundamental shift in the way in which we approach the characterization of cancer. Never before has the make up of cancer tissues and individual cells been so exhaustively researched and characterized. We are now capable of producing molecular "fingerprints" that characterize the expression of all known and unknown genes within tumors and their surrounding tissues. More than 30,000 different genes may be measured in each patient's tumor in a single experiment. Simultaneously, novel therapies that exploit the molecular roadmap have been developed and are now being offered to patients. These novel agents, such as Glivec, Herceptin, Iressa, and others, specifically target individual genes within tumors and can produce dramatic responses in some patients. These drugs are only the forerunners of a coming tidal wave of novel therapeutics that individually target specific molecules within cancer cells—more than 300 such agents are currently in phase I or II clinical trials. This is an exciting time for cancer specialists and patients alike.

However, if we have learned anything from the past 50 or more years of research into cancer, it is that Lord Beaverbrook, in founding the British national health service in the 1950s, was frighteningly prescient when he defined the primary goal of health care to be "Diagnosis, Diagnosis, Diagnosis." Now, more than ever, it is essential that appropriate diagnostic methods and approaches are applied to the selection of patients for treatment. Each of the novel agents above, and those in development, requires, almost by definition, the development of an appropriate molecular test to characterize the patients who are most likely to benefit. For example, Herceptin, which is producing dramatic effects in the treatment of advanced breast cancers, targets the HER2 oncogene. In patients who display this genetic abnormality, response rates are between 25 and 35%, in unscreened breast cancers the predicted response rate would be 3–5%. We are faced, therefore, with the likelihood of an exponential rise in requests for molecular characterization of tumors to identify gene mutations, losses, amplifications, rearrangements, and so on. Experience has shown that many diagnosticians are currently untrained in the specific technical areas critical to this relatively novel field of "Molecular Diagnostics." *Molecular Diagnosis of Cancer* aims to provide not only an academic, but also a fundamentally technical insight into this novel area of diagnostic medicine. We are particularly grateful to those who have taken time to contribute to this volume, their efforts have created a comprehensive overview of current molecular diagnostic approaches and have, by providing detailed technical protocols, produced a laboratory handbook to facilitate the introduction of these techniques.

Although this volume does not seek to cover every possible aspect of molecular research, it does focus on specific molecular techniques that will provide an invaluable aid to those seeking to implement novel technologies into their diagnostic practice. The detailed step-by-step protocols and explanatory notes will, we hope, enable many more laboratories to enter this new and exciting arena.

In addition to those who have contributed to *Molecular Diagnosis of Cancer* we would like to thank those whose assistance and patience have greatly facilitated the production of this book. First, thanks are owed to Patricia Livani, whose hard work and organizational skills kept us on track for a timely publication of this volume. Second, our wives Dorothy and Jacqui and our children who put up with long hours in the evenings when we were closeted with our computers.

John M. S. Bartlett
Joseph Roulston

Contents

Contributors

ELAINE K. ALLAN • *Hemato-Oncology Section, Division of Cancer Science and Molecular Pathology, University of Glasgow, Glasgow, Scotland, UK*

DIANA M. BARNES • *Cancer Research UK Breast Pathology Laboratory, Guy's Hospital, London, UK*

JOHN M. S. BARTLETT • *Division of Cancer and Molecular Pathology, University Department of Surgery, Glasgow Royal Infirmary, Glasgow, Scotland, UK*

JEAN BENHATTAR • *Institute of Pathology, CHUV, Lausanne, Switzerland*

KAREN E. BIJWAARD • *Department of Cellular Pathology and Genetics, Armed Forces Institute of Pathology, Rockville, MD*

ROBERT BROWN • *Department of Medical Oncology, Beatson Laboratories, Glasgow, Scotland, UK*

LUKAS BUBENDORF • *Institute for Pathology, University of Basel, Basel, Switzerland*

PATRICE CAILLAT • *CEA Grenoble, LETI, Department of Microtechnologies, CRCC Val d'Aurelle, Montpellier, France*

K.C. ALLEN CHAN • *Department of Chemical Pathology, The Chinese University of Hong Kong, Prince of Wales Hospital, New Territories, Hong Kong*

MARK W. DRUMMOND • *Hemato-Oncology section, Division of Cancer Science and Molecular Pathology, University of Glasgow, Glasgow, Scotland, UK*

JOANNE EDWARDS • *Division of Cancer & Molecular Pathology, University Department of Surgery, Glasgow Royal Infirmary, Glasgow, Scotland, UK*

AMANDA FORSYTH • *Division of Cancer & Molecular Pathology, University Department of Surgery, Glasgow Royal Infirmary, Glasgow, Scotland, UK*

SANDRA GEBHARD • *Institute of Pathology, CHUV, Lausanne, Switzerland*

GILLIAN GIFFORD • *Department of Medical Oncology, Beatson Laboratories, Glasgow, Scotland, UK*

JAMES J. GOING • *University Department of Pathology, Glasgow Royal Infirmary, Glasgow, Scotland, UK*

BRUNO GRILLI • *Institute for Pathology, University of Basel, Basel, Switzerland*

PETER A. HALL • *Department of Pathology and Cancer Research Center, Queen's University Belfast, The Royal Hospitals, Northern Ireland, UK*

JENNI HAKKARAINEN • *Department of Pharmacology and Toxicology, University of Oulu, Oulu, Finland*

STACEY F. HOARE • *Cancer Research UK Department of Medical Oncology, University of Glasgow, Cancer Research UK Beatson Laboratories, Glasgow, Scotland, UK*
TESSA L. HOLYOAKE • *Hemato-Oncology Section, Division of Cancer Science and Molecular Pathology, University of Glasgow, Glasgow, Scotland, UK*
JORMA ISOLA • *Institute of Medical Technology, University of Tampere, Tampere, Finland*
MARIE JAROSOVA • *Department of Hemato-Oncology, University Hospital, Olomouc, Czech Republic*
YUTAKA KAWAKAMI • *Division of Cellular Signaling, Institute for Advanced Medical Research, Keio University School of Medicine, Tokyo, Japan*
PETER H. KAY • *Department of Pathology, The University of Western Australia, Nedlands, Australia*
W. NICOL KEITH • *Cancer Research UK Department of Medical Oncology, University of Glasgow, Cancer Research UK Beatson Laboratories, Glasgow, Scotland, UK*
WALTER KING • *Vysis/Abbott, Downers Grove, IL*
JACK H. LICHY • *Department of Cellular Pathology and Genetics, Armed Forces Institute of Pathology, Rockville, MD*
THIERRY LIVACHE • *CEA Grenoble, DRFM, CRCC Val d'Aurelle, Montpellier, France*
YUK-MING DENNIS LO • *Department of Chemical Pathology, The Chinese University of Hong Kong, Prince of Wales Hospital, New Territories, Hong Kong*
EVELYNE LOPEZ-CRAPEZ • *Centre de Recherche en Cancérologie, CRCC Val d'Aurelle, Montpellier, France*
MAIKO MATSUSHITA • *Division of Cellular Signaling, Institute for Advanced Medical Research, Keio University School of Medicine, Tokyo, Japan*
MARTINA MIRLACHER • *Institute of Pathology, University Hospital, Basel, Switzerland*
AILEEN J. MONAGHAN • *Cancer Research UK Department of Medical Oncology, University of Glasgow, Cancer Research UK Beatson Laboratories, Glascow, Scotland, UK*
ANDREW PEARCE • *South-East Cytogenetics Service, Lothian Universities Hospital NHS Trust, Edinburgh, Scotland, UK*
EKATERINA PESTOVA • *Vysis/Abbott, Downers Grove, IL*
MICHAEL F. PRESS • *Department of Pathology, Norris Comprehensive Cancer Center, University of Southern California, Los Angeles, CA*
ANTHONY RHODES • *Faculty of Applied Sciences, University of the West of England, Bristol, UK*

Joseph E. Roulston • *Clinical Biochemistry Section, Division of Reproductive and Developmental Sciences, The University of Edinburgh, The Royal Infirmary Edinburgh, Scotland, UK*
Guido Sauter • *Institute of Pathology, University Hospital, Basel, Switzerland*
Michael Scott • *Department of Pathology and Cancer Research Center, Queen's University Belfast, The Royal Hospitals, Northern Ireland, UK*
Ronald Simon • *Institute of Pathology, University Hospital, Basel, Switzerland*
Dominic V. Spagnolo • *Division of Tissue Pathology, The Western Australian Centre for Pathology and Medical Research, Nedlands, Western Australia*
Helen Speirs • *Molecular Endocrinology Unit, Western General Hospital, Edinburgh, Scotland, UK*
Minna Tanner • *Institute of Medical Technology, Tampere, Finland*
Jeremy M. E. Taylor • *Division of Tissue Pathology, The Western Australian Centre for Pathology and Medical Research, Nedlands, Western Australia*
Elizabeth R. Unger • *Centers for Disease Control and Prevention, Atlanta, GA*
Kirsi H. Vähäkangas • *Unit of Toxicology, Department of Pharmacology and Toxicology, University of Kuopio, Kuopio, Finland*
Suzanne D. Vernon • *Centers for Disease Control and Prevention, Atlanta, GA*
Judith A. Welsh • *Laboratory of Human Carcinogenesis, National Cancer Institute, Bethesda, MD*
Linda M. Wasserman • *Division of Medical Genetics, Department of Medicine, University of California, San Diego, La Jolla, CA*
Wen-Hsiang Wen • *Department of Pathology, Norris Comprehensive Cancer Center, University of Southern California, Los Angeles, CA*
Kim Wilber • *Vysis/Abbott, Downers Grove, IL*
Rie Yamazaki • *Division of Cellular Signaling, Institute for Advanced Medical Research, Keio University School of Medicine, Tokyo, Japan*
Daniela Zsoldos • *Apibio, Zone ASTEC, Grenoble, France*

1

Prognostic and Predictive Factors

Michael Scott and Peter A. Hall

1. Introduction

Despite manifold advances in cancer care during recent times, the outlook for many patients with epithelial and mesenchymal malignancies remains poor. Hence, as cancer diagnosis and management moves into the 21st century, cancer has become the paradigm disease of the molecular era, with a burgeoning body of research into aspects of cell biology amenable to earlier molecular diagnosis and efficacious treatment.

An intrinsic component of effective management is the art (or science) of prognostication: the ability to forecast clinical outcome for the benefit of patients and their families. Prognostic factors can, therefore, be defined as objective properties that indicate the likely course or outcome of a disease process.

Given that prognostic factors can, in many instances, determine the course of treatment (ranging from curative to palliative, according to the clinical context), one of the many developing roles of the histopathologist within the multidisciplinary team environment is the assimilation of a spectrum of data arising from traditional morphology in conjunction with relevant immunohistochemical markers and appropriate molecular studies to provide the oncologist with both a tissue diagnosis and a prognostic context into which an individual patient may be placed with confidence and accuracy. Furthermore, the pathologist can now dare to venture beyond the provision of prognosis by providing some degree of prediction of response to various therapeutic modalities.

2. Prognostic Factors in Practice

The concept of prognosis remains at the forefront of oncological theory, but despite the publication of a veritable plethora of articles investigating possible

From: *Methods in Molecular Medicine, vol. 79: Molecular Diagnosis of Cancer*
Edited by: J. E. Roulston and J. M. S. Bartlett © Humana Press Inc., Totowa, NJ

markers of prognosis, only a few have entered common clinical parlance for reasons that will be described in due course. This situation is likely to improve when recent advances in microarray technologies and bioinformatics are fully assimilated into clinical practice.

A key function of a prognostic factor is to provide an estimate of outcome for an individual patient. Conventional prognostic factors in oncology have been well validated over recent years, none more so than stage and histological grade, established indices that provide a convenient means of separating patient subgroups on the basis of differing probabilities of survival as embodied in the familiar concept of the 5-yr survival rate. Amplification of oncogenes such as n-*myc* in neuroblastoma provides extra information with regard to outcome in addition to the conventional parameters of stage and grade ***(1)***. Many such genetic alterations have been described in various tumors, but such detail is outside the scope of this review. A significant limitation of grade and stage is the failure of these criteria to detect patient subgroups likely to relapse or to benefit from adjuvant therapies.

Of similar importance to outcome is the planning of clinical treatment, a sterling example being the widespread adoption of the Nottingham Prognostic Index in breast cancer management ***(2,3)***.

Prognostic factors play an important role in clinical trials by providing criteria with which to define stratified randomized treatment groups, thereby ensuring analytical comparability. A further use is the detection of patients who may benefit from new therapies or adjuvant treatment, simple examples being chemotherapy for lymph node metastasis in colorectal carcinoma and tamoxifen for estrogen-receptor-positive breast carcinomas; new treatments have also been directed against tumors with loss of p53 function ***(4)***. It is evident that a great drive exists within oncology with the ultimate aim of improving outcome by harnessing the knowledge generated by prognostic and predictive factors based on new molecular targets.

To illustrate the level of interest in cancer prognosis, PubMed listed 127,168 articles on "cancer prognosis" on July 8, 2002; only 1681 of these referred to prediction. A multitude of articles exists with regard to prognosis, but as Hall and Going have concluded, "the plethora of prognostic studies leaves one disappointed by how few parameters have been accepted into clinical practice" ***(5)***.

2.1. Tumor Biology: Hidden Complexities

Consideration of reasons for the lack of well-characterized and widely accepted prognostic and predictive factors must begin with the inherent biological complexity of malignancy (compounded by inadequate methodological rigor in many studies). It seems evident that any attempt to predict the behavior of a neoplasm by merely assaying a single molecular entity such as p53 mutations is doomed to fail given the complexity of interactions among a legion of molecular pathways. It is no surprise, therefore, that tumor stage and grade retain their place as the most reliable predictors of outcome by virtue of providing a crude combinatorial bioassay of many molecular events.

Chaos theory, if applied to neoplasia, would suggest that small molecular variations can lead to vastly different patterns of behavior. Such molecular and behavioral heterogeneity is well accepted and provides great impetus for research, particularly when one considers the morphological similarity of many tumors. Urothelial carcinomas can be divided into two broad groups by virtue of histology and behavior, namely superficial (noninvasive) and muscle invasive, the latter having a much worse prognosis. Molecular alterations in bladder cancer clearly associated with adverse outcome include inactivating mutations of p53 and retinoblastoma protein (Rb); hence, the identification of urothelial tumors with the capacity to progress is a current priority and presents a fertile field for prognostic markers ***(6)***.

This molecular heterogeneity of morphologically uniform diagnostic categories is also exemplified in borderline ovarian tumors, a subset of tumors ripe for reclassification by molecular criteria, given the widely differing outcomes seen in this peculiar and poorly understood category where some patients have an excellent prognosis when compared with others who share 5-yr survival rates akin to those with overtly malignant tumors ***(7)***.

The apparent morphological uniformity of such diagnostic categories serves as a motivating force in the search for molecular markers; the developmental concept of the "phenocopy" illustrates this problem, a phenocopy being a mutation having a particular phenotype identical to that caused by a different mutation. Hence, tumors of a particular histological type may be phenocopies but may, therefore, behave very differently given their underlying molecular heterogeneity.

Although a great desire to uncover molecular correlates of tumor behavior undoubtedly exists, our knowledge of genetic events in cancer has made relatively little impact in clinical practice; in breast cancer, none of the described genetic changes have, until recently, defined a subset of patients requiring different therapy ***(8)***. HER-2 amplification is a significant discovery with potential for real clinical impact ***(9)***.

A track record of relatively slow progress points to the need for stronger clinico-pathological frameworks in prognostic studies. There can be no substitute for simple and testable hypotheses, realistic and achievable goals within the context of appropriately designed studies.

It is evident that new molecular techniques will generate vast quantities of data that require interpretation if clinical benefit is to eventuate; there is no place for unfocused data trawling in the absence of a clear hypothesis. The success of the Human Genome Project depends on new bioinformatic technologies to utilize these data in a meaningful way, particularly with regard to gene expression patterns ***(10)***.

2.2. Microarray Technology

DNA microarray technology is an exciting development with almost limitless potential within the context of cancer prognosis studies by means of gene expression profiling in tumors ***(11)*** or population-based polymorphism analysis ***(12)***. The rationale of visualizing these "transcriptome snapshots" is that patterns of gene expression may point toward new genetic targets for therapeutic manipulation or provide an indication of drug resistance.

In essence, DNA microarrays allow simultaneous expression analysis of thousands of genes by hybridization of labeled cDNA (reverse-transcribed from mRNA) to specific cDNA or oligonucleotide substrates. Analysis of hybridized target cDNAs provides data on relative levels of gene expression and the presence of polymorphisms or mutations. Hence, gene profiles can be created for different tumors by analyzing the entire transcriptome of a neoplasm ***(13)***. An effective application of microarray technology has been the genetic profiling of diffuse large B-cell lymphomas with the subsequent identification of two tumor groups with distinct genetic "fingerprints," each group having significantly different prognoses ***(14)***. Global gene expression profiling has more recently been applied to Barrett's esophagus and esophageal adenocarcinoma with intriguing results by hierarchical cluster analysis ***(15)***. Such advances are both encouraging and exciting, with much potential for providing specific treatments for tumor subtypes.

With regard to methodological considerations, DNA microarrays represent a particularly powerful resource given that they provide unbiased detection of genetic variations; such objective means of analysis is a valuable commodity. The focus of prospective researchers can, therefore, be turned upon the selection of clinically robust patient groups for study; without well-characterized study material, microarray technology is in danger of being exploited with the generation of meaningless data. Moreover, experimental data used to suggest a hypothesis must be validated in a second dataset (i.e., data independent of the data that suggests the original hypothesis). Many prognostic studies are severely flawed by such attempts to both suggest and prove a hypothesis by utilizing a single dataset.

Microarray technology is at present expensive and of limited availability. The majority of DNA microarrays have previously utilized RNA from fresh tissue, which is then reverse-transcribed and labeled prior to hybridization; significant advances have been made in the extraction of RNA from formalin-fixed paraffin-embedded tissue with the hope of utilizing archival mRNA for microarray analysis. This would allow the vast potential of archival tissue in pathology departments to be realized in prognostic studies (subject to ethical approval) ***(16)***. Although much progress has been made by the Human Genome Project, most of the identified genes are only partially characterized; many genes with potential for prognostication in cancer probably remain unrecognized. As we have seen, current research efforts are directed toward subclassification of malignancies based on gene expression profiles. Breast cancer is an area of great interest at present in an attempt to refine treatment protocols by molecular characterization ***(17)***.

Tissue arrays are a related development with similar potential for revolutionizing cancer prognosis and predictive studies. Given that cDNA microarrays are expensive and time-consuming to manufacture and that the majority rely on frozen tissue, pathologists have traditionally measured protein expression in formalin-fixed paraffin sections using immunohistochemistry for the evaluation of diagnostic and prognostic markers. Archival tissue also has the advantage of long-term follow-up data in many cases, coupled with the availability of large numbers of cases in surgical pathology departmental archives.

Although conventional immunohistochemistry is widely used in prognostic studies, such approaches can be time-consuming and impractical for high-throughput studies ***(18)***. This has precipitated the development of tissue arrays comprised of small cores from large numbers of paraffin-embedded tumor samples arranged in an ordered array in a new paraffin block ***(19)***. A single section can therefore contain hundreds of individual tumor samples, thereby permitting simultaneous immunohistochemical analysis to be performed on a large sample size; this carries obvious benefits with regard to standardization of test conditions. A primary benefit of this new tool is the rapid characterization of expression patterns of protein targets for new antibodies, allowing comparison with existing markers in the same sample set. Tissue arrays have the potential to take immunohistochemical studies into a new dimension in terms of sample size, scope, and speed of throughput.

Benefits thus far of the microarray revolution include the distinction of a subset of breast carcinomas with a basal epithelial cell phenotype characteristic of poor clinical outcome ***(17)*** and an estrogen-receptor-positive breast cancer subset surprisingly associated with a very poor outcome ***(20)***.

Although this serves to illustrate the power of microarray technology in uncovering markers of molecular heterogeneity with possible prognostic significance, the reader should bear in mind the need to validate gene expression profiling using prospective studies of satisfactory quality. Furthermore, retrospective validation by tissue arrays is a step of major importance in the search for markers that correlate with clinical parameters *(18)*. However, what of conventional analysis methods in situations where microarray capabilities may not yet be available?

2.3. Immunohistochemistry

An important and undisputed role exists for conventional immunohistichemistry in prognostication and prediction; indeed, the majority of practicing histopathologists make use of immunohistochemistry on a regular basis in the context of clinico-pathological multidisciplinary meetings, a useful forum that serves to bring pathologists and oncologists into close collaboration. A comprehensive review by Leong *(21)* surveys the current use of immunohistochemistry in prognosis and describes markers for assessment of basla lamina invasion, micrometastasis to sentinel nodes, hormone receptor status, angiogenesis, and antimetastasis genes, to name but a few. It would appear that immunohistochemistry remains the most amenable method of assessment of these prognostic markers. Indeed, many are now required in the routine histological reporting of tumors such as estrogen receptor status in breast carcinoma.

Prediction of response to various therapies is also within the domain of immunohistochemistry at present; examples include HER-2 overexpression for Herceptin™ treatment in breast cancer *(22)* and multidrug-resistance gene products in the prediction of response to chemotherapy *(23)*.

2.4. Methodology: An Achilles' Heel?

Previous reviews have dealt with performance and reporting of prognostic studies *(24,25)*. In short, studies must be robust, reproducible, and reliable; quantification is the accepted gold standard, although a plethora of semiquantitative studies abounds in the literature. Careful attention must be paid to methodological variables (such as immunohistochemical methods) in order to allow reproduction of assays in other laboratories. Anyone indulging in histological analysis of tumors must consider stereological methods in microscopy *(26,27)*.

Sample size and probability of error are important concepts. Type I error is defined as rejection of a null hypothesis when it is true, whereas type II error is the acceptance of a false null hypothesis. Further considerations are the probability value below which a null hypothesis is rejected (α) and the probability of a null hypothesis being accepted (β). Within this context, we can appreciate the probability of detecting a difference of specified magnitude (expressed as standard difference, or the ratio of the specified difference to the standard deviation of the observations). With a specified number of patients at significance level α, this probability represents the power of the study (which equates to 1–ß), a parameter evaluated by sample size calculations *(28)*. It is essential to perform such pertinent calculations if resources are not to be wasted in the pursuit of a study too small to answer the questions raised.

A problem that can arise is the definition of valid cutoff points between patient groups, particularly in studies of continuous variables; dichotomous variables, by comparison, present fewer issues. Many studies of prognostic or predictive factors are flawed by failure to define how a continuous variable is subdivided into categories. A common but somewhat dangerous approach is to test various cutoff points until statistical significance is attained in a particular case ***(29)***. It is of paramount importance that chosen cutoff points be validated with an independent dataset.

A related error is the acquisition of data on multifarious factors with a subsequent search for "statistically significant" associations. A subtle reminder of the dangers inherent in such multiple testing is illustrated by Bonferroni's correction whereby the *p*-values obtained are multiplied by the number of tests performed ***(30)***, leading to statistical insignificance in many cases.

Incomplete or missing data commonly compromise prospective clinical trials for various reasons, including patient dropout. Retrospective studies lead to problems with case/control selection and the inadvertent introduction of bias into statistical considerations. The choice of study center is also a focus for potential bias in that a tertiary center will very often contain a different spectrum of clinical cases compared with a district general hospital. Moreover, the age-old problem of publication bias still persists, in that positive data are often favored over negative findings. It is therefore worthy of note that similar studies of prognostic factors can have very different outcomes, a situation which may give the reader cause for concern ***(31,32)***. Any discussion of statistics should include a mention of sensitivity, specificity, and positive and negative predictive values; the reader is referred to Altman ***(30)*** for a lucid explanation of these concepts.

2.5. An Analytical Approach to Prognostic Studies

There can be no alternative to a clearly stated and plausible hypothesis, a prerequisite of focused research. The study population should be defined in both retrospective and prospective studies. Study size is of prime significance in relation to the size of effect of the prognostic or predictive factor under investigation. Cutoff points should be clearly defined.

Altman and Lyman ***(33)*** have proposed a prognostic study hierarchy analogous to the study design in clinical drug trials. A clear advantage of such an approach is that it allows a logical exploration and validation of potential prognostic and predictive factors.

Hall and Going have modified these proposals to allow stepwise progression from initial observation and hypothesis formulation through the process

OBSERVATION

Phase I – Exploratory studies

(assay definition, association of variable with diagnostic parameters and established prognostic/predictive data)

HYPOTHESIS

Phase II – Retrospective investigation of clinical utility

(analysis in statistically meaningful cohorts of well-defined patients, test of hypothesis, definition of cut-off points, validation in second dataset)

CLINICAL RESEARCH

Phase III – Prospective confirmation of clinical utility

(demonstration of usefulness in clinical practice, ideally in multicentre trials)

CLINICAL USE

Fig. 1 Stepwise progression from original observation to eventual clinical use. (Adapted from **ref. 5**.)

of research to ultimate clinical use ***(5)*** (*see* **Fig. 1**). The educated reader will appreciate that audit is necessary thereafter to demonstrate continuing clinical relevance.

The purpose of phase I studies is to define assays and allow initial comparisons with diagnostic parameters and established prognostic or predictive factors. Such an approach would permit the generation of testable hypotheses and valid cutoff points. At this juncture, it would be appropriate to test clinical utility in a statistically meaningful cohort of patients in a retrospective manner. Data thus generated could then be validated in a second dataset. Cutoff points should be robust and the assay conditions (and results) should be reproducible by different groups in other centers. The third phase of study would involve a prospective analysis of potential clinical utility, ideally in a multicenter study. Only prognostic or predictive factors passing this test of methodological stringency could be justified for clinical application.

3. Conclusion

It is evident that the published literature is rife with prognostic and predictive studies of very low quality. It appears that the emergence of a new reagent often leads to studies without clear hypotheses or the generation of clinically meaningful data. Indeed, it has been posited that the search for clinically useful prognostic and predictive markers will continue to be difficult because it is a stern task to predict biological behavior, even in a controlled system. There is little doubt that studies of poor quality will continue to diminish the clinical contribution of potential markers.

References

1. Katzenstein, H. M., Bowman, L. C., Brodeur, G. M., et al. (1998) Prognostic significance of age, MYCN oncogene amplification, tumor cell ploidy and histology in 10 infants with stage D (S) neuroblastoma: the Pediatric Oncology Group experience. *J. Clin. Oncol.* **16,** 2007–2017.
2. Sundquist, M., Thorstenson, S., Brodin, L., et al. (1999) Applying the Nottingham Prognostic Index to a Swedish breast cancer population. *Breast Cancer Res. Treat.* **53,** 1–8.
3. Elston, C. W. and Ellis, I. O. (1991) Pathological prognostic factors in breast cancer. I. The value of grade in breast cancer: experience from a large study with long-term follow-up. *Histopathology* **19,** 403–410.
4. Wilman, K. G. (1998) New p53-based anti-cancer therapeutic strategies. *Med. Oncol.* **15,** 222–228.
5. Hall, P. A. and Going, J. J. (1999) Predicting the future: a critical appraisal of cancer prognosis studies. *Histopathology* **35,** 489–494.
6. Knowles, M. A. (2001) What we could do now: molecular pathology of bladder cancer. *J. Clin. Pathol. Mol. Pathol.* **54,** 215–221.
7. Seidmann, J. D., Ronnett, B. M., and Kurmann, R. J. (2000) Evolution of the concept and terminology of borderline ovarian tumors. *Curr. Diagn. Pathol.* **6,** 31–37.
8. Van de Vijver, M. J. (2000) Genetic alterations in breast cancer. *Curr. Diagn. Pathol.* **6,** 271–281.
9. Agrup, M., Stal, O., Olsen, K., et al. (2000) C-erbB2 expression and survival in early onset breast cancer. *Breast Cancer Res. Treat.* **63,** 23–29.

10. Maughan, N. J., Lewis, F. A., and Smith, V. (2001) An introduction to arrays. *J. Pathol.* **195,** 3–6.
11. Schena, M., Shalon, D., Heller, R,. et al. (1996) Parallel human genome analysis: microarray-based expression monitoring of 1000 genes. *Proc. Natl. Acad. Sci. USA* **93,** 10,614–10,619.
12. Hacia, J. G. (1999) Resequencing and mutational analysis using oligonucleotide microarrays. *Nature Genet.* **21 (Suppl.),** 42–47.
13. Berns, A. (2000) Gene expression in diagnosis. *Nature* **403,** 491–492.
14. Alizadeh, A. A., Eisen, M. B., Davis, R. E., et al. (2000) Distinct types of diffuse large B-cell lymphoma identified by gene expression profiling. *Nature* **403,** 503–511.
15. Selaru, F. M., Zou, T., Xu, Y., et al. (2002) Global gene expression profiling in Barrett's esophagus and esophageal cancer: a comparative analysis using cDNA microarrays. *Oncogene* **21,** 475–478.
16. Lewis, F. A., Maughan, N. J., Smith, V., et al. (2001) Unlocking the archive—gene expression in paraffin-embedded tissue. *J. Pathol.* **195,** 66–71.
17. Perou, C. M., Sørlie, T., Eisen, M. B., et al. (2000) Molecular portraits of human breast tumors. *Nature* **406,** 747–752.
18. Alizadeh, A. A., Ross, D. T., Perou, C. M., et al. (2001) Towards a novel classification of human malignancies based on gene expression patterns. *J. Pathol.* **195,** 41–52.
19. Schraml, P., Kokonen, J., Bubendorf, L., et al. (1999) Tissue microarrays for gene amplification surveys in many different tumor types. *Clin. Cancer Res.* **5,** 1966–1975.
20. Sørlie, T., Perou, C. M., Tibshirani, R., et al. (2001) Gene expression patterns of breast carcinomas distinguish tumor subclasses with clinical implication. *Proc. Natl. Acad. Sci. USA* **98,** 10,869–10,874.
21. Leong, A. S.-Y. (2001) Immunohistological markers for tumor prognostication. *Curr. Diagn. Pathol.* **7,** 176–186.
22. Muss, H. B., Thor, A. D., Berry, D. A., et al. (1994) C-erbB2 expression and response to adjuvant therapy in women with node-positive early breast cancer. *N. Engl. J. Med.* **330,** 12,060–12,666.
23. Kartner, N. and Ling, V. (1989) Multi-drug resistance in cancer. *Sci. Am.* **260,** 44–51.
24. Altman, D. G., Lausen, B., Sauerbrei, W., et al. (1994) Dangers of using 'optimal' cutpoints in the evaluation of prognostic factors. *J. Natl. Cancer Inst.* **86,** 829–835.
25. Simon, R. and Altman, D. G. (1994) Statistical aspects of prognostic factor studies in oncology. *Br. J. Cancer* **69,** 979–985.
26. Gunderson, H. J. G., Bagger, P., Bendtsen, T. F., et al. (1988), The new stereological tools: dissector, fractionator, nucleator and point sampled intercepts and their use in pathological research and diagnosis. *Acta Pathol. Microbiol. Scand.* **96,** 857–881.
27. Howard, C. U. and Reed, M. G. (1988) Unbiased stereology, in *Three-Dimen-*

sional Measurement in Microscopy, Bios Scientific Publishers and the Royal Microscopical Society, Oxford.

28. Sokhal, R. R. and Rohlf, F. J. (1981) Estimation and hypothesis testing, in *Biometry: The Principle and Practice of Statistics in Biological Research.* W. H. Freeman, New York, pp. 128–178.
29. Hall, P. A., Richards, M. A., Gregory, W. M., et al. (1988) The prognostic value of Ki67 immunostaining in non-Hodgkin's lymphoma. *J. Pathol.* **154,** 223–235.
30. Altman, D. G. (1991) *Practical Statistics for Medical Research*, Chapman & Hall, London.
31. Hall, P. A. and Lane, D. P. (1994) p53 in tumor pathology: can we trust immunohistochemistry—revisited. *J. Pathol.* **172,** 1–4.
32. Dowell, S. P. and Hall, P. A. (1995) The p53 tumor-suppressor gene and tumor prognosis—is there a relationship? *J. Pathol.* **177,** 221–224.
33. Altman, D. G. and Lyman, G. H. (1998) Methodological challenges in the evaluation of prognostic factors in breast cancer. *Breast Cancer Res. Treat.* **52,** 289–303.

2

Assessment of Predictive Values of Tumor Markers

Joseph E. Roulston

1. Introduction

Reviewing the literature, it would appear that tumor markers have often flattered to deceive. Early promise does not often seem to be borne out in extended trials. Despite apparently high specificity, very few markers are capable of assisting in a screening process.

This brief review attempts to put the roles of tumor markers in perspective and explain how their misapplication has led to misunderstanding of their potential value in a clinical context. It also considers the theoretical basis for their use and highlights how misunderstanding of these can lead to flawed studies and application.

Cancer has been known to mankind since ancient times. There is an early Egyptian papyrus describing how one should differentiate between breast cancer and mastitis. The ancient Greeks and Romans also have left us with writings in which various treatment options are discussed *(1)*. Disease processes and causes were not well understood however; the humoral pathology established by the ancient Greeks of the school of Galen in the 2nd century AD was to survive virtually intact until the mid-19th century. It is perhaps all the more remarkable then that the first tumor marker—Bence Jones' protein in multiple myeloma—should come to light in what was still, by and large, the prescientific medical culture prevailing in 1845.

Multiple myeloma was fully described and named by von Rustizky *(2)* in 1873, but it was Kahler *(3)* who related the disease to Bence Jones' proteinuria and thereby brought a specific tumor marker to medical attention, a marker that is still used to this day to assist in diagnosis.

Despite the lesson of Bence Jones' protein, in which a marker specific for a particular cancer was discovered, many researchers still sought a general test

From: *Methods in Molecular Medicine, vol. 79: Molecular Diagnosis of Cancer*
Edited by: J. E. Roulston and J. M. S. Bartlett © Humana Press Inc., Totowa, NJ

for early diagnosis of all cancers. Homberger ***(4)*** reviewed more than 60 tests that had been suggested in the previous 20 yr (1930–1950). Many of these tests were based upon the physicochemical properties of serum proteins and sought to show a difference between precipitation of serum proteins from normal subjects and cancer patients.

With the benefit of hindsight, it is easy to write off such efforts as misplaced; the biochemical techniques available were crude and not always applied with logic. Bodansky ***(5)*** points out the problems with many early studies. Technically, the tests were deficient because they were based on a gross and nonspecific measurement—the change in a large fraction of the serum protein pool. Second, these investigations were usually carried out in samples from patients with advanced disease, whereas control groups of similarly aged patients with serious nonmalignant diseases were not studied. When these controls were looked at later, the false-positive rate was as high as the true-positive rate in the neoplastic group.

Apart from technical shortcomings, there is also a major assumption in the presupposition that cancers will produce some unique feature that non-neoplastic diseases will not, and for this, there is not a shred of evidence ***(6)***.

As the biochemical tools and techniques available have grown ever more sophisticated, it has enabled more precisely focused studies to be conducted. The advent of immunoassay techniques in the 1960s and their refinement during the following decades with nonisotopic labels and, especially, the development of monoclonal ("hybridoma") technology has brought levels of analytical sensitivity and specificity that were orders of magnitude better than those available to previous generations of researchers.

2. Theoretical Considerations

In order to assess and apply tests in an appropriate and discerning manner, it is necessary to consider what the aims and objectives are and how one monitors and assesses one's efforts. At first thought, it appears very simple. First, it is intended to apply a test to discriminate between the normal and the diseased subject, to assist in diagnosis and possibly to screen populations for occult disease. Second, one may wish to apply a test to monitor the course of the disease in a noninvasive way in order to assess the efficiency of therapy, to watch for drug resistance, and to predict outcome. Third, one may wish to monitor patients in remission to ensure that they remain disease-free and to get a valuable lead time to relapse.

In order to achieve these aims, several points must be made clear. First, one must have confidence in the analytical accuracy and precision of the test(s). However, in order to translate the analytical data into clinically meaningful information, it is essential to be aware of what the objectives are. "Is this result normal?" is a question often asked by a requesting clinician and it is worth considering, at the outset, what the word "normal" may or may not mean.

2.1. What Is "Normal"?

The first problem presenting to workers in clinical medicine is the statistical definition of normal because it is widely misunderstood and even more widely misapplied. Gauss' law of errors applies to repeated measurements on the same subject or object, not a series of measurements of the same analyte in different subjects. Gauss' law proposes that if the same measurement were repeated over and over again in the same subject, the results' spread would fit a bell-shaped distribution symmetrical about the mean. Abnormal results may then be defined as those outside the 95% confidence limit—in other words, the 2.5% of values at the top and bottom end of the range. There is, however, no *a priori* reason why this law of distribution should apply to measurements in more than one subject; it was never derived to describe the distribution of a variable (disease related or otherwise) in a population of subjects. Although it is common practice in laboratories to define a reference range for an analyte as being the limits within which 95% of the healthy population's results fall, these limits *per se* give no indication of morbidity or mortality. Indeed, by definition, 5% of this population will be "abnormal" although disease-free if we assume a 95% (i.e., mean value plus or minus two standard deviations) reference range. It also follows that the more tests performed on each specimen, the greater the likelihood of at least one of the results being "abnormal"—from 5% for 1 test, to 40% for 10 tests (the chance of 10 tests on a sample all being "normal" is 0.95^{10}, which is 0.6 or 60%, leaving a 40% chance for an "abnormal"). The percentage error figure rises to 99% $[(1–0.95^{90}) \times 100\%]$ for 90 tests.

It is for this reason that most laboratories today eschew the phrase "normal range" and prefer the alternatives "reference range" and "referent value," in order to make clear that the range or cutoff cited is not of necessity a range or cutoff that encompasses or defines the limit of the values of the analyte in all disease-free and excludes all diseased subjects. Often, 95% reference ranges, based on the mean value plus or minus two standard deviations, are employed as the reference limits because they have been found empirically to provide cutoffs at clinically useful and discriminant values.

For tumor markers, however, there is less concern whether a reference range based on a symmetric distribution is ideal; in practice, the optimal cutoff value is sought, a point that discriminates "normal" from "elevated." There is no lower limit to the "reference range."

In order to establish this cutoff value empirically, it is necessary to discover the value that discriminates the best between disease and nondisease—in other words, produces the fewest misclassifications. In order to do this, large numbers of measurements in the disease group under study and a *suitably matched* control population must be made. Inevitably, there is an overlap between the range of results produced by the control group and the range produced by the diseased group. There will, therefore, be some false-positive results (elevated analyte in control subject) and some false-negative results ("normal" result in diseased subject), and just how many depends on the test and population in question. In order to proceed further, therefore, it is vital to determine how good the test is in an objective manner.

2.2. How Good Is the Test?

2.2.1. Sensitivity and Specificity

The two most usually applied criteria in order to assess a test are those of sensitivity and specificity. Sensitivity is a measure of how good a test is at picking up the disease in question by giving a positive result. It is expressed in a population with the disease as the number giving a true-positive result divided by the sum of true-positive and false-negative results—in other words, what percentage of the diseased cohort was identified correctly by the test.

It is obvious that a test that is 100% sensitive will score perfectly. A test that is 90% sensitive, however, will generate 10 false negatives in each 100 positives.

As well as correctly identifying the presence of disease, a good test must also correctly classify the disease-free subject by giving a negative result. The measure of a test to so discriminate is called the specificity. This is established by measurements in a disease-free population, and specificity is defined as the number of true negatives divided by the sum of true negatives plus false positives.

It can be seen that sensitivity and specificity are entirely "test-based" parameters; they take no account of the prevalence of the disease in the population, the sensitivity is calculated by study of a group who are all disease positive, and specificity is calculated from a group who are all disease-free. This, as will become apparent, is a serious limitation to the application of these parameters because disease prevalence has serious effects upon the clinical usefulness of tests in certain circumstances.

Furthermore, the choice of cutoff, which effectively determines the sensitivity and specificity, cannot improve both sensitivity and specificity simultaneously; moving the chosen cutoff point to a higher referent value will increase specificity, but correspondingly reduce sensitivity. The optimal choice of cutoff, therefore, depends on whether it is deemed more desirable to optimize sensitivity at the expense of specificity or vice versa, and this consideration, in turn, is influenced by the disease prevalence in the population under study.

2.2.2. Incidence and Prevalence

By definition, incidence relates to the frequency of occurrence of an event and is therefore a rate per unit time. For a disease, the incidence rate is the number of new cases per 100,000 of the population per year. The prevalence, by contrast, is the number of patients per 100,000 of the population who have the given disease at the time of the study; therefore, prevalence is a snapshot of the status quo.

The incidence of epithelial carcinoma of the ovary is of the order of 15 per 100,000 per year. If the average duration of the disease is 5 yr, it follows that the prevalence, assuming a steady-state situation in the population, must be 75 per 100,000. As a general rule, therefore,

Prevalence = Incidence × Duration

The clinical usefulness of a test *in a given situation* will depend on the prevalence of the disease in the cohort under study; high sensitivity and specificity, although vital, are not enough to guarantee "usefulness." For example, a test that was 100% specific and 99% sensitive seems to have impressive credentials, but it would fail dismally as a screening test for ovarian cancer. Screening 100,000 women would yield 99% out of the positives, (i.e., 74 or 75 women), which is an acceptable "pick-up rate," but it would also generate 1% false positives (i.e., 1,000 nondiseased women). Therefore, a positive test result would correctly identify disease presence in less than 7% [75/(1000 + 75) = 6.98%] of the subjects studied. Therefore, it is necessary to use assessment procedures that take into account the prevalence of the disease in the population under study.

2.2.3. Bayes' Theorem and the Predictive Value Model

In 1975, Galen and Gambino ***(7)*** introduced the predictive value model to clinical laboratories. The theoretical basis was hardly new; coming as it did from a posthumous publication in 1763 ***(8)***. What Bayes' theorem allows is the calculation of the *a posteriori* probability of disease being present in an individual given that the patient has a positive test result. By definition, the *a priori* probability that a patient will have the disease (i.e., before the test) is equal to the prevalence of the disease. From prevalence, sensitivity, and specificity, Bayes calculated the *a posteriori* probability—the so-called predictive value of a positive result or positive predictive value.

Let sensitivity be a, specificity be b, and prevalence be p, then one can describe the positive predictive value (PPV) as follows:

$$\mathrm{PPV} = pa/[pa + (1 - b)(1 - p)] \qquad (1)$$

Table 1
Positive Predictive Values as a Function of Prevalence

Disease prevalence (%)	Test sensitivity and specificity = 95% PPV	Test sensitivity and specificity = 99% PPV
0.02	0	2.0
0.1	1.9	9.0
1.0	16.1	50.0
2.0	27.9	66.9
5.0	50.0	83.9
50.0	95.0	99.0

This simplifies to

$$\text{PPV} = \text{True positives/True positives} + \text{False positives}$$

because *pa* is the prevalence of the disease multiplied by the sensitivity of the test for the disease (i.e., the true positive).

Similarly, $(1 - b)(1 - p)$ is the prevalence of nondisease multiplied by the probability of a positive result in such a disease-free person. $1 - b$, which is 1 – specificity is sometimes, albeit incorrectly, referred to as the false-positive rate.

The benefit of the predictive value model is apparent immediately; if a test has a 95% PPV in a given area of use, then the clinician may assume that in a patient with a positive result, there is a 95% chance that the patient has the disease. The same conclusion cannot be made from sensitivity and specificity values, as they take no account of disease prevalence. **Table 1** shows how the predictive value of a positive test varies from virtually zero to 100% as a result of changing disease prevalence *even when sensitivity and specificity are high.* This gives an important insight to screening procedures; where disease prevalence is low, it is necessary to have tests with greater than 99% sensitivity and specificity to achieve an acceptable positive predictive value.

3. Screening for Disease

Screening has been defined as "the presumptive identification of unrecognised disease or defect by the application of tests, examinations, or other procedures that can be applied rapidly" ***(9)***. By definition, therefore, a screening test is applied to asymptomatic subjects and is not diagnostic *per se*, confirmatory tests being required. The idea that early warning leads to a better outcome is not easily translated into a practical program. The economic difficulties of testing large numbers of apparently healthy individuals in order to pick up a small number with the disease are enormous. Second, there are difficult ethical considerations when one is investigating healthy subjects without symptoms or any substantive probability of finding disease.

3.1. Population Screening

The oncology literature contains many reports of apparently promising markers that fail subsequently to claim a routine clinical role. There are many reasons that contribute to this, but the commonest is overextrapolating or illogically applying the results. Consider a study in which an investigator tests a novel tumor marker for a particular cancer that has a prevalence of 100/100,000 in the general population and finds that in 100 patients with the tumor under investigation, 99 have a positive test result; that is, the test has a sensitivity of 99%. Equally, when tested on 100 disease-free subjects, only 1 is test-positive—a specificity of 99%. Owing to this excellent discrimination, it is decided to introduce the test as a screen in the general population in order to detect this tumor at an earlier stage to improve therapeutic efficacy and patient outcome. The results are disastrous; the test appears to have lost its earlier discrimination and is generating lots of false positives—Why?

In the pilot study, the disease prevalence was 50% *by design*; there were 100 patients and 100 controls and the positive predictive value was 99%. In the screening exercise, the prevalence would be 100/100,000, which is 0.1%. Therefore, as well as correctly identifying 99 out of the 100 true positives, the test will also *under these circumstances* misclassify 1000 as false positive, giving us a positive predictive value of 99/(99 + 1000) (i.e., 9.0%). In other words, a test that in the pilot investigation yielded 99% correct results, gives, in a screening situation, a 91% *a posteriori* probability that elevated results are *not* associated with the disease. The marker sensitivity and specificity remain unchanged, the fall in positive predictive value from 99% to 9% was *entirely* caused by the change in prevalence in the cohort under study from 50% to 0.1%.

If a test is genuinely and completely useless (i.e., it yields positive and negative results in a truly random manner), then the positive predictive value will be the same as the prevalence: the *a priori* probability of disease in the patient equals the *a posteriori* probability of disease. Furthermore, for a test to be random, it is not necessary for sensitivity and specificity each to equal 50%; a test may have 90% sensitivity and still give random results if the specificity is only 10%.

Randomness requires only that:

$$\sum(\text{Sensitivity} + \text{Specificity}) = 100\%$$

These findings can be derived simply from Eq. (1):

$$\text{PPV} = pa/[pa + (1 - p)(1 - b)]$$

In a random test, the percentage of true positives in the diseased group will equal the percentage of false positives in the well group—by definition; that is,

$$pa/p = [(1 - p)(1 - b)]/(1 - p)$$

Also, by definition, pa/p is the sensitivity of the test and

$$[(1 - p)(1 - b)]/(1 - p) = (1 - b) = (1 - \text{Specificity})$$

Therefore, in a random test, sensitivity equals 1 – Specificity, which is to say the sum of sensitivity and specificity equals unity (or 100%).

This relationship is of value in the graphical representation of marker performance. When sensitivity is plotted as a function of 1 – Specificity, an immediate visual impression of the marker's discrimination is obtained. This graph is termed the receiver operating characteristic (ROC) plot. A random test will give a straight-line graph at 45° to the axes, whereas a good, highly discriminatory test will give a curve of steep slope from the origin, showing a high sensitivity even at high specificity. Therefore, the greater the area under the curve, the better the test. ROC plots are particularly useful in that they remove the influence of the "cutoff" point from the marker evaluation.

3.2. Optimization

If screening is to be considered, it is necessary to know the disease prevalence and to have tests with high sensitivity and specificity in order to calculate whether an acceptable positive predictive value can be achieved. However, it is impossible to optimize simultaneously both sensitivity and specificity—increasing one automatically decreases the other. Considerations regarding optimization strategies will vary with the natural history of the disease under study (*vide infra*).

The simplest case will be considered; the situation where there is a screening procedure to be optimized and a false-negative result carries an equivalent penalty to a false-positive result. Under these circumstances, we may define our "index of misclassification," f, as the sum of the false-negative and false-positive results.

$$f = \text{FN} + \text{FP} \tag{2}$$

False negatives, FN, can be calculated as the lack of sensitivity $(1 - a)$ multiplied by disease prevalence, p. Similarly, false positives, FP, can be calculated by multiplying lack of disease specificity $(1 - b)$ by the prevalence of nondisease in the population under study. Therefore,

$$f = p(1 - a) + (1 - b)(1 - p) \tag{3}$$

For most cancers, prevalence of disease in a general population screen will be tend to zero. Therefore,

$$f = 1 - b \tag{4}$$

It follows, therefore, that under the conditions and assumptions outlined—very low prevalence and equality of penalty for false-negatives and false-positives—one should increase specificity at the expense of sensitivity to minimize misclassifications.

3.3. Targeted Screening

The most frequently cited example of successful screening using a tumor marker is the use of human chorionic gonadotropin (hCG) in choriocarcinoma, and it is instructive to consider briefly why hCG has worked so wonderfully well when no other tumor markers are as competent.

Choriocarcinoma is rare; it accounts for 0.02% of all cancer deaths and is almost exclusively confined to women who have had a hydatidiform mole, of whom about 8% go on to develop choriocarcinoma. The single key fact that makes the screening program workable is the application of the test to a predetermined group in which the disease is present at a high prevalence.

If we assume that hCG has a sensitivity (a) of 99% and a specificity (b) of 99% and choriocarcinoma has a prevalence (p) of 8% in our screening group, then we can calculate the positive predictive value of hCG in this context:

$$\begin{aligned} \text{PPV} &= pa/[pa + (1 - b)(1 - p)] \\ &= 0.08 \times 0.99/[(0.08 \times 0.99) + (1 - 0.99)(1 - 0.08)] = 89.6\% \end{aligned}$$

By contrast, if one attempted to screen for choriocarcinoma all women whose pregnancies had achieved full term (prevalence 0.01%), the positive predictive value would be vanishingly small:

$$\text{PPV} = 0.0001 \times 0.99/[(0.0001 \times 0.99) + (1 - 0.99)(1 - 0.0001)] = 0.98\%$$

It is, therefore, apparent that for screening to be effective, a high-prevalence group must be identified in order to keep the number of false positives to an acceptable level.

4. Clinical Utility

Clinical effectiveness demands that the early intervention afforded by a successful screen is translated into an increased rate of cure or improved survival time. Objective quantification of improvement in survival time is not quite as simple as it first might appear, as studies are subject to various forms of methodological bias.

4.1. Lead-Time Bias

Survival is measured from the date of diagnosis to death, rather than from the date of inception to death. The date of diagnosis may therefore vary considerably, depending on the methods of detection used, without altering the true length of survival from the date of inception. Lead time generated by screening, or the period from detection while the woman is still asymptomatic until the appearance of clinical symptoms, which would permit conventional diagnosis, may increase the apparent survival without, in fact, the individual having benefited from screening. In such circumstances, the patient has to live longer with the knowledge of the disease.

4.2. Length Bias

A series of cases diagnosed at screening will be atypical of those arising clinically, because it will contain a disproportionate number of patients with slowly developing tumors, probably with a better prognosis. Patients with rapidly progressing tumors are more likely to present with symptoms before the initiation of, or in the interval between, screening tests. This bias is more likely to be manifest at the initiation of screening and is, therefore, especially important in studies of short duration.

4.3. Selection Bias

Selection bias results from entry of a cohort into a screening trial who have a different probability of developing and dying from the disease than the population at large. In self-selected populations, it is common to find a higher than normal proportion of individuals presenting for screening because of a positive family history. These individuals are more motivated to present for screening because they are more educated in this respect and are more likely to benefit from it. This has been well demonstrated in breast and cervical screening programs.

5. Optimization Strategies

It was demonstrated earlier that when prevalence was very low (tending to zero), if false negatives and false positives carried equal penalty, then to minimize misclassifications, one should maximize *specificity*. In addition, one should maximize specificity in situations where the disease is serious but cannot be treated or cured and for which, therefore, any false-positive result would lead to psychological trauma. Some occult cancers would clearly fall into this group, as well as diseases such as multiple sclerosis. Such incurable diseases should not be subject to population screening, as there is usually no benefit to patient or society at large in early diagnosis. In this section, the other available options will be considered and under which circumstances it would be appropriate to use them.

5.1. Sensitivity

Sensitivity should be maximized in situations where although the disease is serious and should not be missed, it *is* treatable and, therefore, false positives are less psychologically damaging. Most treatable infectious diseases would fall into this category, as do phaeochromocytoma and phenylketonuria. Cervical cancer, for which the screening program is effective and confirmatory tests are available prior to an effective therapeutic intervention program, is an example of a malignancy that may fall into this category. Furthermore, the concern caused by the presence of abnormal cells upon a cervical smear can in large measure be offset by the patient being aware of the success of early treatment.

5.2. Positive Predictive Value

The positive predictive value should be maximized in any situation where treatment of a false positive could be seriously damaging. Where the treatment indicated involves major surgery and radiotherapy, such as certain occult carcinomas, instigating treatment in someone who did not have the disease would be a major catastrophe.

5.3. Accuracy (or "Efficiency")

Accuracy of a very high order is required when a disease is both serious and treatable *and* false-positive and false-negative results carry equal penalty. Myocardial infarction has usually been cited as the classical example of where the tests should be optimized for accuracy [(TP + TN)/(TP + TN + FP + FN)]; however, a case for optimizing accuracy could be made in testing for certain leukemias and lymphomas.

6. The Use of Multiple Markers

The idea of using a group of markers in order to complement the sensitivity and specificity of each other seems logical enough and can be extremely beneficial. There are certain rules that can be defined and applied, and certain pitfalls to avoid.

There are two distinct approaches to multiple testing. The first, as described in the above example, is so-called *series* testing; the various tests are performed one after the other depending on the result of the previous test. In series testing, therefore, a "test-positive" patient is one who has scored positive in all of the tests. A secondary consideration here is defining the order in which the tests are to be performed to maximize efficacy, although considerations of cost and patient compliance also need to be included in any trial design. In *parallel* testing, all tests are performed on all patients, a "test-positive" patient in these circumstances is one who is positive on any one (or more) of the tests.

It is usual in a screening exercise for series testing to be preferred because it maximizes specificity at the expense of sensitivity which, as discussed earlier, is a rational approach when disease prevalence is low. Calculation of the PPV for parallel and series regimes bear this out ***(10)***.

For series testing, as not all tests are performed on all samples, there is the option of the order in which the tests are to be performed. There are many considerations: the relative cost of the tests involved, the degree of invasiveness, and the relative sensitivities and specificities of the tests involved. If variables such as cost are set aside, it can be shown that the sensible option is to test in series rather than parallel, as the positive predictive value is far higher and the total number of tests performed is much less. Also, although the PPV is independent of the order of testing, the number of analyses that have to be performed varies considerably, being minimized by application first of the test with the higher (or highest) specificity of those in the panel.

6.1. Series Testing

In an abstract ***(11)***, a research group reported the results of screening 1010 postmenopausal women for epithelial ovarian cancer using the serum marker CA125 followed up by ultrasonography. The group found a level of greater than 30 units/mL (their cutoff level) in 31 women. These 31 were then given ultrasonography; 3 were deemed abnormal and sent for surgery. One had an early-stage ovarian cancer. The authors concluded that CA125 had a high specificity for ovarian cancer, that they could increase the sensitivity by lowering the cutoff from 30 to 23 units/mL (the widely accepted cutoff value is, in fact, 35 units/mL), and that CA125 warranted further investigation for early diagnosis.

Their data are shown in **Table 2.** It is apparent from these data that there is no good reason to lower the cutoff from 30 to 23, as the sensitivity is already 100%. How reliable that figure is, however, is open to question, as there is only one true positive in the study. Furthermore, false negatives—here reported as zero—invariably take longer to emerge from any study and tend to be the most difficult to follow up; for these reasons then, the reported sensitivity may be an overestimate. The one true-positive patient had a CA125 level of 32 units/mL. Therefore, if these workers had followed the axiom of optimizing specificity at the expense of sensitivity, they would, in all probability, have missed the one patient who was to benefit directly from the trial. Their reason for opting for a higher sensitivity in this case was that they had a highly efficient second test

Table 2
Data From 1010 Postmenopausal Women Screened for Epithelial Ovarian Cancer (EOC) Using CA125

	EOC positive	EOC negative	Totals
CA125 positive	1 (TP)	31 (FP)	32 (TP + FP)
CA125 negative	0 (FN)	978 (TN)	978 (TN + FN)
Totals	1 (TP + FN)	1009 (TN + FP)	1010 (all)

Abbr: TP, true positive; TN, true negative; FP, false positive; FN, false negative.
Sensitivity = TP/(TP + FN) = 1/1 = 100%
Specificity = TN/(TN + FP) = 978/1009 = 97%
Prevalence = (TP + FN)/(TP + TN + FP + FN) = 1/1010 = 0.1%
Accuracy = (TP + TN)/(TP + TN + FP + FN) = 979/1010 = 97%
Positive predictive value = TP/(TP + FP) = 1/32 = 3.1%

(ultrasonography) to filter out the majority of the false positives generated by the CA125 alone and did not wish to miss any cases. It can be seen from **Table 2** that despite a sensitivity of 100%, a specificity of 97%, and an overall accuracy of 97%, the PPV was only 3.1% for CA125, hopelessly inadequate as a single selector for exploratory surgery. It is also true to say that knowing the sensitivity and specificity of the test and the disease prevalence, one could have calculated this PPV without having to do the trial, saving considerable expense. ("Since Isaac Newton, we no longer have to chart the fall of each apple"—Sir Peter Medawar.)

However, when ultrasonography is added in as a second-line test, the PPV improves by an order of magnitude to 33% (1/3) which is perhaps an acceptable pickup rate considering the high mortality rate of the disease if not diagnosed early. In effect, the use of CA125 in this and other studies generates a subgroup of the population under study who are at higher risk than the population at large; it defines a high-prevalence group thereby enabling a second-line test of similar sensitivity and specificity to produce a PPV that is far higher.

6.2. Panel Testing

Evaluation of a panel of tests is, of course, subject to all of the same provisions as for the assessment of a single test; particularly, the prevalence of the disease in the study group must be typical of the prevalence in the population to which it is intended to apply the test(s).

In a study of ovarian cancer by Ward et al. *(12)* in 1987, it was reported that by using three markers, the sensitivity in samples from pretreatment patients with stage 1 and 2 disease had increased from 18% using CA125 alone to 64% using human milk-fat globulin II (HMFG2) as the second assay and placental alkaline phosphatase (PLAP) as a third marker. That is to say, CA125 had picked up 2/11 of the diseased group and HMFG2 and PLAP had picked up a further 5 of the CA125 negative group, taking the total to 7/11. However, as all the subjects under study were disease-positive, it can be seen that neither CA125, HMFG2, nor PLAP performed significantly differently from random chance. They also studied the marker panel in patients with advanced disease. In the 26 patients with advanced (stage 3 and stage 4) disease, 25 had elevated CA125 (96%) and the 26th had an elevated PLAP. Therefore, all patients with advanced carcinoma of the ovary were positive for at least one of these three markers. These results are not quite as promising as one might at first believe: Using such a group of patients where prevalence is 100% (whether early-stage or advanced disease), one could achieve apparently excellent sensitivity by four consecutive coin flips at considerably less cost! (Each flip will have a 50% sensitivity; therefore, in series, the cumulative sensitivity will become 50%, 75%, 87.5%, and 93.75%.)

7. Conclusions

Disease prevalence is of fundamental importance in the rational application of tumor marker assays. By and large, cancer prevalence is too low in the population to permit effective screening even if the financial and ethical constraints could be overcome. In ovarian cancer, there is, therefore, a large amount of current research directed at the identification of possible high-risk groups—the so-called cancer families—in which prevalence is significantly higher than in the population at large because of genetic predisposition.

The use of tumor markers to monitor disease progress or remission, to track therapeutic efficacy, or to give a lead time to relapse are much more successful. Here, the markers either are being applied to a group in order to quantify a disease known to be present or to pick up a relapse in a group where relapse and, therefore, disease prevalence will be high. The routine application of tumor markers in a clinical context has been reviewed elsewhere ***(13,14)***.

Acknowledgments

The author is indebted to Dr. Cathie Sturgeon for her critique of this chapter. He is also grateful to Churchill Livingstone for permission to use excerpts from his textbook: *Serological Tumour Markers: An Introduction* ***(10)***.

References

1. Baum, M. (1988) *Breast Cancer; The Facts*. Oxford University Press, Oxford, pp. 1–6.
2. von Rustizky, J. (1873) Multiple myeloma. *Zentralbl. Chirugie (Leipzig)* **3,** 102–111.

3. Kahler, O. (1889) Zur symptomatologie des multiplen myelomas. *Wiener Med. Presse* **30,** 209–253.
4. Homburger, F. (1950) Evaluation of diagnostic tests for cancer. 1. Methodology of evaluation and review of suggested diagnostic procedures. *Cancer* **3,** 143–172.
5. Bodansky, O. (1974) Reflections on biochemical aspects of human cancer. *Cancer* **33,** 364–370.
6. Woodruff, M. (1990) *Cellular Variation and Adaptation in Cancer. Biological Basis and Therapeutic Consequences*, Oxford University Press, Oxford, pp. 1–7.
7. Galen, R. S. and Gambino S. R. (1975) *Beyond Normality: The Predictive Value and Efficiency of Medical Diagnoses*, Wiley Medical, New York.
8. Bayes, T. (1763) An essay toward solving a problem in the doctrine of chance. *Phil. Trans. R. Soc.* **53,** 370–418.
9. Miller, A. B. (1985) Principles of screening and of the evaluation of screening programs, in *Screening for Cancer*, (Miller, A. B., ed.), Academic, New York, pp. 3–24.
10. Roulston, J. E. and Leonard, R. C. F. (1993) *Serological Tumor Markers: An Introduction*, Churchill Livingstone, Edinburgh, pp. 15–34.
11. Jacobs, I. J., Bridges, J., Stabile, I., et al. (1987) CA-125 and screening for ovarian cancer: serum levels in 1010 apparently healthy postmenopausal women. *Br. J. Cancer* **55,** 515.
12. Ward B. G., Cruickshank, D. J., Tucker D. F., et al. (1987) Independent expression in serum of three tumor-associated antigens: CA125, placental alkaline phosphatase and $HMFG_2$ in human ovarian carcinoma. *Br. J. Obstet. Gynæcol.* **94,** 696–698.
13. Bormer, O. P., Paus, E., and Nustad K. (1998) Sensible use of tumor markers in routine practice. *Proc. UK NEQAS Meeting* **3**, 140–145.
14. Hayes, D. F., Bast, R. C., Desch, C. E., et al. (1996) Tumor marker utility grading system: a framework to evaluate clinical utility of tumor markers. *J.N.C.I.* **88**, 1456–1466.

3

Quality Assurance of Predictive Markers in Breast Cancer

Anthony Rhodes and Diana M. Barnes

1. Introduction

It has been estimated that in 2002, 555,500 Americans will have died of cancer, approximating to 1500 people per day *(1)*. In Britain, the figures are similarly high, with 150,200 reported deaths from cancer in the year 2000 *(2)*. Although a considerable proportion of these deaths are linked to environmental factors and arguably could have been reduced by preventative measures, understanding the molecular biological mechanisms that bring about cancer provides a handle by which the scientific and medical community may halt the progression of this disease.

The distinguishing features of tumor cells (i.e., their capacity for invasion, metastasis, unlimited proliferation, angiogenesis, and evasion of apoptosis) are all mediated by complex biological pathways. Many of the genes controlling the molecules in these pathways have been identified and the proteins they encode characterized. With these discoveries, drugs are being developed that target the protein and block or alter a particular molecular pathway with the potential to bring about disease regression. This explosion in molecular-based medicine has the potential to revolutionize the impact that pathology-based assays have on patient management. For example, to date, the majority of immunocytochemical markers employed in the histopathology department have had little direct impact on clinical management and merely assisted the pathologist to arrive at the correct diagnosis. Only a few, of which estrogen receptors (ERs) and HER-2/neu are classical examples, have been able to predict which patients are more likely to respond to a specific therapy. Markers such as ER and HER-2 are forerunners of a likely flood of markers, currently in the research or clinical trial and likely to permeate down to clinical utility in

From: *Methods in Molecular Medicine, vol. 79: Molecular Diagnosis of Cancer*
Edited by: J. E. Roulston and J. M. S. Bartlett © Humana Press Inc., Totowa, NJ

the very near future, some of which require similar quantitation and all of which will require standardization of assay technique. Examples of such markers are testing for BCR-Abl in chronic myeloid leukemia and CD117 in gastrointestinal stromal tumors (GISTs), identifying patients likely to respond to Glivec ***(3)***, and MLH1, MSH2, epithelial growth factor receptor (EGFR), and vascular endothelial growth factor (VEGF) in colorectal and others cancers, identifying patients likely to respond to tyrosine kinase inhibitors ***(4–6)***. One of the stumbling blocks that hinders the passage of all such assays from research to clinical utility is the lack of adequate quality control and reproducibility of assay results, both internally and between different cancer centers ***(7,8)***. Indeed, it is sobering to think that of the numerous potentially valuable predictive and prognostic tumor markers developed over the last 20 yr in breast and colorectal cancer, only ER and progesterone receptor (PR) values to predict benefit to breast cancer patients from endocrine therapy were considered in 1998 by the American Society of Clinical Oncology in 1998 to be clinically useful ***(9)***.

The controversy surrounding the lack of reproducibility of HER-2/neu immunocytochemisty (ICC) assays was in part responsible in the United Kingdom for the delay in transition of the drug Herceptin™ from the clinical trial stage to approved therapy by the National Institute of Clinical Excellence (NICE) ***(10)***. Similarly, a few years ago, there was great excitement about the potential clinical importance of p53 alterations. Multiple assays were used to test for p53, including ICC employing several different antibodies and antigen-retrieval methods, polymerase chain reaction (PCR)/single-strand conformation polymorphism (SSCP) and direct sequencing for p53 mutational status. Subsequently, there was lack of uniformity of the cut point, the method of reporting results, and the criteria to determine a positive result. Consequently, despite a plethora of reports about p53 alterations in various tumors, little in the way of clear evidence of its value as a tumor marker has emerged for any tumor site ***(11)***. The lack of a standardized assay to measure p53 status has contributed to much of this confusion. Grant funding bodies and pharmaceutical companies are keen to ensure that this scenario is not repeated for the new potentially valuable predictive markers currently coming on line. Even so, the quality assurance (QA) arrangements employed by many laboratories participating in the development of new markers and their utilization in clinical trials is often ad hoc, with lack of interlaboratory assay reproducibility of key markers resolved by do-it-yourself (DIY) approaches frequently bolted on at the last moment. Clearly, this is not an effective way of ensuring that the assays on which therapeutic decisions are based are robust, accurate, and have a high level of interlaboratory reproducibility. If this assay reproducibility cannot be assured, then it is likely that promising new therapies that rely on these assays will fall by the wayside and not progress from clinical trial status to approved drug status. This stumbling block in the establishment of robust and reproducible assays for new and potentially valuable predictive markers is deemed to be so important that the US National Cancer Institute (NCI) has specified that stringently quality-assured assays are an essential component in the development of new predictive and prognostic tests. In designing a suitable QA program for new molecular markers, much can be learned from previous experience gained in the QA of breast steroid hormone receptors and HER-2 assays.

2. Estrogen Receptors, Progesterone Receptors, and HER-2/neu

Breast cancer is the commonest form of cancer in women in the United Kingdom, with some 38,000 new cases diagnosed and approx 14,000 patients dying each year from the disease ***(12)***. However, recent statistics also show that breast cancer deaths in the United Kingdom and the United States were down by 25% in the year 2000, compared to death rates from this disease in 1990 ***(13)***. This substantial reduction in national mortality rates has come from the careful evaluation and adoption of many interventions, each responsible in its own way for a moderate reduction in breast cancer mortality. Some of the improvement seen in the breast cancer death rate trend over the last decade has undoubtedly been through the use of adjuvant treatments. Its use has been refined by the greater utilization of steroid hormone receptor assays in patient management—in particular, to predict which patients are most likely to respond to adjuvant tamoxifen treatment ***(14,15)***. Tamoxifen is now used widely as an adjuvant following surgery, and ER status has assumed an important role in identifying patients likely to benefit from such treatment ***(14)***. In turn, the use of ER in the management of breast cancer is one of the first examples of translational research (i.e., the transition of a biological marker from a promising area of research into a routine predictive marker) assayed in laboratories worldwide.

Given the clinical importance of establishing the accurate ER status of women with breast cancer, it was imperative from an early stage that adequate QA was introduced to ensure the reliability of the assays in clinical laboratories. Over the years, an extensive bank of QA data has been established by the European Organisation for the Research and Treatment of Cancer (EORTC) to provide technical validation of the biochemical ligand-binding assay (LBA) performed for ER and PR; these range from information on assay reproducibility, to standardization of the technique, to information relating to the variation in the distribution and frequency of receptor-positive breast carcinomas in different laboratories ***(16)***. More recently, similar validating studies have been made available for the immunocytochemical (ICC) demonstration of hormone receptors, as this assay has now replaced the biochemical based assays in virtually all routine clinical departments ***(17–20)***.

In addition to the proven value of the ER assay in breast cancer as a valuable predictive marker of clinical response to hormonal therapy, evidence has accumulated over the last 15 yr that shows that patients with tumors that have overexpression of the HER-2/neu receptor have a generally poor prognosis ***(21–25)***. This represents around 20–30% of breast cancer patients, the majority of whom tend to have tumors that are ER and PR negative ***(26)***. The HER-2 gene codes for a membrane surface protein related to dimerize and EGFR. Each of the surface receptors in this family have a closely associated intracellular tyrosine kinase that is activated when the receptors then bind to their respective ligands, in turn activating other intracellular signals that are ultimately transmitted to the cell nucleus, resulting in the transcription of genes involved in controlling cellular replication and differentiation ***(27)***. Recently, markers of HER-2/neu have been used to establish predictive assays, as clinical trials show the potential benefits of Herceptin™ (trastuzumab) therapy for patients with invasive breast carcinomas that overexpress the HER-2/neu protein ***(28–30)***. Herceptin therapy, consisting of a humanized monoclonal antibody, targets the HER-2/neu antigen and inhibits the growth of HER-2/neu-overexpressing tumor cells. In order to identify the 20–30% of women with breast cancer who will benefit most from Herceptin therapy, a reliable and reproducible assay is required to detect HER-2/neu overexpression.

Two main types of test have evolved: those directed at detecting amplification of the HER-2/*neu* gene by fluorescent *in situ* hybridization (FISH) and those directed at detecting over expression of the HER-2/neu protein by immunohistochemistry (IHC) ***(27,31)***. Both types of test have the advantage of allowing evaluation of gene amplification (FISH) or protein overexpression (IHC) in relation to tumor morphology, unlike molecular techniques, which require homogenization of the tumor. The rationale behind evaluating gene amplification by FISH and using it as a predictive test lies in the close correlation between HER-2/*neu* gene amplification and HER-2/neu protein overexpression ***(21,32)***. However, the correlation is weak for tumors scored as 2+ by IHC (*see* **Table 1**), with a large proportion of patients tumors scored as 2+ not having gene amplification and, therefore, unlikely to respond to Herceptin therapy (although few clinical outcome data are yet available) ***(33)***. Consequently, in most European countries, the current practice is for 2+ cases identified in an initial screen with the IHC assay to be further tested with FISH to establish the HER-2/*neu* gene amplification status ***(34)***. Patients subsequently shown to have HER-2/*neu* gene amplification are considered for Herceptin therapy, along with the patients categorized as 3+.

Much of the controversy to date on the sometimes apparent lack of concordance between the two assays and, in particular, the emphasis on the large numbers of IHC-positive/FISH-negative results has centered around studies

Table 1
Scoring System Originally Devised for the HER-2/neu Clinical Trials Assay and Now Widely to Assess IHC Staining for HER-2/neu

Score	HER-2/new staining pattern
0	No staining is observed or membrane staining is observed in <10% of invasive tumor cells.
1+	A faint/barely perceptible membrane staining is detected in >10% of invasive tumor cells. The cells are only stained in part of their membrane.
2+	A weak-to-moderate complete membrane staining is observed in >10% of invasive tumor cells.
3+	A strong complete membrane staining is observed in >10% of invasive tumor cells.

that have pooled together both the 2+ cases and the 3+ cases and referred to them as positive results. If the 2+ category is recognized as an equivocal result that requires further study and the 3+ and 0/1+ categories are recognized as unequivocally positive and unequivocally negative results, respectively, then there is excellent correlation between the two techniques. When the data are analyzed in this way, greater than 99% of invasive breast carcinomas categorized as positive (3+) by IHC have HER-2/*neu* gene amplification with FISH, whereas greater than 99% of tumors classified as negative by IHC (0 or 1+) do not have gene amplification with FISH ***(35)***. Current clinical data on invasive breast carcinomas that have 3+ HER/neu overexpression as measured by IHC or HER-2/*neu* gene amplification as measured by FISH show that patients with these tumors have very similar times to progression and response rates ***(36)***. It is worth noting that the UK clinical guidelines on the use of trastuzumab for the treatment of advanced breast cancer currently only recommend patients with tumors expressing HER-2 scored at levels of 3+ as candidates for trastuzumab monotherapy or trastuzumab in combination with paclitaxel ***(10)***. However, these guidelines may well be updated in the future.

2.1. Quality Assurance of Prognostic and Predictive Markers

Quality assurance encompasses all measures taken to ensure the reliability of investigations, starting from satisfactory test sample selection, analyzing it appropriately, to recording the result accurately and reporting it to the clinician for appropriate action, with all procedures being documented for reference ***(37)***. Two of the main features of QA are internal quality control and external quality assessment.

2.2. Internal Quality Control

Internal quality control (IQC) is defined as the set of procedures undertaken by the staff of a laboratory for the continual evaluation of the reliability of the work of the laboratory and its emergent results, in order to decide whether they are reliable enough to be released on a day-to-day basis *(37)*. Most IQC procedures employ analysis of a control material and compare the result with predetermined limits of acceptability *(37)*. As with any laboratory assay, ideally all aspects of the test technique and the preparation of the tissues or cytological preparations on which the assay is performed should be monitored by quality control procedures. Although the following aspects of IQC refer to the considerations required to ensure the effective IQC of a routine clinical laboratory conducting IHC assays, the principles involved are applicable irrespective of the assay employed.

2.3. Quality Control of the Reagents and Procedures Used In the Preparation of Tissue for Assay

Part of the UK's Clinical Laboratory Accreditation (CPA) remit and the requirements of the U.S. Clinical Laboratory Improvement Amendments (CLIA) and the College of American Pathologists (CAP) Laboratory Accreditation Program (LAP) *(38,39)* require that there are written protocols pertaining to the reception of clinical specimens, their handling, and subsequent fixation and processing. All procedures involving the preparation of tissues and the subsequent tests performed require documentation along with detailed "standard operating procedures" (SOPs) of the methods and reagents employed. This allows for subsequent audit trails of the tests performed and the results issued by a laboratory. Batch numbers and sources of all reagents, calibrates, and quality control materials are required to be recorded so that they may be related to those used for an individual assay. The commercial reagents employed in the fixation and processing of tissues to paraffin wax will, themselves, have undergone various quality control procedures by the manufacturers, with stringency depending on the purity and quality of reagents purchased.

2.4. Quality Control of the Reagents Used in the IHC Assay

The primary antibodies, secondary detection systems, and reagents employed in the IHC assay are subject to in-house quality control by the antibody manufacturer, with some manufacturers possessing the International Organisation for Standardisation (ISO) 9001 standard *(40)*.

The quality control of production, marketing, and use of antibodies for use in a clinical setting is currently influenced greatly by the US Food and Drug Administration (FDA). Ruling on the classification and reclassification of immunochemistry reagents and kits took effect November 23, 1999 ***(41,42)***. From this date on, the FDA expected US laboratories not to use antibodies labeled "for research purposes only" in diagnostic tests and that the results of studies using these reagents will not be accepted for reporting in patients' clinical records ***(42)***. Although this is an American ruling, most of the major antibody suppliers and producers in Europe have distribution networks and customers in the United States. Consequently, antibodies and the respective kits produced by some of the major companies, irrespective of their destination, currently conform to the new US FDA requirements. In addition, from 2003 on, European legislation will require European producers of antibodies and ancillary reagents to conform to Directive 98/79/EC ***(43)***. Although this is a self-certification process for most markers, it requires all companies to have in place, from this date onward, quality assurance methods similar to that required for ISO 9000. A few products, however, such as predictive test kits like the DakoCytomation HercepTest™, are likely to require certification from an external body.

2.5. Internal Quality Control of Steps in the Immunocytochemical Assay

Procedure controls are necessary to validate the results of IHC assays. The results of the staining are valid if any interference resulting from nonspecific staining is excluded (i.e., negative controls are not stained) and if the sensitivity of the technique is assured (i.e., positive tissue controls with low expression of the antigen in question are positive). They serve to monitor whether the staining protocols have been followed correctly, whether day-to-day and worker-to-worker variations have occurred, and whether the reagents continue to be in good working order ***(44)***. Procedure controls involve both reagent substitution and tissue controls.

Normal tissues make excellent external control systems for markers that are to be evaluated "qualitatively," where presence or absence of staining is the main contribution to the diagnostic process. For example, a section of reactive tonsil provides an excellent control system for various lymphoid markers such as CD45, CD20, CD3, and so forth. Not only does just about any optimally preserved reactive tonsil exhibit a predictable amount of antigen on the appropriate lymphocytes, but the localization and pattern of staining is also predictably constant, allowing the pathologist or laboratory scientist to easily judge whether or not, on a particular day, the expected pattern and localization of antibody staining was achieved. Consequently, for these markers, the run-to-run, day-to-day quality of staining can be readily ascertained by inspection of these controls.

2.6. Controls for Prognostic and Predictive Assays

The main predictive value of markers such as ER, PR, and HER-2 lies not in the presence or absence of staining in an invasive tumor but in the "quantity" of antigen present, as the amount of expression is predictive of the likelihood of response to therapy. Consequently, for many prognostic and predictive markers, it is not only vital to ensure that localization is appropriate (technical assay *specificity*) but also that the combined "strength" of the assay (technical assay *sensitivity*) is appropriate and does not vary from one day to the next. Technical assay sensitivity is mainly a function of the affinity and avidity of the primary antibody, the sensitivity of the detection system (usually avidin–biotin based), and the efficiency of the antigen retrieval step (e.g., heat-induced epitope retrieval [HIER] in the demonstration of hormonal receptors and HER-2/neu). The importance of the external control cannot be overemphasized, as it functions as a check to ensure that technical assay sensitivity is appropriate and does not vary, as the reported index of antigen expression for a test tumor will ultimately be influenced by not only the actual biological expression of the tumor but also by the sensitivity of the IHC assay. Thus, inadequate or inappropriately high assay sensitivity could result in false-negative or false-positive results, respectively. In this instance, the external control serves as a check to ensure that technical assay sensitivity has remained a constant and, as such, it is imperative that it can detect even slight variations in day-to-day assay sensitivity.

The current recommendations as a sensitive control system for hormone receptors are a composite tissue block comprising receptor-rich, receptor-poor, and receptor-negative invasive breast carcinomas ***(45)***. In addition, normal glands serve as a useful internal positive control, which when stained with an IHC assay for ER or PR appear as single, scattered positive cells surrounded by ER-negative cells ***(46)***.

Similarly, in order to ensure the accuracy and reproducibility of the results for HER-2/neu obtained by IHC, it is necessary to have a standard control by which day-to-day variation in the sensitivity of the assay can be accurately monitored. However, the level of QA required for HER-2/neu is considerably more sophisticated than that required for any other IHC test to date. For ER and PR, it has been shown that interlaboratory variation has been the result of a general lack of assay sensitivity rather than a quantifiable amount and as long as laboratories employed the most sensitive IHC methods, then appropriate and reproducible results were achieved ***(20)***. This is not the case with HER-2/neu; on the contrary, the controversy that has surrounded this important test has focused on assays with too much sensitivity rather than too little ***(47–49)***. However, clearly, too little sensitivity is as just as likely to result in patients receiving inappropriate management as assays for which the sensitivity is set too high. Therefore, for the first time, the importance of setting routine IHC at a defined and standard sensitivity level has been highlighted.

In this respect, the use of QC systems comprised of composite tissue blocks representative of several tumors with varying levels of overexpression for the HER-2/neu protein is not ideal. Tumor material is frequently difficult to acquire and the quantity available for use for quality control (QC) is limited. Consequently, even over a relatively short period of time, a laboratory may need to use several different cases as a control, each with individual variations in tumor expression. Obviously, this is not ideal for a standard by which to stringently gage day-to-day assay sensitivity for HER-2/neu overexpression, as an unpredicted fall or rise in a laboratory's assay sensitivity may not be readably detected ***(50)***.

One way around this problem is to use cell lines fixed and processed in a way similar to histopathological specimens ***(50)***. Although the characteristics of a cell line are liable to change with different treatments or cell passages, a large-scale cell production allows for a single harvest of a large quantity of cells with a specific level of expression ***(51,52)***. Such a harvest of cells of the same phenotype all fixed and processed at the same time allows for a large and long-lasting bank of standard control material. Thus, cell lines have the potential to provide for consistency of antigen expression over a relatively long period of time, not otherwise possible with tumor tissue-based controls.

2.7. Quality Control Systems and Standardization of IHC Assays for Predictive and Prognostic Markers

Different approaches can be used by laboratories to ensure a "standard" result, as a standard result is what is required if patients are to receive appropriate therapy regardless of where they are treated and if data collected from multiple laboratories participating in clinical trials are to be reliable. One approach is for all laboratories to use the exact same test, the exact same tissue preparatory methods, and the exact same system of evaluation. The HercepTest, developed and marketed by DakoCytomation, is one such approach, with the companies insistence that users of the HercepTest kit adhere to strict guidelines on how the tissue is fixed, through to the use of a detailed technical method and interpretation of the results. Individual laboratories are "trained" on both the technical aspects of this FDA-approved methodology and in evaluating the results using the initial clinical trials assay (CTA) scoring system ***(25)***. One would expect, therefore, that the stringent training program and guidelines imposed would result in a greater level of reproducibility among different sites, not only in assay sensitivity but also in the evaluation of the results, when compared to centers not subjected to this stringent training program. Indeed, evidence to date suggests that this is the case (*see* **Table 2**) ***(53)***.

A different approach to achieving the "standard result" is for laboratories to use whatever antibody or method they choose but aim to achieve the same "end point" on a control system that has been calibrated against a standard reference material. Obviously, this depends entirely on the availability of a suitable reference material. An attempt has been made to develop such a system based on four formalin-fixed and paraffin-processed cell lines, one with an expression level for HER-2/neu for each of the scoring categories, 0, 1+, 2+, and 3+ in the CTA scoring system (*see* **Fig. 1**) ***(50)***. The advantage of standardization by this approach is that it may well permit government agencies such as the US FDA to broaden its certification of additional HER-2 reagents, thus allowing laboratories to choose from various commercial suppliers and manufacturers of specific reagents ***(7,8,50)***. This, in turn, will keep costs down and not exclude antibodies and desirable technical innovations that may further improve the reliability of IHC tests. In this respect, it is important that assays other than the DakoCytomation HercepTest continue to be validated, as markers such as the CB11 and TAB 250 clones have recently been shown to have a greater level of concordance with HER-2/*neu* gene amplification as measured by FISH and to have greater statistical significance with respect to patient response rates to combined trastuzumab and paclitaxel therapy ***(54)***.

The value of a standard reference material therefore is that it provides a biological "constant" against which the "variable" of immunohistochemical assay sensitivity for HER-2/neu can be accurately gaged, regardless of which antibody, antigen-retrieval system, detection system, or method of evaluation is employed. It allows the same laboratory and multiple laboratories to check that they are achieving the same sensitivity level on a run-to-run, day-to-day, year-to-year, laboratory-to-laboratory basis.

Any standard reference material should be extensively analyzed to establish staining patterns with the most commonly used markers (e.g., the HercepTest, clones CB11 and TAB 250 for HER-2/neu assays). In addition, the HER-2/neu amplification status should be established by FISH as should ideally the numbers of receptors per cell, as preclinical observations have suggested that a HER-2 receptor density in excess of 100,000 receptors per cell is required for maximal trastuzumab benefit ***(25)***.

It has been suggested that a control system such as this would have to be fixed under identical conditions to the test specimen in order that it be subjected to the same variations in fixation and processing ***(55)***. The argument is that only then can it be assured that the same amount of antigen retrieval and the same assay sensitivity would reveal the same antigen expression in both control system and test specimen. However, providing that laboratories follow

Table 2
Comparison of the Proportion of Appropriate Results With Different IHC Assays for HER-2/neu by 78 Laboratories Participating at Two Consecutive Assessment Runs, Utilizing a Cell Line Standard Reference Material

	Appropriate results*			
Antibody and supplier†	1st	2nd	x^2	p
DAKO HercepTest	15/22 (68%)	19/25 (76%)	0.735	0.391
DAKO Polyclonal code A0485	10/34 (29%)	17/31 (55%)	10.052	0.002
Novocastra clone CB11	2/14 (14%)	6/15 (40%)	8.422	0.004
Other	1/8 (13%)	5/7 (71%)	21.129	<0.001
Total	**28/78 (36%)**	**47/78 (60%)**	**19.919**	**<0.001**

*The proportion of laboratories achieving the following scores on the four cell lines; SKOV-3 (3+), MDA-MB-453 (2+), BT-20 (0 or 1+), MCF-7 (0 or 1+).

†DAKO (Ely, Cambridgeshire, UK), Novocastra Laboratories Ltd. (Newcastle upon Tyne, UK). Others include clone CB11, Biogenex (San Ramon, CA); clone 3B5, Immunotech (Beckman Coulter, Inc., Fullerton, CA); clone 3B5 Oncogene Research Products (CN Biosciences, UK), clones CBE-1 and TAB 250, Zymed Laboratories Inc. (San Francisco, CA).

Source: Reprinted from **ref. *53*** with permission from the *American Journal of Clinical Pathology.*

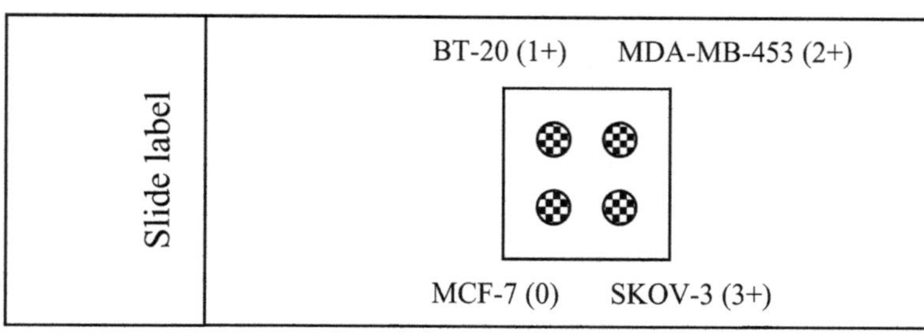

Fig. 1. A diagram of a cell line standard for HER-2/neu, showing the names of the four-cell lines, the position of the cell lines in the paraffin section mounted on a glass slide, and the expected and most appropriate results (in parentheses) following IHC assay and evaluation with the CTA scoring system. (Reprinted from **ref. *50*** with permission from the *American Journal of Clinical Pathology.*)

generally approved guidelines on formalin fixation and processing, this may not be important. The fact that different authors have used the same cell lines but grown at different sites and fixed using varying fixation regimes and yet still report similar HER-2/neu overexpression levels suggest that this is the case ***(50,56,57)***. In any event, the rate of penetration and crosslinking of a formalin fixative on free cells suspended in agar is unlikely to be the same as that of invasive tumor cells set in a connective tissue matrix, even if the cell line control and specimen are fixed and processed simultaneously and under identical conditions. Furthermore, evidence from reference centers with standardized assays analyzing tumors for ER and HER-2 from nonreferral laboratories with varying fixation regimes shows that the main reason for interlaboratory variation in results is not the result of differences in fixation and preparatory methods but to poor quality assays ***(18,36)***. Therefore, a robust and standard assay appears to be reproducible even on referral material having undergone differences in fixation and processing. Consequently, the main limiting factor in assay reproducibility is assay quality, not slight variations in fixation. From this, it can be deduced that slightly different formalin fixation of a standard reference material from than that of the test specimen is unlikely to result in significantly different HER-2/neu antigen exposure and demonstration by the same assay.

Similar standard reference materials (SRMs) could be developed for other predictive markers in addition to HER-2/neu. The most appropriate level of IHC assay sensitivity will be established from clinical response data, ultimately the "gold standard" by which the power of all predictive tests are evaluated. However, it is perceived that SRMs will be extremely valuable tools in ensuring that day-to-day, month-to-month, and laboratory-to-laboratory assay sensitivity remain a constant while clinical data accumulates to establish the value of new and established predictive tests. Government-backed agencies such as the National Institute of Science and Technology (NIST) and professional groups in the United States are currently exploring this approach. In Europe, evidence to date suggests that even after limited exposure to an SRM composed of cell lines, significant improvement in IHC assay reproducibility is seen between multiple HER-2/neu testing laboratories (*see* **Table 2**) ***(53)***. Although SRMs may provide the much needed QC materials upon which a "standard result" is possible, comprehensive quality assurance programs will almost certainly be required to provide educational guidance to laboratories on how to achieve the most appropriate results on these control systems and their own "in-house" tumors.

2.8. External Quality Assessment

The principal advantage of external quality assessment (EQA) is that it is able to detect differences of quality between laboratories and provide guidance on how to achieve the standards deemed to be universally "acceptable." EQA is defined by the World Health Organisation and the European Committee for Clinical Laboratory Standards as a system of retrospectively and objectively comparing results from different laboratories by means of an external agency ***(58,59)***. Whereas IQC controls the precision of investigations, EQA provides an assessment of their accuracy with respect to other test sites. This is done

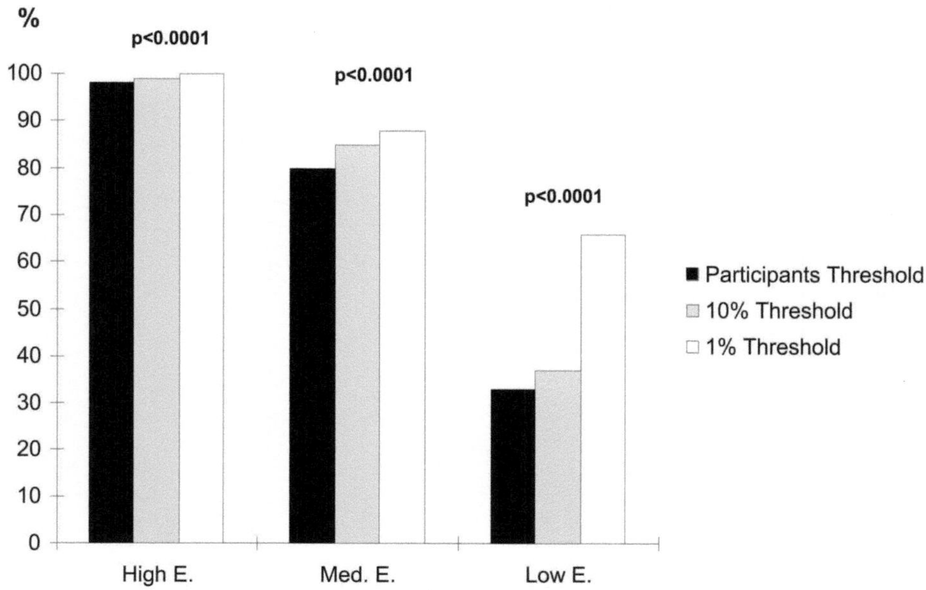

Fig. 2. The proportion of 200 laboratories whose immunohistochemical assays reliably demonstrated three tumors with high, medium, and low ER expression, respectively, using different threshold values. *p*-Values are two-tailed. (Reprinted from **ref.** ***17*** with permission from the *BMJ* Publishing Group.)

periodically and retrospectively, hence the term "assessment" rather than "control" ***(37)***. Participation in a relevant EQA scheme is now a prerequisite for clinical laboratories in the United Kingdom wishing to gain Clinical Laboratory Accreditation (CPA).

Prior to the introduction of IHC assays for ER and PR, the majority of ICC markers employed in the histopathology department had little direct impact on clinical management and merely assisted the pathologist to arrive at the correct diagnosis, in much the same way as "special stains" had done for many years. Consequently, markers such as those to ER heralded a new type of marker and a new challenge with respect to ensuring adequate QA of such techniques. Evidence gradually accumulated from EQA programs to show that assays of relatively low sensitivity could achieve adequate demonstration in breast cancers with large amounts of ER expression as determined by the "gold standard" LBA. However, when this assay sensitivity was applied to tumors with relatively few ER receptors, as determined by the LBA, a significant proportion of laboratories produced false-negative results even when employing their own threshold value to determine a positive result (*see* **Fig. 2**) ***(17)***. This suboptimal assay sensitivity on EQA material was subsequently shown to correlate strongly with the results achieved by participating laboratories on "in-house"

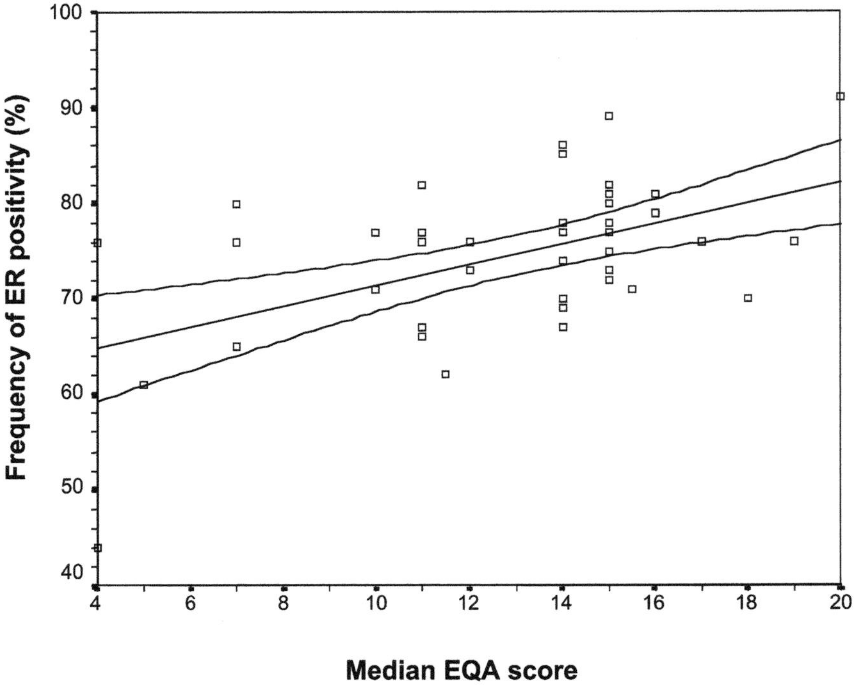

Fig. 3. Scatter diagram to show the relationship between frequency of ER positivity of in-house breast tumors over an 18-mo period in 42 different laboratories with the median EQA score (range: 4–20) achieved over the same time period. A least-squares linear regression line is shown with a 95% confidence interval, giving the best fit for all the data points. Spearmans coefficient = 0.346, $p = 0.019$ (two-tailed). (Reprinted from **ref.** ***19*** with permission from the *BMJ* Publishing Group.)

tumors (*see* **Figs. 3** and **4**) ***(18,19)***. Furthermore, it was possible to show that the main reason for the lower proportion of positive tumors in participants' laboratories achieving low scores at EQA was the result of suboptimal IHC assays and that this was independent of other variables such as the method of scoring or threshold value used ***(17,19)***. Consequently, it could be shown that EQA results were an accurate indicator of "in-house" laboratory performance and, therefore, useful in monitoring assay sensitivity in multiple laboratories performing clinical tests for ER and PR. In addition, this variability in results for important predictive markers between multiple laboratories provided evidence to support a message that had been espoused by experts in the field for some time, this being that QA and standardization of IHC is essential if erroneous results are to be avoided and patients are to receive the most appropriate therapy ***(55,60,61)***.

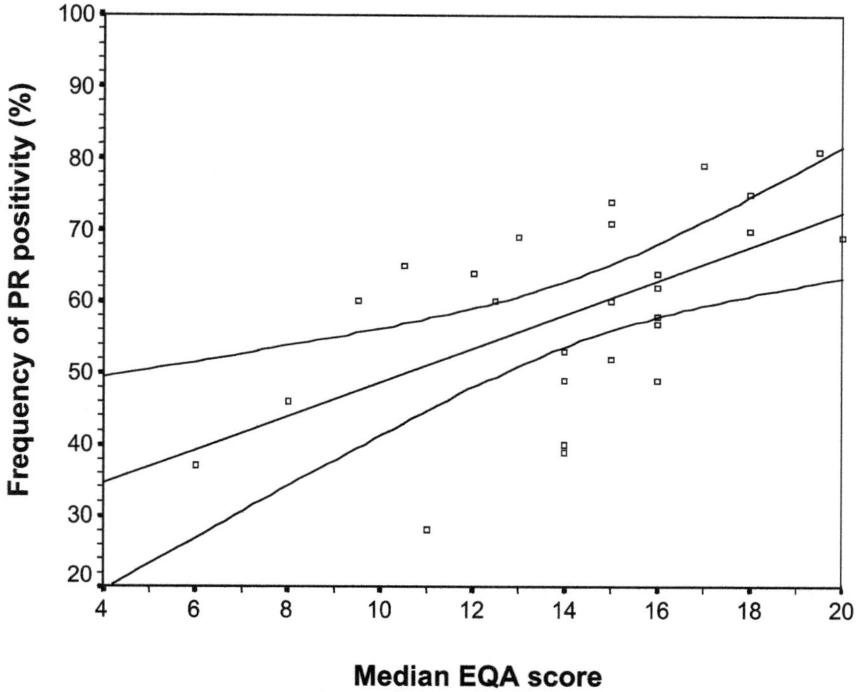

Fig. 4. Scatter diagram to show the relationship between frequency of PR positivity of in-house breast tumors over an 18-mo period in 42 laboratories and the median EQA score (range: 4–20) achieved over the same time period. A least-squares linear regression line is shown with a 95% confidence interval, giving the best fit for all the data points. Spearmans correlation coefficient = 0.561, p = 0.003 (two-tailed). (Reprinted from **ref.** ***19*** with permission from the *BMJ* Publishing Group.)

Although much of the QA for the IHC assay implemented to date has relied on the distribution of sections of invasive breast tumors to each participating laboratory where they are immunostained and returned for assessment, a different approach to QA has been to look at the frequency of positive tumors in a group of laboratories using the IHC assay to ER and PR ***(19)***. This sought, in part, to emulate previous work carried out by a study group of the EORTC that investigated the distribution of ER and PR in a large number of cases from seven European laboratories, as determined by enzyme immunoassay (EIA) and the LBA ***(62)***. The authors worked on the assumption that if the natural history of breast cancer is the same in different geographical areas, then similar frequencies of receptor positivity would be expected in different laboratories. As well as determining the variation of ER and PR distributions between the different laboratories, the study provided useful data on the expected frequency of receptor positivity in the populations studied. The accumulative frequency data on the receptor status of tumors in the participating institutions using IHC assays showed good correlation with that of the studies by Romain et al. and other workers utilizing LBA and EIA assays to establish these values *(19,62)*. In addition, with data on over 4000 cases from 42 mainly European laboratories, it was also possible, for the first time, to stratify ER/PR IHC positivity into different patient age groups (*see* **Table 3**) *(19)*. The value of this dataset is that it is a useful QA tool, against which any laboratory can compare their current IHC receptor assay positivity rates. The data can be further refined by including only that from laboratories that were recorded as achieving optimal results in an EQA program over the same period of time (*see* **Table 4**).

However, external quality assurance entails more than monitoring and reporting variability of results between different laboratories. In effect, if EQA served to do no more than this, then, essentially, it would be just an external form of "internal" quality control (IQC) that would detect errors in the system but not claim to be able to do anything about them, either by troubleshooting to identify the problem area or to provide the tools required to correct the problem once identified. EQA, therefore, entails identifying laboratories that have suboptimal assays, identifying the underlying reason for the suboptimal results, and then assisting these laboratories adjust their assays in order to achieve optimal results. This process not only helps ensure appropriate results but also helps to standardize the assays used by the participating laboratories. As such, this process has already been shown to be effective in the QA of ER and can be used as a template for other predictive and prognostic markers.

2.9. Evidence to Show That EQA Can Effectively Improve Interlaboratory Standards for Hormonal Receptor Assays

The IHC assay consists of a number of technical variables; the main ones being antigen retrieval, choice of primary antibody and detection system as well as automation. When these 4 variables were investigated using data from the same 105 European laboratories participating in an EQA program over a 2-yr period, it was found that inefficient antigen-retrieval techniques were the main cause of poor results (*see* **Table 5** and **Fig. 5**). When laboratories achieving suboptimal results addressed this factor, significant improvement was seen and maintained at future assessment runs *(20)*.

The type and duration of fixation had been proposed as major variables affecting the reliability of IHC assay for ER and PR. However, providing fixation is prompt and occurs without delay following surgical removal of tissue to prevent destruction of the labile receptor epitopes and providing fixation is in a predominantly formalin-based fixative, such as 10% formalin or neutral-buffered formalin, for approx 24 h, fixation does not appear to be a limiting factor *(18)*.

Table 3
ER and PR Status of the 4053 Cases From the 42 Laboratories That Provided Data on Both Receptors, With Respect to Patient Age

Age (yr)	ER+ve, PR+ve	ER–ve, PR–ve	ER+ve, PR–ve	ER–ve, PR+ve	Total no. in each age group
21–30	18 (45.0%)	17 (42.5%)	3 (7.5%)	2 (5.0%)	40 (1.0%)
31–40	134 (45.9%)	97 (33.2%)	45 (15.4%)	16 (5.5%)	292 (7.2%)
41–45	195 (57.9%)	88 (26.1%)	35 (10.4%)	19 (5.6%)	337 (8.3%)
46–50	319 (58.6%)	116 (21.3%)	83 (15.3%)	26 (4.8%)	544 (13.4%)
51–55	378 (53.5%)	114 (21.9%)	112 (21.5%)	16 (3.1%)	520 (12.8%)
56–60	239 (51.0%)	102 (21.8%)	111 (23.7%)	16 (3.4%)	468 (11.6%)
61–65	271 (55.3%)	98 (20.0%)	113 (23.1%)	8 (1.6%)	490 (12.1%)
66–70	251 (57.2%)	85 (19.4%)	94 (21.4%)	9 2.1%)	439 (10.8%)
71–75	194 (57.6%)	60 (17.8%)	76 (22.6%)	7 (2.1%)	337 (8.3%)
>75	323 (55.1%)	119 (20.3%)	132 (22.5%)	12 (2.1%)	586 (14.5%)
Total (receptor status)	2222 (54.8%)	896 (22.1%)	804 (19.8%)	131 (3.2%)	4053 (100%)

Source: Reprinted from **ref. *19*** with permission from the *BMJ* Publishing Group.

Table 4
ER and PR Status of the 1985 Cases From the 16 Laboratories With High Assay Sensitivity for Both ER and PR, With Respect to Patient Age

Age (yr)	ER+ve, PR+ve	ER–ve, PR–ve	ER+ve, PR–ve	ER–ve, PR+ve	Total no. in each age group
21–30	5 (38.5%)	6 (46.2%)	1 (7.7%)	1 (7.7%)	13 (1.0%)
31–40	77 (42.4%)	43 (29.3%)	20 (13.65)	7 (4.8%)	147 (7.4%)
41–45	106 (60.9%)	44 (25.3%)	15 (8.6%)	9 (5.2%)	174 (8.8%)
46–50	165 (61.6%)	46 (17.2%)	44 (16.4%)	13 (4.9%)	268 (13.5%)
51–55	153 (59.1%)	47 (18.2%)	52 (20.1%)	7 (2.7%)	259 (13.1%)
56–60	128 (54.9%)	48 (20.6%)	51 (21.9%)	6 (2.6%)	433 (11.7%)
61–65	149 (62.3%)	39 (16.3%)	49 (20.5%)	2 (1.0%)	239 (12.0%)
66–70	122 (59.8%)	35 (17.2%)	43 (21.1%)	4 (2.0%)	204 (10.3%)
71–75	100 (64.5%)	20 (12.9%)	31 (20.0%)	4 (2.6%)	155 (7.8%)
>75	169 (57.7%)	51 (17.4%)	68 (23.2%)	5 (1.7%)	293 (14.8%)
Total (receptor status)	1174 (59.1%)	379 (19.1%)	374 (18.8%)	58 (2.9%)	1985 (100%)

Source: Reprinted from **ref. *19*** with permission from *BMJ* Publishing Group.

Table 5
Comparison of the Main Types of Antigen-Retrieval System Used by Laboratories Shown to Have Sensitive and Reproducible Immunohistochemical Assays for ER and PR With That Used by All Other Laboratories Participating in EQA Over the Same 2-yr Period

	Proportional use by laboratories (%)					
	With reproducible assays ($n = 24$)		Without reproducible assays ($n = 42$)			
System of antigen retrieval	Mean	95% CI	Mean	95% CI	Mann–Whitney U-test	p (two-tailed)
Microwave oven	34	28–40	60	54–66	0.000	0.001
Pressure cooker	54	50–58	26	23–30	0.000	0.001

Source: Reprinted from **ref. *20*** with permission from the *American Journal of Clinical Pathology.*

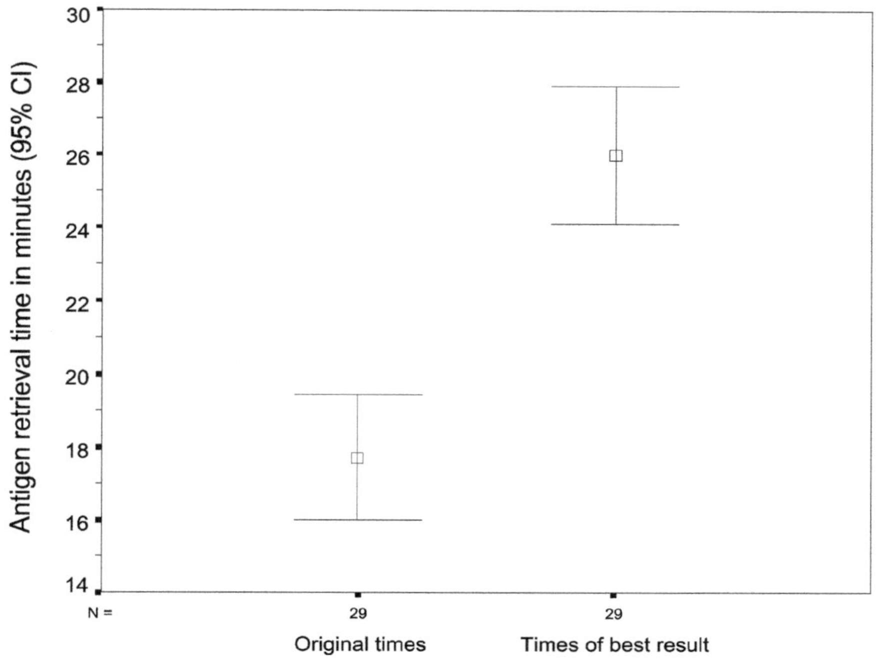

Fig. 5. Comparison of the original microwave antigen-retrieval times by 29 laboratories initially getting poor results at assessment using an immunohistochemical assay for ER, with the time, subsequently giving the best result for these laboratories, on the same cases. (Data reprinted from **ref. *20*** with permission from the *American Journal of Clinical Pathology.*)

Table 6
Methods of Evaluation for ER Used by UK NEQAS–ICC Participants

Threshold value	Frequency	%
10% or greater of tumor nuclei demonstrated	106	50.0%
Histo ("H") score	17	8.1%
20% or 25% and greater of tumor nuclei demonstrated	13	6.1%
5% or greater of tumor nuclei demonstrated	10	4.7%
"Quick" score	6	2.8%
1% or greater of tumor nuclei demonstrated	3	1.4%
Category score	2	0.9%
50% or greater of tumor nuclei demonstrated	2	0.9%
Values known but each account for less than 0.9% of total	8	3.8%
Unknown (information not provided by participant)	45	21.2%
Total	212	100%

Source: Reprinted from **ref. *17*** with permission from the *BMJ* Publishing Group.

2.10. Scoring of IHC Assays for ER, PR, and HER-2/neu

Of equal importance in ensuring appropriate results of ER and PR assays is the accuracy of the scoring systems employed to assess the receptor status (positive or negative) of a breast tumor and the establishment of an appropriate cutoff point, below which the likelihood of patients responding to tamoxifen is unlikely and for whom alternative first-line therapy would be more appropriate. Although there is still great variation in the scoring systems used to establish receptor status in Europe (*see* **Table 6**), a method in which the proportion of positive tumors is added to the intensity of staining is currently recommended in the United Kingdom (*see* **Table 7**). Various authors have testified to the good level of interobserver and intraobserver agreement using this Quick score method ***(63–65)***.

A recent article emphasized the need for a consensus on both the scoring system employed and the cutoff value used ***(15)***. However, such aspirations sometimes lack sufficient understanding of all the issues involved in establishing a standard scoring system and cutoff value. For example, unless all laboratories are achieving identical assay sensitivity on tumors fixed and processed in their own laboratories, the adoption of a single scoring system and cutoff value is pointless and likely to generate more false-positive and false-negative results than if every laboratory established its own scoring system and cutoff point. This highlights the importance of stringent QA of the technical aspects of assays for important predictive and prognostic markers, as, ultimately, the

Table 7
Recommended System for Scoring IHC Assays in the UK

Score for proportion staining	Score for staining intensity
0 = no nuclear staining	0 = no staining
1 = <1% nuclei staining	1 = weak staining
2 = 1–10% nuclei staining	2 = moderate staining
3 = 11–33% nuclei staining	3 = strong staining
4 = 34–66% nuclei staining	
5 = 67–100% nuclei staining	

Note: Adding the two scores together gives a maximum score of 8.
Source: Reprinted from **ref. *45*** with permission from the *BMJ* Publishing Group.

reliability of interpretation of the results of these assays relies considerably on the technical quality with which the assay sensitivity is performed. For example, on the same tumor, an assay of relatively high assay sensitivity will ultimately result in a higher "score" when the staining is interpreted than an assay from a different laboratory with lower sensitivity, regardless of how well the scoring is performed ***(18,64)***. This is important because the current recommendations predict that patients with higher scores are more likely to show a more favorable response to hormone therapy than those with lower scores. Another point to consider in establishing a useful threshold is whether the assay is being performed for purposes of predicting response to tamoxifen therapy or for prognosis, as the most appropriate cutpoint for both may well be different. Also, whether the test is being performed on tumors from premenopausal or postmenopausal women needs to be considered, as the tumors of premenopausal women will tend to have lower amounts of ER than postmenopausal women and, therefore, a different cutpoint may be appropriate.

A wide range of methods and threshold values have been employed in the scoring of assays for hormonal receptors (*see* **Table 6**), for the assessment of HER-2/neu IHC results the original CTA scoring system is employed in the vast majority of laboratories (*see* **Table 1**). Some studies have shown greater reproducibility of scoring when HER-2/neu is evaluated using an automated cellular imaging system than when using manual microscopy ***(66,67)***. For the investigation of the reproducibility of manual and automated scoring systems, the use of validated cell line standards in addition to tumor material has a number of advantages ***(50)***. First, it is possible to verify the level of gene amplification with FISH techniques on the whole cells as compared to tissue sections. This makes the subsequent counts of signals representing the amplified genes easier and, therefore, more reliable. Second, the presence of misleading fixation and processing artifacts frequently present in tissue samples has been eliminated. Confusion about which is the most representative area to score is therefore avoided, as all the cells are equally fixed and evenly distributed. Third, cell lines are the material on which the CTA scoring system was initially established and are currently used as procedure controls to ensure the reliability of the HercepTest staining, prior to evaluation of the results on the tumor test material ***(25,68)***. Consequently, for the HercepTest, it is important to ensure the reproducibility of the scoring system on both cell lines and tissue samples, as the evaluation of both will ultimately influence the reliability of the results. If there is a weakness in the scoring system, comparison of the evaluations performed by laboratories on cell lines and tumor samples may help identify whether the problem lies in the heterogeneity of the tumors and their fixation and processing, or purely in the difficulties encountered in accurately defining cell membrane staining intensity using a four-point scoring system.

When such a cell line system was used to investigate scoring reproducibility among evaluators employing the HercepTest and other HER-2/neu IHC assays, it was found that the stringent training program and guidelines imposed on users of the HercepTest resulted in a greater level of reproducibility between different sites in the evaluation of the results when compared to centers not subjected to this stringent training program ***(53)***. The results showed that agreement in scoring between laboratories employing the HercepTest was excellent both on cell lines and "in-house" tumors ($\kappa = 0.81$). In comparison, the level of agreement between laboratories using IHC assays other than the HercepTest was poor and the proportion of evaluations showing complete agreement was significantly lower on both tumors ($\kappa = 0.48$) and cell lines ($\kappa = 0.53$) (*see* **Table 8**). This discordance among non-HercepTest users would have resulted in tumors being erroneously reported as being unequivocally positive or unequivocally negative in 10/58 (17%) of the cases ***(53)***.

The level of agreement between the laboratories in evaluating the cell lines tended to reflect the level of agreement recorded for the evaluation of the in-house tumors. Consequently, this study suggested that lack of reproducibility of the CTA scoring system among multiple laboratories was not primarily because of the heterogeneity of the tumors being evaluated or the different ways in which they have been fixed and processed but because of how stringently the scoring criteria had been being applied ***(53)***. The findings suggests that when the CTA scoring system is strictly adhered to, it gives excellent agreement in scoring among different laboratories, both in the evaluation of tumors and in the evaluation of cell lines stained for HER-2/neu. Therefore, future work should focus on promoting the use of a standard scoring system

Table 8
Level of Agreement Between the EQA Assessor Scores and the Participating Laboratories' Scores When Using the CTA Scoring System on the Cell Lines SKOV-3, MDA-MB-453, BT-20, MCF-7, and Breast Tumors JHC Stained for HER-2/neu

Agreement	N[a]	κ	*95% CI*
All laboratories on the cell lines	268	0.64	0.57–0.71
All laboratories on breast tumors	103	0.62	0.50–0.74
Laboratories using the HercepTest on cell lines	104	0.81	0.72–0.90
Laboratories using IHC assays other than HercepTest on cell lines	164	0.53	0.43–0.63
Laboratories using the HercepTest on breast tumors	45	0.81	0.67–0.95
Laboratories using IHC assays other than HercepTest on breast tumors	58	0.48	0.30–0.65

[a]*N* = the total number of evaluations.

Source: Data reprinted from **ref. *53*** with permission from the *American Journal of Clinical Pathology*.

and introducing educational programs to ensure that the criteria defining the scoring system are strictly followed.

2.11. Quality Assurance of FISH for HER-2/neu

The main advantage of utilizing the FISH technique to establish the HER-2/neu status of patients with breast cancer is that it allows for quantitative evaluation of HER-2/*neu* gene amplification. As previously mentioned, because of the finding that significant numbers of patients tumors scored as 2+ by IHC have been shown not to have gene amplification by FISH and therefore not likely to respond to Herceptin therapy, current recommendations in the United Kingdom are that all 2+ cases identified in an initial screen with the IHC assay should be further tested with FISH to establish their HER-2/*neu* gene amplification status ***(34)***. Similar practice exists in most other European countries and has been recommended in the United States ***(33)***.

However, it remains to be seen whether the interlaboratory variation in assay results seen with the IHC assay also occurs when the results of large numbers of laboratories employing the FISH assay are analyzed. Persons et al. looked at the interlaboratory reproducibility of FISH results of five different institutions on three different assay days and found a high level of reproducibility ***(69)***.

Initial reports from the College of American Pathologists (CAP) Laboratory Improvement Program showed excellent agreement when 63 laboratories assayed an amplified case and a nonamplified case. However, only 78% of participants submitted results for the nonamplified tumor (as opposed to 92% for the amplified case), suggesting that 14% of laboratories were unsure of their negative results ***(70)***. In an ongoing adjuvant Herceptin clinical trial (National Surgical Adjunctive Breast and Bowel Project B31) in the United States, patients were tested by IHC in a local laboratory, with 3+ cases on HercepTest being sent to a central laboratory for review by both HercepTest and FISH. If the local laboratory was a reference laboratory and used HercepTest, the central laboratory's findings were in 96% agreement (a reference laboratory being defined as one with an average of 100 HER-2/neu cases per month for 6 mo). If the local laboratory was a nonreference laboratory using the HercepTest, the level of agreement fell to 81%, and if the local laboratory was a nonreference laboratory using other antibodies, the concordance rate fell to 52–65% ***(36)***. In a second trial (the Breast Intergroup N9831 study), there was 75% concordance between samples testing 3+ by IHC in a local laboratory and by a central testing laboratory. However, for FISH, the concordance rates for local versus central testing was even lower, 67% ***(36)***. These results suggest that if FISH were to become as widely used as IHC, similar levels of interlaboratory variation would be likely, emphasizing the need for stringent QA assurance programs for *in situ*-based assays.

3. The Future

Genes coding for specific molecules involved in the control of crucial pathways in the normal and malignant cell have been identified and continue to be identified following sequencing of the human genome. Running in tandem with these discoveries, scientists involved in translational research are working hand-in-hand with pharmaceutical companies to develop new therapies that specifically target overexpression of these molecules in carcinogenesis. This will result in a flood of potentially valuable predictive markers in the very near future, all of which will require robust and reproducible laboratory assays if they are to fulfill their potential and provide hope and improved quality of care to cancer patients. As gene amplification or protein overexpression status requires, at the very least, semiquantitative analysis, the reliability of these assays is totally dependent on stringent QA, to include provision of both standard reference materials and expert guidance to ensure the reproducibility and accuracy of results between different laboratories. This need for QA is evident at all stages; from the initial research investigation of a potential predictive marker through to its development in clinical trials and eventual use as a nationally approved assay. Only then can we be sure that valuable markers do not fall by the wayside because of spurious results caused by diverse and inappropriate methodologies, that pooled data from clinical trials involving multiple centers is reliable, and, ultimately, that patients receive the most appropriate therapy irrespective of where they are treated.

References

1. American Cancer Society. http://www.cancer.org/docroot/STT/stt_0_2002.asp?sitearea=STT&level=1. Accessed February 28, 2003.
2. Cancer Research UK. Statistics, mortality. http://www.cancerresearchuk.org/aboutcancer/statistics. Acessed December 15, 2002.
3. Kindblom, L. G., Remotti, L. G., Adlenborg, F., et al. (1998) Gastrointestinal pacecmaker cell tumor (GIPACT): gastrointestinal stromal tumors show phenotypic characteristics of the intestinal cells of Cajal. *Am. J. Pathol.* **152,** 1259–1269.
4. Redston, M. (2001) Carcinogenesis in the GI tract: from morphology to genetics and back again. *Mod. Pathol.* **14,** 236–245.
5. Goldstein, N. S. and Armin, M. (2001) Epidermal growth factor receptor immunohistochemical reactivity in patients with American Joint Committee on cancer stage IV colon adenocarcinoma. *Cancer* **92,** 1331–1346.
6. Takahashi, Y., Kitadai, Y., Bucana, C. D., et al. (1995) Expression of vascular endothelial growth factor and its receptor, KDR, correlates with vascularity, metastasis and proliferation of human colon cancer. *Cancer Res.* **55,** 3964–3968.
7. Wick, M. R. and Swanson, P. E. (2002) Targeted controls in clinical immunohistochemistry; a useful approach to quality assurance. *Am. J. Clin. Pathol.* **117,** 7–8.
8. Moskaluk, C. A. (2002) Standardisation of clinical immunohistochemistry: why, how and by whom? *Am. J. Clin. Pathol.* **118,** 669–671.
9. ASCO. (1998) 1997 Update of recommendations for the use of tumor markers in breast can colorectal cancer. Adopted on November 7, 1997 by the American Society of Clinical Oncology. *J. Clin. Oncol.* **16,** 793–795.
10. National Institute for Clinical Excellence (NICE). (2002) Guidance on the use of trastuzumab for the treatment of advanced breast cancer. Technology appraisal No. 34. Available at www.nice.org.uk.
11. Hammond, M. E. H. and Taube, S. E. (2002) Issues and barriers to development of clinically useful tumor markers: a development pathway proposal. *Semin. Oncol.* **29,** 213–221.
12. The Cancer Research Campaign. Common cancers: breast cancer. http://www.crc.org.uk (June 24, 2002).
13. Peto, R., Boreham, J., Clarke, M., et al. (2000) UK and USA breast cancer deaths down by 25% in year 2000 at ages 20–69 years. *Lancet* **355,** 1822.
14. Early Breast Cancer Trialists' Collaborative Group. (1998) Tamoxifen for early breast cancer: an overview of the randomized trials. *Lancet* **351,** 1451–1467.
15. Wishart, G. C., Gaston, M., Poultsidis, A. A., et al. (2002) Hormone receptor status in primary breast cancer—time for a consensus? *Eur. J. Cancer* **38,** 1201–1203.

16. Geurts-Moespot, J., Leake, R., Benraad, Th. J., et al. (2000) Twenty years of experience with the steroid receptor External Quality Assessment program—the paradigm for tumor biomarker EQA studies (review). *Int. J. Oncol.* **17,** 13–22.
17. Rhodes, A., Jasani, B., Barnes, D. M., et al. (2000) Reliability of immunohistochemical demonstration of oestrogen receptors in routine practice: inter-laboratory variance in the sensitivity of detection and evaluation of scoring systems. *J. Clin. Pathol.* **53,** 125–130.
18. Rhodes, A., Jasani, B., Balaton, A. J., et al. (2000) Immunohistochemical demonstration of oestrogen and progesterone receptors: correlation of standards achieved on 'in house' tumors with that achieved on external quality assessment material in over 150 laboratories from 26 countries. *J. Clin. Pathol.* **53,** 292–301.
19. Rhodes, A., Jasani, B., Balaton, A. J., et al. (2000), Frequency of oestrogen and progesterone receptor positivity by immunohistochemical analysis in 7,016 breast carcinomas: correlation with patient age, assay sensitivity, threshold value and mammographic screening. *J. Clin. Pathol.* **53,** 688–696.
20. Rhodes, A., Jasani, B., Balaton, A. J, et al. (2001) Study of interlaboratory reliability and reproducibility of estrogen and progesterone receptor assays in Europe: documentation of poor reliability and identification of insufficient microwave antigen retrieval time as a major contributory element of unreliable assays. *Am. J. Clin. Pathol.* **115,** 44–58.
21. Slamon, D. J., Clark, G. M., Wong, S. G., et al. (1987), Human breast cancer: correlation of relapse and survival with amplification of the HER-2/neu oncogene. *Science* **235,** 177–182.
22. Ross, J. S. and Fletcher, J. A. (1998) The HER-2/neu oncogene in breast cancer: prognostic factor, predictive factor, and target for therepy. *Stem Cells* **16,** 413–428.
23. Andrulis, I. L., Bull, S. B., Blackstein, M. E., et al. (1998) Neu/erbB-2 amplification identifies a poor-prognosis group of woment with node-negative breast cancer. Toronto Breast Cancer Study Group. *J. Clin. Oncol.* **16,** 1340–1349.
24. Press, M. F., Bernstein, L., Thoma, P. A., et al. (1997) HER-2/neu gene amplification characterized by fluorescence in situ hybridization: poor prognosis in node-negative breast carcinomas. *J. Clin. Oncol.* **15,** 2894–2904.
25. Mass, R. (2000) The role of HER-2 expression in predicting response to therapy in breast cancer. *Semin. Oncol.* **27,** 46–52.
26. Harris, J., Lippman, M., Veronesi, U., et al. (1992) Breast cancer. *N. Engl. J. Med.* **327,** 473–480.
27. Wisecarver, J. L. (1999) HER-2/neu testing comes of age. *Am. J. Clin. Pathol.* **111,** 299–301.
28. Pegram, M. D., Lipton, A., Hayes, D. F., et al. (1998) Phase II study of receptor-enhanced chemosensitivity using recombinant humanized anti-p185$^{HER2/neu}$ monoclonal antibody plus cisplastin in patients with HER2/neu-overexpressing metastatic breast cancer refactory to chemotherapy treatment. *J. Clin. Oncol.* **16,** 2659–2671.
29. Slamon, D., Leyland-Jones, B., Shak, S., et al. (1998) Addition of Herceptin

(humanized anti-Her2 anitbody) to first line chemotherapy for Her2 over-expressing metastatic breast cancer (Her2+/MBC) markedly increases anticancer activity: a randomized multinational controlled phase III trial. *Proc. ASCO* **17,** 98A (abstract 377).

30. Cobleigh, M. A., Vogel, C. L., Tripathy, D., et al. (1999) Multinational study of the efficacy and safety of humanized anti-HER2 monoclonal antibody in women who have HER2–overexpressing metastatic breast cancer that has progressed after chemotherapy for metastatic disease. *J. Clin. Oncol.* **17,** 2639–2648.
31. Tubbs, R. R. and Stoler, M. H. (2000) The quality of Her-2/Neu predictive immunohistochemistry: something FISHy? *Mod. Pathol.* **13,** 1–3.
32. Slamon, D. J., Godolphin, W., Jones, L. A., et al. (1989) Studies of the HER-2/neu proto-oncogene in human breast cancer and ovarian cancer. *Science* **244,** 707–712.
33. Tubbs, R. R., Pettay, J. D., Roche, P. C., et al. (2001) Discrepancies in clinical laboratory testing of eligibility for trastuzumab therapy: apparent immunohistochemical false-positives do not get the message. *J. Clin. Oncol.* **19,** 2714–2721.
34. Ellis, I. O., Dowsett, M., Bartlett, J., et al. (2000) Recommendations for HER2 testing in the UK. *J. Clin. Pathol.* **53,** 890–892.
35. Dowsett, M., Ellis, I. O., Bartlett, J. M. S., et al. (2001) Correlation between immunohistochemistry and FISH for HER-2 in 441 breast carcinomas from multiple hospitals. *J. Pathol.* **195(Suppl.),** 5A.
36. Check, W. (2002) Making the call on HER2 testing methods. *CAP TODAY.* Available at http:/www.cap.org/CAPToday/current/feature.
37. UK NEQAS. (1998) *Report and Directory*, 3rd ed. NEQAS Sheffield, UK, pp. 4–25.
38. Burnett, D., Blair, C., Haeney, M. B., et al. (2002) Clinical Pathology Accreditation: Standards for the Medical Laboratory. *J. Clin. Pathol.* **55,** 729–733.
39. College of American Pathologists. (1998) *Laboratory Accreditation Programs—Checklists & Commentaries*. CAP, Northfield, IL.
40. British Standards Institution. (1987) BS.5750: Part 1 Specification for design/development, production, installation and servicing (ISO 9001, 1987, Quality Systems—Model for Quality Assurance in Design/Development, Production, Installation and Servicing).
41. Taylor, C. R. (1999) FDA issues final rule for classification of reclassification of immunochemistry reagents and kits. *Am. J. Clin. Pathol.* **111,** 443–444.
42. Swanson, P. E. (1999) Labels, disclaimers and Rules (Oh, My!): analyte-specific reagents and practice of immunohistochemistry. *Am. J. Clin. Pathol.* **111,** 445–448.
43. European Law 34. (1999) Directive 98/79/EC: regulation of *in-vitro* medical diagnostic devices.
44. Balaton A. (1999) Defining objectives for technical quality in immunohistochemistry. *J. Cell Pathol.* **4(3),** 69–77.
45. Leake, R., Barnes, D., Pinder, S., et al., on behalf of the UK Receptor Group, UK NEQAS, the Scottish Breast Cancer Pathology Group and the Receptor and

Biomarker Study Group of the EORTC. (2000) Immunohistochemical detection of steroid receptors in breast cancer: a working protocol. *J. Clin. Pathol.* **53:** 634–635.

46. Shoker, B. S., Jarvis, C., Sibson, D. R., et al. (1999) Oestrogen receptor expression in the normal and pre-cancerous breast. *J. Pathol.* **188,** 237–244.
47. Jacobs, T. W., Gown, A., Yasiji, H., et al. (1999), Specificity of HercepTest in determining the HER-2/neu status of breast cancers using the United States Food and Drug Administration-approved scoring system. *J. Clin. Oncol.* **17,** 1983–1987.
48. Lebeau, A., Deimling, D., Kaltz, C., et al. (2001) HER-2/neu analysis in archival tissue samples of human breast cancer: comparison of immunohistochemistry and fluorescence *in situ* hybridisation. *J. Clin. Oncol.* **17,** 354–363.
49. Pauletti, G., Dandekar, S., Rong, H.-M., et al. (2000) Assessment of methods for tissue-based dectection of the HER-2/neu alteration in human breast cancer: a direct comparison of fluorescence *in situ* hybridisation and immunohistochemistry. *J. Clin. Oncol.* **18,** 3651–3664.
50. Rhodes, A., Jasani, B., Couturier, et al. (2002) A formalin-fixed, paraffin processed cell line standard for quality control of immunohistochemical assay of HER-2/neu expression in breast cancer. *Am. J. Clin. Pathol.* **117,** 81–89.
51. Ruby, S. G. and McNally, A. C. (1995) Quality control of imprint and tissue section DNA ploidy analysis in image analysis systems utilizing cell culture-based control materials. *Am. J. Clin. Pathol.* **104(2),** 167–171.
52. Ruby, S. G. and McNally, A. C. (1996) Quality control of prolilferation marker (MIB1) in image analysis systems utilizing cell culture-based control materials. *Am. J. Clin. Pathol.* **106(5),** 634–639.
53. Rhodes, A., Jasani, B., Anderson, E., et al. (2002) Evaluation of HER-2/neu immunohistochemical assay sensitivity and scoring on formalin fixed and paraffin processed cell lines and breast carcinomas: a comparative study involving results from laboratories in 21 countries. *Am. J. Clin. Pathol.* **118,** 408–417.
54. Seidman, A. D., Fornier, M. N., Esteva, F. J., et al. (2001) Weekly trastuzumab and paclitaxel therapy for metastatic breast cancer with analysis of efficacy by HER2 immunophenotype and gene amplification. *J. Clin. Oncol.* **19,** 2587–2595.
55. Riera, J., Simpson, J. F., Tamayo, R., et al. (1999) Use of cultured cells as a control for quantitative immunocytochemical anlalysis of estrogen receptor in breast cancer. The quicgel method. *Am. J. Clin. Pathol.* **111,** 329–335.
56. Tanner, M., Gancberg, D., Di Leo, A., et al. (2000) Chromogenic *in situ* hybridisation: a practical alternative to fluorescence *in situ* hybridisation to detect HER-2/neu oncogene amplification in archival breast cancer samples. *Am. J. Pathol.* **157,** 1467–1472.
57. Jacobs, T. W., Gown, A. M., Yaziji, H., et al. (2000) HER-2/neu protein expression in breast cancer evaluated by immunohistochemistry: a study of interlaboratory agreement. *Am. J. Clin. Pathol.* **113,** 251–258.
58. WHO. (1981) *External Quality Assessment of Health Laboratories*. WHO Regional Office for Europe, Copenhagen.

59. Leblanc, A., Woodford, F. P., Gardener, P. S., et al. (1985) *Standard for Quality Assurance. Part 1. Terminology and Principles.* Beckenham, Kent, UK.
60. Allred, D. C. (1993) Should immunohistochemical examination replace biochemical hormone receptor assays in breast cancer? *Am. J. Clin. Pathol.* **99,** 1–2.
61. Taylor, C. R. (1994) An exultation of experts: concerted efforts in the standardization of immunohistochemistry. *Hum. Pathol.* **25,** 2–11.
62. Romain, S., Laine Bidron, C., Martin, P. M., et al. on behalf of the EORTC Receptor Study Group. (1995) EORTC Receptor Study Group Report. Steroid receptor distribution in 47 892 breast cancers. A collaborative study of 7 European laboratories. *Eur. J. Cancer* **31A(3),** 411–417.
63. Barnes, D. M., Harris, W. H., Smith, P., et al. (1996) Immunohistochemical determination of oestrogen receptors: comparison of different methods of assessment of staining and correlation with clinical outcome of breast cancer patients. *Br. J. Cancer* **74,** 1445–1451.
64. Rhodes, A. and Jasani, B. (2001) Immunohistochemical demonstration of oestrogen and progesterone receptors. *J. Clin. Pathol.* **54,** 78–79.
65. Harvey, J. M., Clark, G. M., Osbourne, C. K., et al. (1999) Estrogen receptor status by immunohistochemistry is superior to the ligand binding assay for predicting response to adjuvant endocrine therapy in breast cancer. *J. Clin. Oncol.* **17,** 1474–1481.
66. Wang, S., Saboorian, M. H., Frenkel, E. P., et al. (2001) Assessment of HER-2/neu status in breast cancer: automated cellular imaging (ACIS)-assisted quantitation of immunohistochemical assay achieves high accuracy in comparison with fluorescence in situ hybridisation assay as the standard. *Am. J. Clin. Pathol.* **116,** 495–503.
67. Bloom, K. S., and De La Torre-Beuno, J. (2000) Comparison of HER-2/*neu* analysis using FISH and IHC when HercepTest is scored using conventional microscopy and image analysis. *Breast Cancer Res. Treat.* **64,** 99.
68. Genentech (1998) Herceptin (trastuzumab) (package insert), Genentech, San Francisco, CA.
69. Persons, D., Bui, M. M., and Lowery, M. C. (2000) Fluorescence *in situ* hybridisation (FISH) for detection of HER-2/neu amplification in breast cancer: a multicenter portability study. *Ann. Clin. Lab. Sci.* **30,** 41–48.
70. Cell Markers and Cytogenetics Committees, College of American Pathologists. (2002) Clinical laboratory assays for Her-2/neu amplification and overexpression: quality assurance, standardization, and proficiency testing. *Arch. Pathol. Lab. Med.* **126,** 803–808.

4

Extraction of Nucleic Acid Templates

John M. S. Bartlett and Helen Speirs

1. Introduction

The following series of short technical descriptions covers the extraction of DNA and RNA from various starting materials. We have gathered these together to provide an easy reference. The techniques described in the rest of this volume are, in the main, worked laboratory methods giving detailed examples of the procedures used by the authors in their own research. However, the aim is to provide the reader with a method that may be translated into their own research.

Extraction of nucleic acids is a fundamental precursor to many of the techniques described within this volume. Isolation of RNA and DNA from blood and fresh tissues can be performed using a variety of techniques that also form the basis of methods of extraction of these substrates from other sources. The sensitivity of polymerase chain reaction (PCR) methods is now such that extraction of DNA and RNA from tissues fixed in formaldehyde and buffered formalin is considered routine and we are now able to extract DNA from ancient tissues, feces, and many other sources. It has not proven desirable nor feasible to be exhaustive in our approach to DNA/RNA extraction protocols and we have, therefore, restricted these to major methods in use in many laboratories. Further references that provide detailed reviews of methods for nucleic acid extraction and some recommended websites are provided *(1–7)*.

There are many differing protocols used for the extraction of DNA from whole blood and a large number of commercially available kits. The procedure described in **Subheading 3.1.** is one we use routinely in both research and clinical service provision and is inexpensive and robust. It can also be applied to cell pellets from dispersed tissues or cell cultures (omitting the red blood lysis step).

From: *Methods in Molecular Medicine, vol. 79: Molecular Diagnosis of Cancer*
Edited by: J. E. Roulston and J. M. S. Bartlett © Humana Press Inc., Totowa, NJ

The method for RNA extraction from whole blood (**Subheading 3.2.**) is based on the method of Chomczynski and Sacchi *(8)* and is an extremely reliable method without the requirement for centrifugation over CsCl gradients. As with any RNA protocol, extreme care should be taken to exclude RNAse contamination, the greatest source of which will be the sample itself. All disposables and reagents should be RNAse-free. The use of diethyl pyrocarbonate (DEPC) pretreatment of solutions and glassware may be useful in preventing RNAse contamination (*see* **Subheading 3.4.**).

The protocol for tissue extraction of DNA (**Subheading 3.3.**) is one of the longest established methods of DNA extraction and works well with a wide range of solid tissues. Proteins are digested with proteinase K and extracted with phenol chloroform. DNA is then precipitated with ethanol. The resultant DNA (10–50 μg) is of high molecular weight and is a suitable template for long PCR and other applications.

Protocols for RNA extraction from tissues (**Subheading 3.4.**) or tissue sections (**Subheading 3.5.**) require that tissue be stored frozen and not be processed for optimum histology. There are two different methods of preparing tissue for histology: paraffin embedding and freeze embedding. Each has its advantages and drawbacks. Paraffin-embedded tissues (PET) produce optimum morphology but have comparatively poor molecular preservation and recovery. Although frozen sections have poorer histology, they allow excellent recovery of DNA and RNA for analysis.

Formalin, one of the most popular fixatives, crosslinks nucleic acids to protein, thus making the molecules rigid and susceptible to mechanical shearing. The duration of formalin fixation also appears to be important. Studies that have demonstrated DNA recovery around 200 basepairs recommend a period of fixation from 16 to 24 h, but not any longer ***(9–11)***.

RNA is a more labile species than DNA, and the paraffin-embedding process has been shown to greatly harm it. Many studies have shown that formalin fixation has the worst effects among commonly used fixatives, and ethanol-based fixatives have the best RNA preservation. As a general rule, however, if RNA is to be isolated from tissues, any fixative should be avoided.

It is sometimes desirable to extract both RNA and DNA from the same sample, especially when the sample is small. This can be achieved (*see* **Subheading 3.6.**) by isolating a total nucleic acid fraction that is then divided into two portions that are treated differentially with either Dnase I (to remove DNA and recover RNA) or with RNase A (to selectively recover the DNA); however, this wastes half of the DNA and RNA. An alternative approach is to sequentially isolate the RNA and DNA fractions from the same sample. This protocol, based on one reported by Chevillard ***(10)***, begins by extracting RNA as in **Subheading 3.4.**, but then re-extracts the DNA from the collected organic phases. The method described is for the extraction of both DNA and RNA from tissue but can be modified for either blood or cell lines (*see* **Notes 17** and **18**).

There are occasions when the only material available on a patient is stored plasma or serum samples. In normal individuals, the amount of DNA in these samples is very low, but sufficient to serve as template for PCR reactions. Moreover, increased amounts of circulating DNA have been found in a variety of disorders, including cancer, autoimmune disease, and infection. Additionally, small amounts of fetal DNA have been detected in maternal plasma/serum during gestation. We have used the protocol described in **Subheading 3.7.** to successfully genotype archival plasma samples.

2. Materials

2.1. DNA Extraction from Blood

This method uses standard chemicals that can be obtained from any major supplier; we use Sigma:

1. Water bath set at 65°C.
2. 15-mL Centrifuge tubes (Falcon).
3. 1.5-mL Microfuge tubes.
4. Tube roller/rotator.
5. Glass Pasteur pipets, heated to seal the end and curled to form a "loop" or "hook" for spooling DNA.
6. 0.5 *M* EDTA, pH 8.0: Add 146.1 g of anhydrous EDTA to 800 mL of distilled water. Adjust pH to 8.0 with NaOH pellets (will require about 20 g). Make up to 1 L with distilled water. Autoclave at 15 psi for 15 min.
7. 1*M* Tris-HCl, pH 7.6: Dissolve 121.1 g of Tris base in 800 mL of distilled water. Adjust pH with concentrated HCl (requires about 60 mL). Caution: Addition of acid produces heat. Allow to cool to room temperature before finally correcting pH. Make up to 1 L with distilled water. Autoclave at 15 psi for 15 min.
8. Reagent A (red blood cell lysis): 0.01*M* Tris-HCL, pH 7.4, 320 m*M* sucrose, 5 m*M* MgCl2, 1% Triton X-100.
9. Add 10 mL of 1*M* Tris-HCL (*see* **step 7**), 109.54 g sucrose, 0.47 g $MgCl_2$, and 10 mL Triton X-100 to 800 mL distilled water. Adjust pH to 8.0; make up to 1 L with distilled water. Autoclave at 10 psi for 10 min (*see* **Note 3**).
10. Reagent B (cell lysis): 0.4*M* Tris-HCl, 150 m*M* NaCl, 0.06*M* EDTA, 1% sodium dodecyl sulfate (SDS), pH 8.0. Take 400 mL of 1*M* Tris-HCl (pH 8.0; *see* **step 7**), 120 mL of 0.5 *M* EDTA (pH 8.0), 8.76 g NaCl; adjust pH to 8.0. Make up to 1 L with distilled water. Autoclave 15 min at 15 psi. After autoclaving, add 10 g SDS.
11. 5*M* Sodium perchlorate: Dissolve 70 g sodium perchlorate in 80 mL distilled water. Make up to 100 mL.
12. TE buffer, pH 7.6: Take 10 mL of 1*M* Tris-HCl, pH 8.0, 2 mL of 0.5*M* EDTA.

Adjust pH to 7.6; make up to 1 L with distilled water. Autoclave 15 min at 15 psi.

13. Chloroform prechilled to 4°C.
14. Ethanol (100%) prechilled to 4°C.

2.2. RNA Extraction From Blood

1. 1.5 mL Microfuge tubes.
2. Ice bucket
3. Microfuge.
4. Red cell lysis buffer: 1.6*M* sucrose, 5% Triton X-100, 25 m*M* $MgCl_2$, 60 m*M* Tris-HCl pH 7.5; stored at 2–8°C and used cold.
5. Extraction buffer: 5.25*M* guanidinium thiocyanate, 50 m*M* Tris-HCl, pH 6.4, 20 m*M* EDTA, 1% Triton X-100, 0.1*M* β-mercaptoethanol (add immediately prior to use).
6. 2*M* Sodium acetate, pH 4.0.
7. Phenol: Saturated with 1*M* Tris-HCl, 0.1*M* EDTA, pH 8.0.
8. Chloroform:isoamyl alcohol (24:1)
9. Isopropyl alcohol.
10. 70% Ethanol.
11. RNAse-free distilled water.

2.3. DNA Extraction From Tissue

1. 1.5-mL Microfuge tubes.
2. Shaking water bath or incubator with rotisserie.
3. Microfuge.
4. DNA digestion buffer: 50 m*M* Tris-HCl, 100 m*M* EDTA, 100 m*M* NaCl, 1% SDS, pH 8.0.
5. Proteinase K: 0.5 mg/mL in DNA digestion buffer.
6. Phenol:chloroform:isoamyl alcohol (25:24:1, v/v/v).
7. 100% EtOH.
8. 70% EtOH.
9. TE buffer: 10 m*M* Tris-HCl, 1 m*M* EDTA, pH 8.0.

2.4. RNA Extraction From Frozen Tissue

All chemicals, unless otherwise noted, are molecular biology grade and obtained from Sigma UK (Poole, Dorset). All glassware was pretreated with DEPC. All deionized distilled water was pretreated with DEPC and autoclaved (DEPC water). DEPC is a potent anti-RNAse agent.

2.4.1. DEPC Treatment of Glassware/Distilled Water

Add 0.1% DEPC to distilled deionized water and glassware filled and leave to stand overnight. The water was decanted and autoclaved (DEPC-treated water) and glassware sterilized at 220°C for 2 h (DEPC-treated glassware). DEPC is driven off by both procedures.

2.4.2. RNA Extraction From Tissue

1. Braun microdismembranator and Teflon vessels (Braun GmBH, Germany).
2. 3*M* Lithium chloride, 6 *M* urea: Dissolve in 800 mL DEPC water and make up to 1 L. Store at 4°C for 3–6 mo.
3. 10 m*M* Tris-HCl, 0.5% SDS, pH 7.5. Prepare stock solutions of 10% SDS, 0.5*M* Tris-HCl (pH 7.5) in DEPC water. Stocks are stable at room temperature for up to 12 mo.
4. Proteinase K: Prepare 1 mg/mL (w/v) DEPC water stock, store at –20°C for up to 12 mo. Dilute in 10 m*M* Tris-HCl/0.5% SDS as required; discard unused diluted enzyme.
5. Phenol:chloroform:isoamyl alcohol: Phenol is presaturated with 10 m*M* Tris-HCl, pH 7.5. Prepare a mixture of 25:24:1 phenol:chloroform:isoamyl alcohol (v/v/v). Store at room temperature for up to 6 mo; shield from light.

2.5. RNA Extraction From Tissue Sections

1. 1.5-mL Microfuge tubes.
2. Ice bucket
3. Microfuge.
4. Extraction buffer: 5.25*M* guanidinium thiocyanate, 50 m*M* Tris-HCl, pH 6.4, 20 m*M* EDTA, 1% Triton X-100, 0.1*M* β-mercaptoethanol (add immediately prior to use).
5. Glycogen (10 mg/mL) in distilled water.
6. 2*M* Sodium acetate, pH 4.0.
7. Phenol: Saturated with 1*M* Tris-HCl, 0.1*M* EDTA, pH 8.0.
8. Chloroform:isoamyl alcohol (24:1).
9. Isopropyl alcohol.
10. 70% Ethanol.
11. RNAse-free distilled water.

2.6. Dual DNA RNA Extraction

All chemicals, unless otherwise noted, are molecular biology grade and obtained from Sigma UK (Poole, Dorset). All glassware was pretreated with DEPC. All deionized distilled water was pretreated with DEPC and autoclaved (DEPC water). DEPC is a potent anti-RNAse agent.

2.6.1. DEPC Treatment of Glassware/Distilled Water

Add 0.1% DEPC to distilled deionized water and glassware filled and leave to stand overnight. The water was decanted and autoclaved (DEPC-treated water) and glassware sterilized at 220°C for 2 h (DEPC-treated glassware). DEPC is driven off by both procedures.

2.6.2. RNA Extraction

1. Braun microdismembranator and Teflon vessels (Braun GmBH, Germany).
2. 3 *M* Lithium chloride, 6 *M* urea: Dissolve in 800 mL DEPC water and make up to 1 L. Store at 4°C for 3–6 mo.
3. 10 m*M* Tris-HCl, 0.5% SDS, pH 7.5. Prepare stock solutions of 10% SDS, 0.5*M* Tris-HCl (pH 7.5) in DEPC water. Stocks are stable at room temperature for up to 12 mo.
4. Proteinase K: Prepare 1 mg/mL (w/v) DEPC water stock, store at –20°C for up to 12 mo. Dilute in 10 m*M* Tris-HCl/0.5% SDS as required, discard unused diluted enzyme.
5. Phenol:chloroform:isoamyl alcohol: Phenol is presaturated with 10 m*M* Tris-HCl, pH 7.5. Prepare a mixture of 25:24:1 phenol:chloroform:isoamyl alcohol (v/v/v). Store at room temperature for up to 6 mo; shield from light.
6. TE buffer, pH 7.6: Take 10 mL of 1*M* Tris-HCl, pH 8.0, 2 mL of 0.5*M* EDTA, make up to 1 L with distilled water. Adjust pH to 7.6. Autoclave 15 min at 15 psi.

2.6.3. DNA Extraction (as for RNA Plus)

1. Dual-extraction buffer: 0.1*M* NaCl, 10 m*M* Tris-HCl, pH 8.0, 1 m*M* EDTA, 1% SDS. Adjust to pH 12.0 with 5 *N* NaOH immediately prior to use.
2. 7.5*M* Ammonium acetate.

2.7. DNA Extraction From Plasma and Serum

1. 10X SDS/protein K: 10 g/100 mL lauryl sulfate (SDS), 5 mg/mL proteinase K.
2. TE (Tris-EDTA) buffer: 10 m*M* Tris-HCl, 1 m*M* EDTA, pH 8.0.
3. Phenol:chloroform (1:1, v/v).
4. Glycogen (10 mg/mL).
5. 7.5*M* Ammonium acetate.
6. 100% Ethanol.
7. 70% Ethanol.

3. Methods

3.1. DNA Extraction From Blood

3.1.1. Blood Collection

Collect blood in either a heparin- or EDTA-containing vacutainer by venipuncture (*see* **Note 4**). Store at room temperature and extract within the same working day.

3.1.2. DNA Extraction

To extract DNA from cell cultures or disaggregated tissues, omit **steps 1–3**.

1. Place 3 mL whole blood in a 15-mL Falcon tube.
2. Add 12 mL reagent A.

3. Mix on a rolling or rotating blood mixer for 4 min at room temperature.
4. Centrifuge at 3000*g* for 5 min at room temperature.
5. Discard supernatant without disturbing cell pellet. Remove remaining moisture by inverting the tube and blotting onto tissue paper.
6. Add 1 mL reagent B and vortex briefly to resuspend the cell pellet.
7. Add 250 µL of 5*M* sodium perchlorate and mix by inverting tube several times.
8. Place tube in water bath for 15–20 min at 65°C.
9. Allow to cool to room temperature.
10. Add 2 mL ice-cold chloroform.
11. Mix on a rolling or rotating mixer for 30–60 min (*see* **Note 5**).
12. Centrifuge at 2400*g* for 2 min.
13. Transfer upper phase into a clean Falcon tube using a sterile pipet.
14. Add 2–3 mL ice-cold ethanol and invert gently to allow DNA to precipitate (*see* **Note 6**).
15. Using a freshly prepared flamed Pasteur pipet, spool the DNA onto the hooked end (*see* **Note 7**).
16. Transfer to a 1.5-mL Eppendorf tube and allow to air-dry (*see* **Note 8**).
17. Resuspend in 200 µL TE buffer (*see* **Notes 9** and **10**).

3.2. RNA Extraction From Blood

1. In a microfuge tube mix, 100 µL anticoagulated blood with 1 mL red cell lysis buffer (*see* **Notes 11–13**).
2. Leave at room temperature with occasional shaking until the red cells have lysed and the solution translucent (usually within 5 min).
3. Microfuge for 30 s at 13,000*g* to pellet the white blood cells. Remove and discard supernatant.
4. Add 200 µL extraction buffer and resuspend cell pellet by drawing through narrow-gage needle several times.
5. Add 20 µL of 2*M* sodium acetate and mix gently by inversion.
6. Add 220 µL phenol and mix gently by inversion.
7. Add 60 µL chloroform:isoamyl alcohol (24:1) and vortex vigorously.
8. Place on ice for 15 min.
9. Microfuge at 12,000*g* for 5 min and transfer the upper phase to a new microfuge tube.
10. Add 200 µL ice-cold isopropanol mix and store at –20°C for 30 min.
11. Microfuge at 12,000g for 15 min and discard supernatant.
12. Resuspend pellet in 200 µL extraction buffer.
13. Repeat **steps 3–9**.
14. Wash pellet with 400 µL cold 70% ethanol.
15. Microfuge at 12,000*g* for 5 min and discard supernatant.
16. Carefully remove last traces of ethanol from tube (folded sterile swab or Kimwipe works well).
17. Resuspend in 100 µL distilled water and incubate at 50°C for 15 min to dissolve RNA (*see* **Note 14**).

3.3. DNA Extraction From Tissue

1. Place 0.1–0.5 g of tissue into polypropylene microfuge tube (*see* **Note 15**).
2. Add 0.5 mL DNA digestion buffer with proteinase K (*see* **Note 16**).
3. Incubate overnight at 50–55°C with gentle shaking.
4. Spin tubes for 5 s at 500*g* to collect mix in bottom of tube.
5. Add 0.7 mL phenol:chloroform:isoamyl alcohol (25:24:1, v/v/v).
6. Mix by inversion for 1 h (do not vortex).
7. Microfuge at 12,000*g* for 5 min and transfer 0.5 mL of the upper phase to new microfuge tube.
8. Add 1 mL of 100% ethanol at room temperature and gently invert until DNA precipitate forms (approx 1 min).
9. Microfuge at 12,000*g* for 5 min and discard supernatant.
10. Add 1 mL of 70% ethanol (–20°C) and invert several times. This ethanol wash removes excess salt, which may otherwise interfere with PCR.
11. Microfuge at 12,000*g* for 5 min and discard supernatant.
12. Spin tubes for 5 s to collect any remaining ethanol in bottom of tube. Remove last drops of ethanol with fine pipet.
13. Air-dry at room temperature for 10–15 min (any longer will render DNA difficult to redissolve).
14. Resuspend in 100 μL TE and incubate at 65°C for 15 min to dissolve DNA (*see* **Note 14**).

3.4. RNA Extraction From Whole Tissues

1. Tissues should ideally be collected fresh from theatre and stored in liquid nitrogen. Routinely, samples are collected on ice and transported for freezing within 30–60 min.
2. Tissues are disaggregated using a Braun microdismembranator. Teflon vessels and steel ball bearings are cooled in liquid nitrogen prior to use. Frozen tissue (50–500 mg) is placed in the vessel with a single ball bearing and agitated at 1000 cycles/s for 60 s. The vessel is then recooled in liquid nitrogen. This process is repeated until tissue is powdered (usually two times; *see* **Note 17**).
3. Immediately after disaggregation of tissue, tissue material is resuspended from frozen in 1.5 mL LiCl/urea and transferred to a separate tube. The vessel is washed a further two times with 1.5 mL LiCl/urea and the washing combined with the original sample. The resuspended medium is made up to 6 mL in LiCl/urea and sonicated for 2 × 30 s at maximum power using a probe sonicator. The sonicated samples are stored overnight at 4°C (*see* **Note 18**).
4. Centrifuge at 15,000*g*, 4°C for 30 min. The supernatant is discarded and the pellet washed with a further 6 mL of lithium chloride/urea, recentrifuged (15,000*g*, 4°C for 30 min), and the supernatant again discarded.
5. The pellet is resuspended in 6 mL Tris-HCl/SDS with 50 μg/mL proteinase K (Boehringer Mannheim, UK) and incubated at 37°C for 20 min.
6. Samples are extracted with 100% phenol, followed by phenol:chloroform:isoamyl

alcohol. Following each extraction, the sample is centrifuged at 2000*g* at room temperature for 10 min and the aqueous phase recovered.

7. Following the final extraction, 300 µL of 8*M* LiCl and 2.5 vol absolute alcohol are added and samples stored at –20°C for 30 min or overnight.
8. RNA is pelleted by centrifugation at 4000*g*, 4°C for 45 min. The supernatant is discarded and the RNA pelleted dried and resuspended in DEPC-treated distilled water.
9. Concentrations are estimated by optical density at 260 nm/280 nm.

3.5. RNA Extraction From Tissue Sections

1. The extraction is initiated by incubating tissue sections or microdissected cells in 500 µL extraction buffer for 5 min at room temperature with gentle agitation, inverting several times.
2. Add 20 µL of 2*M* sodium acetate and mix gently by inversion.
3. Add 220 µL phenol and mix gently by inversion.
4. Add 60 µL chloroform:isoamyl alcohol (24:1) and vortex vigorously.
5. Place on ice for 15 min.
6. Microfuge at 12,000*g* for 5 min and transfer the upper phase to a new microfuge tube.
7. Add 1–2 µL of glycogen (10 mg/mL). Glycogen is a carrier that is used if RNA quantities are less than 1 µg. It also facilitates visualization of the pellet.
8. Add 200 µL ice-cold isopropanol mix and store at –20°C for 30 min.
9. Microfuge at 12,000*g* for 15 min and discard supernatant.
10. Resuspend pellet in 200 µL extraction buffer.
11. Repeat **steps 3–9**.
12. Wash pellet with 400 µL cold 70% ethanol.
13. Microfuge at 12,000*g* for 5 min and discard supernatant.
14. Carefully remove last traces of ethanol from tube (folded sterile swab or Kimwipe works well).
15. Resuspend in 100 µL RNAse-free distilled water and incubate at 50°C for 15 min to dissolve RNA (*see* **Note 14**).

3.6. Dual DNA/RNA Extraction

3.6.1. RNA Extraction

1. Tissues should ideally be collected fresh from the theatre and stored in liquid nitrogen. Routinely, samples are collected on ice and transported for freezing within 30–60 min.
2. Tissues are disaggregated using a Braun microdismembranator. Teflon vessels and steel ball bearings are cooled in liquid nitrogen prior to use. Frozen tissue (50–500 mg) is placed in the vessel with a single ball bearing and agitated at 1000 cycles/s for 60 s. The vessel is then recooled in liquid nitrogen. This process is repeated until tissue is powdered (usually two times) (*see* **Note 17**).
3. Immediately after disaggregation of tissue, material is resuspended from frozen

in 1.5 mL LiCl/urea and transferred to a separate tube. The vessel is washed a further two times with 1.5 mL LiCl/urea and the washing combined with the original sample. The resuspended medium is made up to 6 mL in LiCl/urea and sonicated for 2 × 30 s at maximum power using a probe sonicator. The sonicated samples are stored overnight at 4°C (*see* **Note 18**).

4. Centrifuge at 15,000*g*, 4°C for 30 min. The supernatant is discarded and the pellet washed with a further 6 mL of lithium chloride/urea, recentrifuged (15,000*g*, 4°C for 30 min), and the supernatant again discarded.
5. The pellet is resuspended in 6 mL Tris-HCl/SDS with 50 µg/mL proteinase K (Boehringer Mannheim, UK) and incubated at 37°C for 20 min.
6. Samples are mixed with an equal volume of phenol:chloroform:isoamyl alcohol and mixed by inversion several times.
7. Following mixing, the sample is centrifuged at 2000*g* at room temperature for 10 min and the aqueous phase recovered for RNA extraction; the organic phase is retained for DNA extraction.
8. Repeat **steps 6** and **7**.
9. Following the final extraction, 300 µL of 8*M* LiCl and 2.5 vol absolute alcohol are added and samples stored at –20°C for 30 min or overnight. RNA is pelleted by centrifugation at 4000*g*, 4°C for 45 min.
10. The supernatant is discarded and the RNA pelleted dried and resuspended in 50 µL TE. Concentrations are estimated by optical density at 260 nm/280 nm.

3.6.2. DNA Extraction

1. Combine the organic phases including the interfaces from **step 7** of **Subheading 3.6.1.** (both times) in a 15-mL polypropylene tube.
2. Add an equal volume of extraction buffer, vortex for 1 min, and place on ice for 10 min.
3. Centrifuge for 20 min at 10,000*g*, 4°C.
4. Transfer aqueous phase to fresh tube and add 1/15 vol of 7.5*M* NH_4OAc and 2 vol ice-cold EtOH. Incubate at –20°C for at least 1 h.
5. Centrifuge for 20 min at 10,000*g*, 4°C.
6. Carefully decant the supernatant and wash the pellet with 1 mL of 70% ethanol.
7. Centrifuge briefly to ensure that the pellet remains attached.
8. Carefully remove the supernatant and air-dry the pellet for 10–15 min.
9. Resuspend the DNA pellet in 50 mL TE. Heat 5 min at 55°C and then vortex thoroughly to dissolve the DNA.

3.7. DNA Extraction From Plasma and Serum

1. Place 1.5 mL serum or plasma into a 15-mL centrifuge tube.
2. Add 1.5 mL of 1X SDS/proteinase K solution in the tube containing the serum and mix well.
3. Digest overnight at 55°C in water bath.
4. Add 3 mL phenol:chloroform solution.

5. Vortex for 30 s and centrifuge for 10 min at 1000*g* using a swing-out rotor.
6. Transfer aqueous layer to fresh tube and repeat **steps 4** and **5**.
7. Transfer aqueous layer to fresh tube and add 5 µL glycogen (10 mg/mL), 1 mL of 7.5*M* ammonium acetate, and 8 mL of 100% ethanol.
8. Mix by inverting and centrifuge at 2500*g* for 40 min.
9. Carefully remove supernatant and wash pellet in 10 mL of 70% ethanol.
10. Centrifuge at 2500*g* for 10 min. Carefully remove last traces of ethanol and allow to air-dry for 10 min before redissolving in 100 µL TE.

4. Notes

1. For extraction from cell lines, scrape cells into 1.5 mL lithium chloride/urea and then proceed from **step 3** of the RNA extraction in **Subheading 3.3.**
2. Extraction of DNA/RNA from blood can be achieved by collecting blood in either a heparin- or EDTA-containing vacutainer by venipuncture (*see* **Note 4**). Store at room temperature and extract within the same working day. Three milliters of whole blood are placed in a 15-mL polypropylene tube and mixed with 12 mL of red blood cell lysis solution (0.01*M* Tris-HCl, pH 7.4, 320 m*M* sucrose, 5 m*M* $MgCl_2$, 1% Triton X-100). Blood is then mixed on a rolling or rotating blood mixer for 4 min at room temperature. Lymphocytes are recovered by centrifugation at 3000*g* for 5 min at room temperature. Then proceed with RNA extract at **step 3** above.
3. Autoclaving sugars at high temperature can cause caramelization (browning), which degrades the sugars.
4. As will all body fluids, blood represents a potential biohazard. Care should be taken in all steps requiring handling of blood. If the subject is from a known high-risk category (e.g., intravenous drug abusers), additional precautions may be required.
5. Rotation for under 30 min or over 60 min can reduce the DNA yield.
6. DNA should appear as a mucuslike strand in the solution phase.
7. Rotating the hooked end by rolling between thumb and forefinger usually works well. If the DNA adheres to the hook, break it off into the Eppendorf and resuspend DNA before transferring to a fresh tube.
8. Ethanol will interfere with both measurements of DNA concentration and PCR reactions. However, overdrying the pellet will prolong the resuspension time.
9. The small amount of EDTA in TE will not affect PCR. We routinely use 1 µL per PCR reaction without adverse affects.
10. DNA can be quantified and diluted to a working concentration at this point or simply use 1 µL per PCR reaction; routinely, we expect 200–500 ng/µL DNA to be the yield of this procedure.
11. Blood stored at room temperature or 4°C should be mixed thoroughly prior to aliquots being removed.
12. Frozen blood samples should be allowed to thaw completely and mixed thoroughly prior to aliquots being removed. Although freezing lyses red blood cells,

the red cell lysis step should still be performed to efficiently remove hemoglobin from the sample. Repeated freeze–thaw cycles should be avoided.

13. Buffy coat contains two to four times the amount of white blood cells per volume compared to fresh blood. Therefore, it is advisable to use only 50 μL of buffy coat diluted with 50 μL phosphate-buffered saline as starting material for this protocol.
14. Repeat pipetting through a narrow-gage tip can help this process.
15. Some tissues contain large amounts of connective tissue and are difficult to digest. These can be ground frozen in liquid nitrogen, and ground in a mortar and pestle before being digested with proteinase K.
16. Proteinase K solution can be kept for several days at 4°C.
17. Disaggregation is critically dependent on tissue structure. Most tissues are readily disaggregated in 2 × 60 s bursts. Other tissue types (e.g., fibrous tissues) may require longer periods to disrupt tissue. If a mechanical dismembranator is not available, other methods of tissue homogenization work equally well, either using a mortar and pestle or blade homogenizers.
18. Other methods can be used to lyse cells, such as passage through a syringe needle and so forth. Extraction of RNA from solid tissues can be problematic, many of the commercial systems available for RNA extraction are validated for extraction of RNA from cell culture material or blood lymphocytes. These kits have often been less successful with tissue-derived material.

References

1. US Department of Commerce Molecular Biology Techniques Forum. http://research.nwfsc.noaa.gov/protocols/methods/.
2. http://www.stratagene.com/.
3. http://www.promega.com/tbs/.
4. http://www.highveld.com/protocols.
5. http://www.dynal.no/.
6. Sambrook, J., Fritsch, E. F., and Maniatis, T. (1989) *Molecular Cloning: A Laboratory Manual.* Cold Spring Harbor Laboratory Press, Cold Spring Harbor, NY.
7. Bartlett J. M. S., ed. (2000) *Ovarian Cancer: Methods & Protocols.* Methods in Molecular Biology. Volume 39. Humana, Totowa, NJ.
8. Chomczynski, P. and Sacchi, N. (1987) Single-step method of RNA isolation by acid guanidinium thiocyanate-phenol-chloroform extraction. *Anal. Biochem.* **162,** 156–159.
9. Foss, R., et al., (1994) Effects of fixative and fixation time on the extraction and polymerase chain reaction amplification of RNA from paraffin-embedded tissue. *Diagn. Mol. Pathol.* **3(3),** 148–155.
10. Chevillard, S. (1993) A method for sequential extraction of RNA and DNA from the same sample, specially designed for a limited supply of biological material. *Biotechniques* **15(1),** 22–24.

5

Microdissection and Extraction of DNA From Archival Tissue

Joanne Edwards, James J. Going, and John M. S. Bartlett

1. Introduction

Microdissection of cells with distinct histological features from tissue sections has become important because of the development of sensitive genetic techniques. This is of particular importance when analyzing genetic differences in tumor tissue compared to normal tissue. Failure to separate normal and tumor cell types can result in masking of results, false results, and discrepancies between repeat experiments. For example, use of polymerase chain reaction (PCR) to identify loss of heterozygosity or mutations in tumor cell DNA may be missed without use of microdissection, as the DNA from normal cell population may dilute out the DNA from the tumor cells.

In recent years, multiple methods of microdissection have emerged. They vary from crude methods of simply identifying large areas of a cell type and scraping them from the slide to single-cell selection and dissection using laser-assisted methods. Because of the high resolution associated with laser microdissection, single-cell dissection is possible even if cells are dispersed in complex tissue. The term "laser microdissection" covers two different techniques; the first type employs ultraviolet light at a high flux density (excimer laser), to cut the section without any associated heat. For large-scale throughput, this may be automated, where cells for dissection may be selected using computer software. Although this method is highly selective, the equipment is expensive compared to a manual micromanipulator. There is also controversy about the quality of DNA obtained by this method. The second method is when a tissue section is overlain by a thermoplastic film. Low-wattage, long-wavelength laser light is then passed through the section in areas of tissue to be recovered. Because of heating of the thermoplastic film, the areas for analysis

From: *Methods in Molecular Medicine, vol. 79: Molecular Diagnosis of Cancer*
Edited by: J. E. Roulston and J. M. S. Bartlett © Humana Press Inc., Totowa, NJ

stick to the film, but unwanted tissue remains on the glass slide. With this method, precision is poor and DNA may be damaged as a result of the high temperatures involved.

Laboratories without a laser microdissector can microdissect using a manual micromanipulator and light microscope. Although this method is more time-consuming, it can be used to accurately dissect one cell type from a heterogeneous cell population. The equipment necessary (manual micromanipulator and light microscope) is relatively inexpensive and the DNA retrieved is of high quality. This chapter will discuss in detail a mechanical microdissection utilizing a micromanipulator and light microscope.

2. Materials

All reagents should be of molecular biology quality.

1. Xylene.
2. 99%, 95%, and 70% Industrial methylated spirits (IMS).
3. Distilled water.
4. 005% Toluidine blue.
5. Proteinase K (Signa, St Louis, MO), 20 mg/mL stock solution. Store 50 μL aliquots at –20°C; thaw and dilute to 1 mL with digestion buffer containing 1% Tween-80 to give working stock solution of proteinase K of 1 mg/mL.
6. Digestion buffer, pH 8.3 (1.8 m*M* Tris-HCl and 0.9 m*M* EDTA).
7. Leica micromanipulator (Leica, UK; model no. 117562).
8. Light microscope (*see* **Note 1**).
9. 0.5-mm-Diameter tungsten wire for dissection needles.
10. Bacteriological loop holders for mounting needles in micromanipulator.
11. Facility for electrolytic sharpening of tungsten needles (*see* **Subheading 3.3.**).
12. Microfuge tubes.
13. Water bath.
14. Desktop centrifuge.
15. PCR block.

3. Methods

Tissue is microdissected from 5- to 6-μm sections mounted on glass slides.

3.1. Dewaxing and Staining Sections

1. Immerse sections in xylene for 6 min and repeat to remove wax from the tissue.
2. Rehydrate by taking sections through graded alcohol solutions. Immerse sections in 99% IMS for 2 min, 99% IMS for 2 min, 95% IMS for 1 min, 70% IMS for 1 min, then transfer into distilled water.
3. Stain tissue by immersing in 0.05% toluidine blue for 30 s (*see* **Note 2**).
4. Wash in distilled water (*see* **Note 3**).

3.2. Microdissection Tools

1. Sharpen and polish 25 mm of tungsten wire (0.5 mm in diameter) to a fine point using a electrolysis sharpening, to produce a needle with tip radius of several microns.
2. Mount the needle in a collect-type bacteriological loop holder.
3. Mount the loop holder in the tool holder of the micromanipulator and angle it downward at 25–30° (*see* **Note 4**).

3.3. Making the Electrolysis Sharpening Tool

1. Obtain approx 10 cm of platinum wire and make a circular loop in it, just small enough to fit inside a standard 20-mL universal container, with a tail 2–3 cm long.
2. Drill a 1-mm hole in the side of universal container near the base and thread the platinum wire tail through it, with the loop neatly placed at the base of the container. Seal the hole inside and out with an epoxy resin glue (e.g., Araldite).
3. Almost fill the cell with 0.1*M* KOH.
4. Connect the platinum wire cathode to the negative terminal of a standard 9-V battery (dry cell) and make the tungsten wire mounted in the bacteriological loop holder the anode.
5. Complete the circuit by dipping 5–10 mm of the tungsten wire vertically into the KOH solution. Hydrogen bubbles appear at the platinum cathode and nascent oxygen removes tungsten from the anode, which sharpens to a fine, polished point.
6. New needles are made in this way and damaged needles may be refurbished (*see* **Note 4**).

3.4. Performing Microdissection

1. Take a section for dissection from the water bath immediately before it is needed, drain it, and blot any surplus water from around the section with a disposable, lint-free tissue without touching the section.
2. Place the section on the microscope stage (*see* **Note 1**) and cover with a pool of digestion buffer from a disposable sterile Pasteur pipet. Spread the pool of buffer until it extends 3–4 mm beyond all edges of the section and is as deep as possible.
3. Center the area of cells in the section to be retrieved for subsequent analysis in the microscope field at an appropriate magnification.
4. Using the coarse motion controls of the micromanipulator, place the needle over the area to be dissected.
5. Lower the needle gently at the edge of the area to be dissected until its tip just touches the slide. Stop lowering the needle when a small lateral deflection of the needle tip occurs.
6. Microdissection techniques vary for different specimens. In general, attempt to develop cleavage between groups of cells. Work around the area to be dissected, developing a split between the area to be kept and the area to be removed. Then,

use the point of the needle gradually to undermine the area to be recovered, pushing and pulling with the tip and side of the needle until the area to be retrieved has been peeled from the slide and floats freely in the buffer pool.

7. If it is not clear whether the fragment is still attached to the section, gently agitate the slide. Attached fragments do not move freely.
8. Sometimes, a tissue fragment remains attached by a few strands of collagen; a second tungsten needle in a bacteriological loop holder, used freehand may be used to detach it.
9. Using the second tungsten needle, place the dissected tissue into a microfuge tube containing 12.5 μL of 1 m*M* proteinase K in digestion buffer with detergent.
10. Wash the tissue to the bottom of the tube using a further 12.5 μL of 1 m*M* proteinase K in digestion buffer.
11. Several areas may be dissected in this manner and placed in one tube to increase DNA content or multiple tubes if the section is large.
12. Once dissection is complete the slide may be dehydrated by taking sections through graded alcohol solutions. Immerse sections in 70% IMS for 1 min, 95% IMS for 1 min, 99% IMS for 1 min, and xylene for 1 min. Cover slip to provide a permanent record of areas dissected (*see* **Note 5**).

3.5. DNA Extraction

1. Incubate tubes containing tissue and proteinase K at 37°C in a water bath for 4–7 d to digest protein.
2. Centrifuge at 1000*g* to spin sample to the bottom of the tube.
3. Following digestion, inactivate proteinase K by heating to 95°C for 10 min in a PCR block. Failure to inactivate proteinase K might lead to digestion of *Taq* polymerase and failed PCRs.
4. Centrifuge at 1000*g* to spin sample to the bottom of the tube.
5. Specimens may be stored short term at 4°C. Store for longer periods at –20°C.
6. Extracted DNA is suitable for use in PCR reactions if PCR products required are less than 350 basepairs. However, in some cases, it is necessary to further purify the DNA, as the blue dye from the toludine blue can interfere with some reactions (e.g., real-time PCR or fluorescent sequencing reactions). It may also be necessary in some cases to increase the concentration of the DNA extracted. In either case, this problem may be solved by precipitating the DNA and resuspending it in DNA/RNAse-free water.

4. Notes

1. Any microscope can be used if there is enough space between the objective and stage for access to the specimen. Ordinary or inverted standard microscopes can be used, but a stereo dissecting microscope with relatively high maximum magnification (up to ×120) is ideal.
2. Staining reveals tissue structure, but unstained sections may be dissectable, especially if a serial section is available for reference. Staining often makes dissection easier. Toludine blue staining is easy and does not appear to interfere with

subsequent PCR, although this should be verified for particular applications (e.g., real-time PCR).

3. Stained sections can be stored in distilled water for about 3 h until dissection. Refrigeration at 4°C in water overnight causes some destaining and sections may lift from the slide. Stained sections can be stored dry, but it is best not to dewax and stain more sections than can be used in a single dissection session.
4. Bacteriological loop holders and tungsten wire are inexpensive. Either prepare enough needles in advance to use a new needle for each microdissection if necessary or briefly repolish the needle between samples, which exposes a new tungsten surface. The risk of DNA carryover on the needle from one specimen to the next appears largely theoretical
5. A serial hematoxylin and eosin section shows what has been removed. A magnified photocopy or digital image of such a serial section can be annotated on hard copy or digitally to record the dissection. Photocopy histological sections through an acetate sheet to avoid scratching the photocopier glass or smearing it with mounting medium.

6

Fluorescence *In Situ* Hybridization

Technical Overview

John M. S. Bartlett

1. Introduction

Fluorescence *in situ* hybridization (FISH) is now widely applied to the detection of specific normal and aberrant DNA sequences in both intact cells, either in interphase or metaphase, and isolated chromosomes. A logical extension of early *in situ* hybridization (ISH) techniques, simply exploiting the ability to label DNA with high-energy fluorophores, FISH is now applied in an increasing number of molecular diagnostic areas, including karyotype analysis, gene mapping, disease diagnosis, and therapeutic targeting. FISH has advantages over ISH, which are critical to its implementation in diagnostic medicine, particularly in reduced exposure time over radioactive ISH methods. Furthermore, FISH is perceived to be safer and has the added advantage that multiple fluorochromes can be used to discriminate different targets simultaneously.

Although over 30 yr have elapsed since the description of the first ISH experiments ***(1)***, yet it is less than 50 yr since the correct number of human chromosomes was identified in 1956 ***(2)***. Progress in molecular techniques over this period has been dramatic, with the introduction of interphase cytogenetics in the early 1980s and nonisotopic methods in the late 1980s and early 1990s ***(3)***. However, it is only with the relatively recent advent of FISH methods, applicable to both freshly prepared and formalin-fixed preparations, that the true diagnostic potential of ISH is becoming apparent. The application of FISH to detect gene amplification [HER2 in breast cancer ***(4)***], gene rearrangements (BCR-Abl in leukemias) ***(5)***, microdeletions ***(6)***, chromosomal duplication, and viral infections (i.e., human papilloma virus [HPV]) demonstrates the broad

From: *Methods in Molecular Medicine, vol. 79: Molecular Diagnosis of Cancer*
Edited by: J. E. Roulston and J. M. S. Bartlett © Humana Press Inc., Totowa, NJ

applicability of this methodology in molecular diagnostic medicine. Wider research applications, such as karyotyping and gene mapping ***(7,8)*** are providing further impetus to the application of diagnostic FISH. However, experimental extensions of FISH such as comparative genomic hybridization (CGH) and spectral karyotyping (SKY), have yet to be widely applied within the diagnostic arena ***(9,10)***.

In the chapters following this overview are included examples of some of the current applications for FISH technology within diagnostic medicine. There is no place within a volume of this size to supply exhaustive protocols for even those diagnostic applications outlined earlier; however, representative methods from each of the key diagnostic areas are included, that may be readily adapted for use within the reader's discipline. In this overview, it is my intention to try to highlight some of the key lessons learnt in our experience with FISH.

1.1. Probes

For FISH to be applied, the first requirement is the availability of a DNA probe with homology to the target region. In many cases, such probes are now commercially available, greatly facilitating the development of diagnostic assays. In cases where probes must be synthesized, pure DNA is required, which must then be labeled by either nick translation, random priming, or polymerase chain reaction (PCR). The production of such "in-house" probe preparations for diagnostic procedures should be rigorously quality controlled. Our recommendation is that wherever possible, commercial probes be utilized. In all cases, probes must be supplemented by the addition of Cot-1 DNA (usually supplied with commercial probes). Cot-1 DNA represents repetitive sequences of the human genome and addition to the probe mix suppresses crosshybridization to the large quantities of such DNA present in normal and abnormal cells. If unlabeled Cot-1 DNA is not included in the hybridization mix, a frequent effect is the appearance of nonspecific hybridization, which can mask signals in a wash of background noise ***(11)***.

Repetitive sequence probes have proven to be of great value in the development of diagnostic FISH applications. These probes target regions of the genome rich in repetitive DNA sequences, typically telomeres and centromeres. Alpha satellites are tandom arrays of approx 171 basepair repeats found at the centromeric region of human chromosomes ***(12,13)*** Sequence variations between chromosomes allow specific centromeric markers to be provided for the majority of human chromosomes. Other repeat sequences in similar regions ("classical" satellites or type II and III satelites) are also used to generate chromosome-specific probes ***(14)***.

1.2. Sample Preparation

Diagnostic FISH methodologies are most commonly applied either to isolated cells from whole blood or other body fluids (*see* Chapters 8 and 9), frozen-tissue sections, or, increasingly over the past few years, tissues that have been preserved by formalin fixation (*see* Chapters 7 and 12). Where required, metaphase chromosome spreads can be prepared from cultured cells using a spindle inhibitor (e.g., colcemid) to cause cell arrest during mitosis ***(11)***.

For unfixed cells and tissues, the challenge is to sufficiently pretreat samples so that the FISH protocol, which involves high-temperature and high-salt washes, does not damage the sample to be evaluated. Typically, this involves the use of charged slides (silane or, less commonly, polylysine coated; *see* Chapter 7) and a brief fixation (30–60 s) with acid ethanol or, exceptionally, formalin buffers (*see* Chapter 12).

However, for the majority of applications involving tissue biopsies, access to fresh or frozen (i.e., unfixed) material is limited and diagnostic applications must be adapted to take account of the effects of fixation, particularly with formalin-based fixatives, that are the most commonly used, on the tissue sample. Therefore, although charged slides are also used for FISH applications on formalin-fixed (archival) tissue specimens, the technical challenge of applying FISH to such tissue is far greater. The majority of laboratories use neutral-buffered formalin as a tissue fixative because of its well-proven ability to preserve tissue architecture and provide an excellent platform for assessment of tissue morphology. Tissues are generally then mounted in paraffin wax to provide a support for sectioning for subsequent sectioning and evaluation. In order to achieve this, tissue samples are dehydrated (into 100% alcohol) and then saturated in liquid paraffin wax, which is then allowed to permeate the tissue and solidify to provide a solid support. This process causes further protein denaturation over and above the effects of formalin. Neutral-buffered formalin is a oxidizing agent (an aldehyde) and, as such, causes extensive protein–protein and protein–nucleic acid crosslinks, facilitating the formation of disulfide bonds and other covalent linkages between macromolecules within cells during the fixation process.

The combined effects of prolonged exposure to formalin and the dehydration and heating steps required to preserve tissue architecture is to markedly alter intracellular proteins and nucleic acid, producing an hydrophobic and highly crosslinked network that experience shows provides a significant barrier to the entry of macromolecules, such as FISH and ISH probes, into the cell. In effect, the nucleic acids within the cell are masked, or shielded, by the denaturation of proteins and other effects of the fixation process. In order to facilitate the entry of probes into the cell, so that they may find and link with their targets, two steps are required: rehydration of the tissue section and permeabilization by means of breaking down protein–protein and protein–DNA crosslinks. Ideally, these steps should be achieved with minimal tissue damage to enable tissue morphology to be correlated with genetic aberrations. Despite these limitations, formalin is preferred as a preservative for FISH-based experimentation ***(15,16)***. We are currently unaware of FISH protocols that work well following use of Bouins fixation.

1.3. Rehydration

The first of these steps, rehydration, is common to most staining protocols, including hematoxylin and eosin staining and immunohistochemical techniques. Following sectioning and mounting on charged slides, the section is treated to remove paraffin wax and passed through graded alcohols (*see* Chapter 7).

Following rehydration, a number of different steps may be used to increase permeabilization of the tissue section and allow probe access, each of these will, when taken to extremes, cause significant tissue damage and loss of morphology. Ultimately, overtreatment of tissue sections prior to *in situ* analysis may cause complete loss of tissue structure and loss of nuclei, essentially causing the technique to fail. Conversely, undertreatment will reduce, perhaps to undetectable levels, the amount of probe that reaches and binds to the target nucleic acid. Therefore, each step, in the pretreatment protocol must be critically evaluated for the benefit it provides toward reaching a successful experimental or diagnostic outcome. In particular, within clinical diagnostic practice, where failures may cause treatment delay, a robust pretreatment protocol is required.

Although a number of different pretreatment protocols have been described, those most frequently used contain one or more steps whose purpose is to permeabalize tissue and this is followed by a protease digestion step that serves to break down the cellular proteins and both enhance probe penetration and reduce autofluorescence ***(16)***. Steps used for tissue permeabilization include treatment with acid, detergents, and reducing agents.

1.4. Acid Permeabilization

Most commonly, incubation in 0.2 *N* HCl is used to deproteinize tissues, increasing probe access ***(1,17)***; incubation in acid is thought to reverse some of the effects of formalin fixation, which is pH dependent, and proceeds more rapidly at high pH ***(18)***.

1.5. Reducing Agents

Both sodium metabisulfite *(3)* and sodium thiocyanate *(4,19)* are used in protein disulfide bonds formed by formalin fixation *(20)* and both facilitate protease digestion and increase nuclear accessibility.

By use of acids and reducing agents, the exposure of tissues to proteolytic enzymes can be reduced and this minimizes the amount of tissue damage produced by these pretreatment steps.

1.6. Protease Digestion

This must be achieved with minimal tissue damage, to enable tissue morphology to be correlated with genetic aberrations. Optimum maintenance of cell and tissue morphology following unmasking of nucleic acids is achieved by varying digestion times and assessment of tissue sections following proteolytic digestion prior to hybridization. The duration of exposure of the slides to protease is perhaps the most critical step in ensuring adequate pretreatment of formalin-fixed tissues prior to application of DNA probes for FISH. The extent of treatment required varies according to the tissue and, to a far lesser extent, to the degree of fixation (*see* Chapter 7) *(4,21,22)*. In our experience one of the main reasons for the failure of a laboratory to establish FISH methods is overrigid adherence to an inadequate digestion period; we therefore recommend that digestion times be evaluated in each laboratory to optimize results *(16)*. The importance of ensuring adequate digestion cannot therefore be underestimated *(16)* and we routinely ensure, by visual examination (*see* **refs.** ***4,16,21,*** and *22*), that slides be adequately digested prior to proceeding with probe hybridization. The concentration and activity of protease will also affect the duration of this step and, therefore, digestion times should be reassessed each time the protease batch is changed. Although we have used both proteinase K and pepsin in the past *(4,21,22)*, we currently recommend the use of pepsin for the majority of procedures.

2. Hybridization/Posthybridization

2.1. Probe Hybridization to Target DNA

Once samples are adequately prepared for hybridization, the aspects of FISH most likely to influence efficiency and specificity are (in order or importance) probe sequence, hybridization temperature (and posthybridization washes), and the buffer system.

2.1.1. Probe Sequence

The probe is, by far, the most critical component of ensuring specificity of hybridization. Both with in-house probes and those commercially available, it is essential that a clear understanding of the hybridization target be available before proceeding with any diagnostic application. For microdeletion and gene amplification assays, care must be taken to ensure that crossover with neighboring genes is eliminated when it may compromise the result.

2.1.2. Denaturation and Hybridization

Unlike PCR, the hybridization temperature in FISH assays is less critical, as with other hybridization techniques. It is possible to calculate the theoretical probe hybridization temperature (T_m) using a number of different approaches. However, in practice, hybridization temperatures are designed to ensure maximum binding of the probe to DNA. In general, sample DNA is denatured for 5–10 min at 95°C, whereas Cot-1 and probe DNA are heated for approx 5 min. Hybridization between the probe DNA and the target DNA is performed, usually on a flat-bed-heated stage, for anywhere between 12 and 72 h. Again, as with Northern and Southern blotting, specificity is largely determined by the stringency of the posthybridization washes.

2.1.3. Stringency

Most problems encountered with FISH specificity relate to the specific hybridization of the probe and subsequent detection. The stringency (i.e., an arbitrary measure of specificity) of probe hybridization cellular DNA and of posthybridization washes is governed by salt and formamide concentrations and by temperature ***(3)***. Increasing temperature and formamide concentration will decrease hybridization (i.e., increase stringency), whereas decreasing salt concentration will have the same effect; each of these has the effect of destabilizing the hydrogen bonds required for probe binding to DNA. The use of formamide can enable high-stringency washes to be performed at relatively low temperatures. The optimum DNA:DNA hybridization temperature can be defined by:

$$T = 81.5°C + 16.6(\log_{10}[Na^+]) + 0.41(\%G{+}C) - 820/l - 0.6(\%F) - 1.4(\%mismatch)$$

In this formula, $[Na^+]$ is the molar salt concentration, l is the probe length (bases), %F is the % formamide, and % mismatch is % noncomplementary basepairs between hybridizing strands ***(13,14)***. As stated earlier, it is common to use a relatively low stringency during probe hybridization and then to increase in a stepwise manner the degree of stringency in a series of posthybridization washes.

3. Scoring/Interpretation of Results

Signals are visualized by use of a fluorescence microscope using a light source, usually a mercury or xenon vapor lamp of 100 W power, which emits photons that excite the fluorophores. The specific emission wavelengths of different fluorophores is then focused through detection filters, which can be either single or multiple bandpass. The increasing use of image analysis to capture, document, and, more recently, evaluate FISH results is an important ongoing development in this area.

There remains a wide variation in methods for quantifying the results of FISH, based on subjective and objective approaches. However, although variations between laboratories are acceptable in the research context, for the technique to be applied in a diagnostic setting, a clear protocol is required. Individual tests will differ in the criteria for detecting abnormalities. The detection of aneuploid cells in urine, for example (*see* Chapter 9), requires different criteria than those applied to the detection of gene/chromosomal deletions and amplifications. The identification of gene-fusion products (*see* Chapter 8), embodies further constraints. Furthermore, unlike fresh preparations of cells from urine, blood, or other sources, scoring of tissue sections is limited by the phenomenon of nuclear truncation, making it essential that (1) control genes are used for loss of signals or signal amplification and (2) some correction or control is applied.

We have used FISH to assess chromosomal copy number, aneuploidy in urines, and gene amplification and deletion ***(4,21–24)***. We have studied the effects of both intraobserver and interobserver variation, coupled with the number of cells scored to achieve an accurate and reliable result ***(23,25,26)***. We have developed a rigorously quality controlled quantitation method ***(23)***, using normal tissues as a reference for normosomic signals to circumvents previous variations in methodology and provides straightforward guidelines.

3.1. Scoring Criteria and Use of Normal Controls

It is probably not relevant to lay down strict criteria for the scoring of widely differing assays in an overview such as this. However, certain principles do hold true for most situations. First, in order to correctly define the presence of an abnormality, whether a translocation/fusion or deletion/amplification, considerable experience with the appearance of normal cells is required. This is particularly relevant to the scoring of tissue sections, where nuclear truncation by sectioning and reduced hybridization efficiencies may affect results. As an illustration, it is our experience ***(21,23,26)*** that in normal tissue sections (disomic), the average chromosomal copy number detected ranges between 1.4 and 1.7 copies per cell, significantly lower than the predicted value of 2.0. Indeed, chromosome copy numbers around 2.0–2.2 are frequently indicative of a trisomy. As a consequence, we recommend that in detection of cellular abnormalities, careful characterization of normal tissues, often by two observers (*see* **Subheading 3.2.**), be performed to define the "normal range" (we use the mean ± 3 standard deviations derived from normal tissues). Once this is identified, the detection of abnormalities is greatly facilitated. Clearly, such restraints apply much less to whole-cell preparations (e.g., urines and bloods). However, in the latter context, discrimination between diseased and nondiseased cells may require that larger numbers of cells be scored and a low proportion of abnormal cells is still indicative of abnormalities.

Scoring of gene deletions and amplifications imposes further constraints. Particularly in cancer, where the majority of such deletions/amplifications occur, there may be a significant risk of loss or gain of the entire chromosome. Therefore, a method is required to discriminate between, for example, gene duplication (where the chromosome is aneusomic, increasing gene copy number) and gene amplification (where an excess of gene copies over chromosome copies is observed). In this instance, the use of a chromosomal control (such as a specific telomeric or centromeric satellite markers) is essential as an aid to accurate diagnosis. For tests of gene amplification (such as the HER2 test described in Chapter 7), an increase in gene:chromosome ratio to >2.0 is usually taken as indicative of amplification. Conversely, a decrease in ratio to 0.5 or less might be a useful criterion for detection of deletions. In each case, careful correlation with normal samples should also be performed.

3.2. Intraobserver and Interobserver Variation

Currently, almost all diagnostic FISH assays rely on a manual interpretation of results. As with all subjective assessment methods, this can lead to errors between observers as a result of inexperience or subjective bias. Evidence that assesses the impact of both intraobserver and interobserver scoring on results of FISH assays is still relatively sparse. Our own experience, garnered over many years, would suggest that within the normal diagnostic range (i.e., in discrimination between disomy and aneusomy or amplification/deletion), intraobserver and interobserver variations are of the order of 10% ***(4,21–24)***. This result holds true for many different assays and observers. It is also apparent that as the number of signals/cell increases, particularly when >10 signals/nucleus are seen in gene amplified samples, so does the interobserver variation ***(4,25)***. In terms of both accuracy and reproducibility, therefore, dual-observer scoring is a valuable method of achieving close concordance of results and validation of what is otherwise a purely objective interpretation of results. Where close concordance between observers is achieved and maintained, the number of cells scored for a clear diagnosis can be reduced. Ultimately, however, the use of objective systems, such as image analysis, will reduce the error rate and also the eye strain associated with most current FISH diagnostic procedures.

4. Quality Assurance

The development of internal and external quality assurance often lags behind the implementation of novel diagnostic tests. For example, at present, there is no United Kingdom or, to my knowledge, European external quality assurance (EQA) program in place for HER2 FISH diagnoses. Although this oversight is likely to be rectified in the near future, individual service managers may wish to be proactive in the development of EQA schemes within their own areas. Internal quality assurance is often much simpler to establish and we routinely use both normal and abnormal quality assurance samples selected around the diagnostic interval for all our diagnostic and research assays. These provide a constant measure of both observer and methodological errors that might otherwise arise unchecked.

5. Conclusion

Many of the technical issues surrounding the application of FISH to molecular diagnostic techniques have been resolved over recent years. The assessment of a wide range of genetic disorders is now dependent of FISH-based assays and the number is likely to expand rapidly in the coming years both in oncology and other branches of medicine. The need for standardized and robust protocols, scoring systems, and quality assurance schemes is highlighted here and in Chapters 7–11.

References

1. Warford, A. (1994) An overview of *in situ* hybridisation, in *A Guide to* In Situ, Hybaid UK, pp. 15–17.
2. Tijo, J. H. and Levan, A. (1956) The chromosome number in man. *Hereditas* **42,** 1–6.
3. Wolfe, K. Q. and Herrington, C. S. (1997) Interphase cytogenetics and pathology: a tool for diagnosis and research. *J. Pathol.* **181,** 359–361.
4. Bartlett, J. M. S., Going, J. J., Mallon, E. A., et al. (2001) Evaluating HER2 amplification and overexpression in breast cancer. *J. Pathol.* **195,** 422–428.
5. Nolte, M., Werner, M., Ewig, M., et al. (1996) Megakaryocytes carry the fused bcr-abl gene in chronic myeloid leukaemia: a fluorescence *in situ* hybridization analysis from bone marrow biopsies. *Virchows Arch.* **427,** 561–565.
6. Lavarino, C., Corletto, V., Mezzelani, A., et al. (1998) Detection of TP53 mutation, loss of heterozygosity and DNA content in fine-needle aspirates of breast carcinoma. *Br. J. Cancer* **77,** 125–130.
7. Bell, S. M., Zuo, J., Myers, R. M., et al. (1996) Fluorescence *in situ* hybridization deletion mapping at 4p16.3 in bladder cancer cell lines refines the localisation of the critical interval to 30 kb. *Genes Chromosomes Cancer* **17,** 108–117.
8. Hu, R. J., Lee, M. P., Connors, T. D., et al. (1997) A 2.5-Mb transcript map of a tumor-suppressing subchromosomal transferable fragment from 11p15.5, and isolation and sequence analysis of three novel genes. *Genomics* **46,** 9–17.

9. Bryndorf, T., Kirchhoff, M., Rose, H., et al. (1995) Comparative genomic hybridization in clinical cytogenetics. *Am. J. Hum. Genet.* **57,** 1211–1220.
10. Houldsworth, J. and Chaganti, R. S. K. (1994) Comparative genomic hybridization: an overview. *Am. J. Pathol.* **145,** 1253–1260.
11. Haar, F. M., Durm, M., Aldinger, K., et al. (1994) A rapid FISH technique for quantitative microscopy. *Biotechniques* **17,** 346–348, 350–353.
12. Warburton, P. E., Greig, G. M., Haaf, T., et al. (1991) PCR amplification of chromosome specific alpha satellite DNA: definition of centromeric STS markers and polymorphic analysis. *Genomics* **11,** 324–333.
13. Weier, H. U. G., Kleine, H. D., and Gray, J. W. (1991) Labeling of the centromeric region on human chromosome 8 by *in situ* hybridization. *Hum. Genet.* **87,** 489–494.
14. Vorsanova, S. G., Yurov, Y. B., Soloviev, I. V., et al. (1994) Rapid identification of marker chromosomes by *in situ* hybridization under different stringency conditions. *Anal. Cell. Pathol.* **7,** 251–258.
15. Sauter, G., Moch, H., Carroll, P., et al. (1995) Chromosome-9 loss detected by fluorescence *in situ* hybridization in bladder cancer. *Int. J. Cancer* **64,** 99–103.
16. Watters, A. D. and Bartlett, J. M. S. (2002) Fluorescence *in situ* hybridization in paraffin tissue sections: a pretreatment protocol. *Mol. Biotechnol.* **20,** 1–4.
17. Wolman, S. R. (1994) Fluorescence *in situ* hybridisation; a new tool for the pathologist. *Hum. Pathol.* **25,** 586–590.
18. Pahphlatz, M. M. M., de Wilde, P. C. M., Poddighe, P., et al. (1995) A model for evaluation of *in situ* hybridisation spot-count distributions in tissue sections. *Cytometry* **20,** 193–202.
19. Pycha, A., Mian, C., Haitel, A., et al. (1997) Fluorescence *in situ* hybridization identifies more aggressive types of primarily noninvasive (stage pTa) bladder cancer. *J. Urol.* **157,** 2116–2119.
20. Visscher, D. W., Wallis, T., and Ritchie, C. A. (1995) Detection of chromosome aneuploidy in breast lesions with fluorescence *in situ* hybridization: comparison of whole nuclei to thin tissue sections and correlation with flow cytometric DNA analysis. *Cytometry* **21,** 95–100.
21. Bartlett, J. M., Watters, A. D., Ballantyne, S. A., et al. (1998) Is chromosome 9 loss a marker of disease recurrence in transitional cell carcinoma of the urinary bladder? *Br. J. Cancer* **77,** 2193–2198.
22. Edwards, J., Krishna, N. S., Mukherjee, R., et al. (2001) Amplification of the androgen receptor may not explain development of androgen independent prostate cancer. *Br. J. Urol.* **88,** 1–10.
23. Watters, A. D., Ballantyne, S. A., Going, J. J., et al. (2000) Aneusomy of chromosomes 7 and 17 predicts the recurrence of transitional cell carcinoma of the urinary bladder. *BJU Int.* **85,** 42–47.
24. Watters, A. D., Stacey, M. W., Going, J. J., et al. (2001) Genetic aberrations of *NAT2* and chromosome 8; their association with progression in transitional cell carcinoma of the urinary bladder. *Urol. Int.,* **67,** 235–239.
25. Going, J. J., Mallon, L., Reeves, J. R., et al. (2000) Inter-observer agreement in

assessing c-erbB-2 status in breast cancer: immunohistochemistry and fish. *J. Pathol.* **190,** 19A-19A.

26. Bartlett, J. M. S., Adie, L., Watters, A. D., et al. (1999) Chromosomal aberrations in transitional cell carcinoma that are predictive of disease outcome are independent of polyploidy. *BJU Int.* **84,** 775–779.

7

HER2 FISH in Breast Cancer

John M. S. Bartlett and Amanda Forsyth

1. Introduction

The assessment of *HER2/c-erbB-2/neu* (hereafter *HER2*) gene amplification and protein expression has become one of the central debating points in current breast cancer diagnosis and biology. The debate around whom to test, when testing should be offered, and, most importantly, which method to use is represented at most current conferences where breast cancer pathology is under discussion.

Overexpression of the p185^{HER2} protein product of *HER2/neu* is closely related to gene amplification in breast cancer ***(1–6)***. Slamon et al. first described the biological importance of HER2 in breast cancer in 1987 ***(7)*** and many subsequent publications ***(8)*** confirm the prognostic significance of HER2 amplification and overexpression in breast cancer ***(9–12)***. There has been controversy regarding node-negative carcinomas ***(10–12)***, but some of the reported differences may be methodological ***(13–15)***. *HER2* is one of four homologous receptors that together make up the HER (or type I or erbB) family of transmembrane receptor tyrosine kinases. These receptors form homodimers or heterodimers following ligand binding to their external domains and activate a complete series of intracellular signaling pathways via autophosphorylation of tyrosines on their intracellular domains.

Recent clinical trials implicating HER2 in modified responses to antiestrogens and anthracyclins ***(9,16–23)*** have stimulated interest in accurate and reliable identification of patients with carcinomas driven by HER2 amplification and overexpression ***(17)***. Most critically, the recent Food and Drug Administration (FDA) approval for the first anti-HER2 therapy, Herceptin™, and the wide licensing of this agent throughout the world, coupled with the

From: *Methods in Molecular Medicine, vol. 79: Molecular Diagnosis of Cancer*
Edited by: J. E. Roulston and J. M. S. Bartlett © Humana Press Inc., Totowa, NJ

likelihood of further targeted therapies, have thrown the need for HER2 testing into sharp relief and has intensified the debate.

Fluorescence *in situ* hybridization (FISH) is a technique used to study gene and chromosome copy number *in situ*. It has found clinical application in the assessment of gene rearrangements in leukemia and lymphoma ***(24)*** and recently forms part of the routine diagnostic assessment of amplification of the gene *HER2/neu* in breast cancer ***(25–30)***.

2. Materials

2.1. Slide Pretreatment

2.1.1. Manual Protocol

Many of the reagents required for this protocols form part of the Abbott/ Vysis Paraffin Pretreatment Reagent Kit (cat. no. 32-801200); alternatively, they can be made up as follows:

1. Silanized microscope slides (*see* **Note 1**).
2. Control sections (*see* **Note 2**); for example, "Probe check" quality control slides (Abbott Inc., UK).
3. Water baths set at 80°C and 37°C.
4. 0.2*N* HCl, pH 2.0.
5. Pretreatment reagent: Sodium thiocyanate 8% (w/v) in distilled water.
6. Pepsin (Fluka or Sigma, UK): Prepare a 10% (w/v) stock solution in 0.2*N* HCl, aliquot and store at –20°C for up to 4 mo (*see* **Note 3**), then dilute to 25 mg/50 mL of 0.2*N* HCl immediately prior to use or use protease from Vysis slide pretreatment kit (25 mg lyophilized aliquot in 50 mL of 0.2 *N* HCl).
7. Two staining dishes with 100% xylene.
8. Two staining dishes with 100% methanol.
9. Wash buffer: 2X SSC, pH 7.0: Dissolve 175.3 g NaCl and 88.2 g sodium citrate in 800 mL distilled water, adjust pH to 7.0 with 10*M* NaOH; make up to 1 L with distilled water and autoclave. Dilute 1:10 with distilled water for 2X SSC.
10. Staining dish with 70% methanol.
11. Staining dish with 85% methanol.
12. DAPI in Vectashield: Vectashield (Vectorlabs, UK) with 200 ng/mL of 4,6-diamidino-2 phenylindole-2 hydrochloride (DAPI) (Sigma, UK) added,
13. 100-W Epifluorescence microscope with appropriate filters (*see* **Note 4**).

2.1.2. Automated Slide Pretreatment

When large numbers of FISH samples are being analyzed, we have found that the use of the VP2000 tissue processor produces significant advantages in both tissue processing time and consistency of results.

1. VP2000 Tissue processing robot (Vysis Inc., Chicago, IL).
2. 2X SSC, pH 7.0: Dissolve 175.3 g NaCl and 88.2 g sodium citrate in 800 mL

distilled water, adjust pH to 7.0 with 10 *M* NaOH; make up to 1 L with distilled water and autoclave. Dilute 1:10 with distilled water for 2X SSC.

3. Silanized microscope slides (*see* **Note 1**).
4. Control sections (*see* **Note 2**); for example, "Probe check" quality control slides (Abbott Inc., UK).
5. Xylene.
6. 95% Ethanol.
7. Distilled water.
8. 0.2 *N* HCl, pH 2.0.
9. Pretreatment reagent: Sodium thiocyanate 8% (w/v) in distilled water.
10. Pepsin (*see* **Note 3**): 250 mg in 500 mL of 0.2*N* HCl (Vysis protease buffer).
11. 10% Neutral-buffered formalin.
12. 70% Ethanol.
13. 85% Ethanol.
14. DAPI in Vectashield: Vectashield (Vectorlabs, UK) with 200 ng/mL of 4,6-diamidino-2 phenylindole-2 hydrochloride (DAPI) (Sigma, UK) added.
15. 100-W Epifluorescence microscope with appropriate filters (*see* **Note 4**).

2.2. Denaturation and Probe Hybridization

1. Omnislide hybridization platform (Thermo-Hybaid) with dark plastic lid.
2. 2X SSC, pH 5.3: Dissolve 175.3 g NaCl and 88.2 g sodium citrate in 800 mL distilled water, adjust pH to 5.3 with 10*M* HCl; make up to 1 L with distilled water and autoclave. Dilute 1:10 with distilled water for 2X SSC, pH 5.3. Alternatively, take 66 g of 20X SSC salts (provided with Pathvysion™ kit) and dissolve in 200 mL distilled water, adjust pH to 5.3 with 10 *M* HCl, and make up to a final volume of 250 mL with distilled water.
3. Denaturing solution, pH 7.0–8.0: 49 mL Ultrapure formamide (Fluka UK), 7 mL 2X SSC, pH 5.3 and 14 mL distilled water. Check that pH is between 7.0–8.0 before each use (*see* **Note 5**).
4. Temporary "coverslips": Cut Parafilm into temporary coverslips (*see* **Note 6**).
5. Staining dish with 70% alcohol.
6. Staining dish with 85% alcohol.
7. Staining dish with 100% alcohol.
8. HER2/chromosome 17 probe mixture (from Pathvysion™ kit).
9. Rubber cement (*see* **Note 7**).

3. Methods

3.1. Manual Pretreatment of Slides

Note: This method has been adapted from the Pathvysion pretreatment protocol (Abbott Diagnostics and Vysis, Inc.).

1. Cut 5-µm tissue sections onto silanized slides (*see* **Note 1**) and bake at 56°C overnight. Store at room temperature until required (*see* **Note 8**).

2. Prepare two water baths, one at 85°C and one at 37°C, place one Coplin jar per five slides to be treated in each water bath. Fill those at 80°C with 8% sodium thiocyanate and those at 37°C with 0.2 *N* HCl for protease digestion (do not add protease at this time).
3. Immerse slides to be analyzed in xylene for 10 min to remove wax (*see* **Note 9**).
4. Repeat **step 3** with a fresh xylene bath.
5. Transfer slides into 100% methanol for 5 min.
6. Repeat **step 5**.
7. Place slides in 0.2*N* HCl for 20 min (*see* **Note 10**) at room temperature.
8. Wash slides in distilled water for 3 min at room temperature.
9. Wash in wash buffer for 3 min at room temperature.
10. Place slides in 8% sodium thiocyanate (Vysis, UK or Sigma, UK) in distilled water at 80°C for 30 min (*see* **Note 11**).
11. Wash in distilled water for 1 min at room temperature.
12. Wash in wash buffer for 5 min at room temperature.
13. Repeat **step 12** with fresh wash buffer and remove excess fluid before proceeding (*see* **Note 12**).
14. Place in protease buffer at 37°C for 22 min (*see* **Note 13**).
15. Immerse slides in 2X SSC buffer for 5 min at room temperature.
16. Repeat **step 15** with fresh wash buffer.
17. Place slides in 70% alcohol for 1 min at room temperature.
18. Place slides in 85% alcohol for 1 min at room temperature.
19. Place slides in 100% alcohol for 1 min at room temperature.
20. Allow slides to air-dry.
21. Apply DAPI in mountant and apply cover slips.
22. Assess the extent of tissue digestion with a 100-W fluorescence microscope that incorporates a filter block specific for the excitation and emission wavelengths of DAPI (*see* **Note 14**). If digestion is optimal, proceed to **step 23**. If sections are underdigested, proceed to **step 23** and then replace sections in protease buffer (**step 14**) for 2–20 min depending on the extent of underdigestion. Repeat **steps 15–21** and reassess digestion. If sections are overdigested, discard and repeat with new section, reducing the incubation time in protease (**step 14**).
23. Place slides in 2X SSC, pH 7.0, buffer until the cover slips fall off; then, dry in an oven at 45°C before proceeding with *in situ* hybridization.

3.2. Automated Pretreatment of Slides

The VP2000 is an automated tissue processing station with a robotic arm, which moves slides (up to 50) among 12 reagent basins, up to 3 temperature-controlled water baths, a rinse bath (with circulating distilled water), and a drying station. Movement of slides is controlled by a computer with steps programmable for position and duration in each wash. The temperature-controlled baths can also be agitated. The protocol describes the use of the system for pretreatment of batches of breast tumors.

1. Switch on the VP2000 and computer control station (*see* **Note 15**). Lift the protective plastic covering from each side of the VP2000 processor and remove any metal lids covering solutions. Check the levels of each solution in basins marked 4–15. The plastic containers have a fine groove at approx 700 mL; containers should be topped up to this line with the appropriate solution every time the machine is run.
2. Basins 1–3 are the temperature-controlled water baths. Basin 1 contains the pretreatment solution and basin 3 contains the protease buffer. The pretreatment solution should be topped up to 500 mL with distilled water before each use (*see* **Note 16**).
3. If required, top up the protease buffer in basin 1 to 500 mL with fresh protease buffer (*see* **Note 17**); do not add protease at this time.
4. Allow the water bath to fill with distilled water from the reservoir.
5. Place slides (up to 50) into the slide holder and mount on the robotic arm.
6. Allow the water baths to reach target temperatures (80°C and 37°C), add protease to protease buffer (**step 16**), and select a program, for HER2 FISH pretreatment, we use the following:
7. Xylene (basin 4), 5 min at room temperature.
8. Xylene (basin 5), 5 min at room temperature.
9. Xylene (basin 6), 5 min at room temperature.
10. 95% Ethanol (basin 7), 1 min at room temperature.
11. 95% Ethanol (basin 8), 1 min at room temperature.
12. 0.2 *N* HCl (basin 9), 20 min at room temperature.
13. Water rinse (water bath set to recirculate), 3 min at room temperature.
14. Pretreatment reagent (basin 1), 30 min at 80°C.
15. Water rinse (water bath set to recirculate), 3 min at room temperature.
16. Protease digestion (basin 3), 18 min (*see* **Note 18**) at 37°C.
17. Water rinse (water bath set to recirculate), 3 min at room temperature.
18. Fix in 10% neutral-buffered formalin (basin 11), 10 min at room temperature.
19. Water rinse (water bath set to recirculate), 3 min at room temperature.
20. 70% Ethanol (basin 12), 1 min at room temperature.
21. 85% Ethanol (basin 13), 1 min at room temperature.
22. 95% Ethanol (basin 14), 1 min at room temperature.
23. Air-dry (drying station) at 28°C for 3 min.
24. At this point, digestion should be checked using **steps 21–23** (*see* **Note 14**) of **Subheading 3.1.** before proceeding to denaturation and probe hybridization (**Subheading 3.3.**).

3.3. Denaturation and Probe Hybridization

1. Ensure that pretreated slides from **Subheadings 3.1.1.** or **3.1.2.** are dry.
2. Check pH of denaturing solution and apply 100 μL to each slide in a fume hood (*see* **Note 5**). Cover with a temporary cover slip (*see* **Note 6**). Place slides on the Omnislide in a rack with light shielding.
3. Denature slides for 5 min at 72°C using the Omnislide.

4. Remove slide rack from the Omnislide and remove temporary coverslips in a fume hood.
5. Place in 70% alcohol in a fume hood for 1 min at room temperature.
6. Place in 85% alcohol for 1 mim at room temperature.
7. Place in 100% alcohol for 1 min at room temperature.
8. Remove slides, remove excess ethanol, and allow to air-dry.
9. Apply 10 μL of HER2/chromosome 17 probe mixture to a 22 × 26-mm cover slip. Invert the slide and lower gently onto cover slip.
10. Seal the slide with rubber cement.
11. Repeat for each slide to be analyzed and place on the Omnislide.
12. Hybridize slides overnight at 37°C on the Omnislide shielded from light (*see* **Note 19**).

3.4. Posthybridization Wash

1. Place a Coplin jar containing 50 mL of posthybridization wash buffer into a water bath set at 72°C. Prepare a staining dish with posthybridization wash buffer at room temperature.
2. Remove slides from the Omnislide hybridization station.
3. Using forceps, remove rubber cement from each slide and place in posthybridization wash buffer at room temperature to allow the cover slip to float off.
4. Check that temperature of 72°C posthybridization wash buffer is 72±1°C before proceeding.
5. Remove slides from room-temperature wash; carefully remove excess buffer (*see* **Note 12**).
6. Place slides into posthybridization wash at 72°C for 2 min. Do not add more than five slides per jar (*see* **Note 20**).
7. Allow slides to air-dry shielded from light (*see* **Note 21**).
8. Mount slide in mountant with 0.2 ng/mL DAPI and seal with nail polish (*see* **Note 22**).

3.5. Quantitation of Hybridization Signals

The following description relates specifically to the scoring scheme used in our laboratory for scoring of HER2 gene amplification; alternative systems for scoring chromosome copy and androgen-receptor amplification are described elsewhere (refs).

1. Identify regions for analysis by FISH using adjacent hematoxylin and eosin-stained sections for each case (*see* **Note 23**).
2. Count signals for HER2 (orange) and chromosome 17 in 60 nonoverlapping tumor cell nuclei in the control and carcinoma sections (*see* **Note 24**). Record the individual results on the sheet in **Fig. 1**, noting the case number, coordinates, batch number of probe, date, and observer code. Score 20 nuclei each from separate tumor areas within the slide when possible (*see* **Note 25**).

Case Number		Probe Batch No:	Date	
		Protease batch Number	Observer	

AREA 1: Ordinates			AREA 2			AREA 3		
	Green	Orange		Green	Orange		Green	Orange
1			1			1		
2			2			2		
3			3			3		
4			4			4		
5			5			5		
6			6			6		
7			7			7		
8			8			8		
9			9			9		
10			10			10		
11			11			11		
12			12			12		
13			13			13		
14			14			14		
15			15			15		
16			16			16		
17			17			17		
18			18			18		
19			19			19		
20			20			20		
TOTAL			TOTAL			TOTAL		

Fig. 1. Scoring template for HER2 FISH.

3. Calculate the total number of HER2 and chromosome 17 signals observed for each area by summing the counts for each cell on the spreadsheet in **Fig. 1**.
4. Calculate the HER2:chromosome 17 ratio for each area by entering the individual counts for HER2 and chromosome 17 onto the results spreadsheet shown in **Fig. 2**. This spreadsheet can be set up in programs such as Excel or Lotus to automatically calculate variation between area scores and between observers (*see* **Note 26**).

Pathology Number:			Batch No:	
			Date	

Observer 1	Observer 2	

	Chromosome 17	HER-2	Ratio	Chromosome 17	HER-2	Ratio	Mean Ratio
Area 1	50	190					
Area 2	45	180					
Area 3	48	195					
	Score Obs 1			Score Obs2			

Inter-Observer variation

Overall c-erbB2 ratio is		

Tumour is **Amplified** **Normal** (circle 1)

Fig. 2. Result spreadsheet for HER2 amplification (giving worked example).

4. Notes

1. Silanized slides can be purchased from several suppliers (e.g., Sigma, UK) or prepared as described in **Subheading 2.1.1.**
2. In performing diagnostic FISH analysis, it is essential to include internal and external quality controls. We routinely include sections from amplified and nonamplified controls within each diagnostic run. In addition, we currently participate in a local external quality control scheme. The UK National External Quality Assurance Scheme is currently being expanded to include HER2 FISH testing. We would recommend participation in this or another equivalent scheme. In addition, a negative control section, omitting the probe cocktail controls for hybridization efficiency and nonspecific staining.
3. Pepsin activity can be highly variable between suppliers and batches; therefore, activity should be tested prior to use of a new batch. Pepsin is also highly labile and activity declines rapidly once diluted. Pepsin should be added to digestion buffer immediately prior to starting digestion and fresh pepsin added for each batch of slides to be digested. If more than 30 min are required for digestion, additional pepsin should be added.
4. The use of a 100-W epiflourescence microscope is essential if good results are to be obtained. Filters specific for DAPI, Spectrum Orange, and Spectrum Green are required, along with a triple bandpass filter for all fluors. We would also recommend the use of a dual-bandpass Spectrum Orange/Spectrum Green filter

for the HER2 test. For other fluors, appropriate filters will need to be purchased. For many applications a ×40 or ×63 objective is sufficient; however, when scoring FISH, we prefer to use a ×100 objective.

5. The denaturing solution contains formamide, which is toxic and should be handled within a fume cabinet.
6. The use of temporary "coverslips" in conjunction with a humidified hybridization chamber, such as that present on the Omnislide, provides a convenient alternative to glass coverslips. Temporary "coverslips" are made by cutting Parafilm to the appropriate size. Following addition of the denaturation solution, the Parafilm is used to cover the slide during the 5-min denaturation period.
7. Routlinely, we use rubber cement supplied for cycle puncture repair, as it is provided in easy-to-use tubes.
8. Unlike some immunohistochemistry procedures, we have not observed any deterioration of slides when stored for prolonged periods (6–24 mo) prior to FISH analysis. However, we recommend the use of slides within a period of 6 mo of cutting.
9. Xylene should be used with care and within a fume hood. The solution should be changes periodically to avoid wax buildup in the wash bath. The use of nonorganic solutions such as Hemo-de (ref source), when available, may provide a useful alternative to xylene.
10. The 0.2*N* HCl is thought to act by acid deproteination of tissue, thus increasing probe penetration possibly resulting from a partial reversion of the fixation process. The use of a pretreatment permeabilization step reduces the requirement for prolonged incubation in proteases and allows preservation of better tissue morphology.
11. Sodium thiocyanate acts as a reducing agents to break the protein–protein disulfide bonds formed by formalin and facilitate subsequent proteolytic digestion.
12. Fluid can be removed by gently touching the slide edgewise onto a pad of absorbant tissues.
13. The duration of exposure of the slides to protease is perhaps the most critical step in ensuring adequate pretreatment of formalin-fixed tissues prior to application of DNA probes for FISH. The extent of treatment required varies according to the tissue and, to a far lesser extent, to the degree of fixation. We recommend that digestion times be evaluated in each laboratory to optimize results. In our laboratory and in many others, the optimal protease digestion time for breast cancer specimens is between 22 and 28 min. This is significantly longer than that described within the Pathvysion protocol. In our experience, one of the main reasons for the failure of a laboratory to establish FISH is overrigid adherence to an inadequate digestion period. Therefore, the importance of ensuring adequate digestion cannot be underestimated. When performing FISH for the first time, we recommend performing a digestion series on representative samples using the digestion assessment protocol described in **steps 15–23**. Selected slides, with optimal morphology, can then be identified for hybridization with probes. The duration of exposure of tissue sections to pepsin required for adequate digestion

will vary from tissue type to tissue type and also, to a far lesser degree, within tissues. In our experience, tissues such as breast require digestion times between 18 and 22 min, whereas tissues from bladder cancers require digestion times of 25–30 min. The concentration and activity of pepsin will also affect the duration of this step (*see* **Note 3**); therefore, digestion times should be reassessed each time the pepsin batch is changed.

14. When assessing the nuclei for extent of digestion, the staining intensity resulting from the intercalation of DAPI with DNA in the nucleus is a good indicator. Nuclei that stain gray to gray/blue are underdigested and, once the coverslip is removed, can be reintroduced to a fresh batch of pepsin/HCl for up to 15 min. Nuclei that stain blue with clearly visible nuclear borders are suitably digested. When nuclear borders are lost, these sections are overdigested and are discarded. The digestion is repeated with different sections for 30 min. It is important to examine areas from different parts of the slide when dealing with thin sections that have been formalin fixed and paraffin processed, as there will inevitably be variations in the fixation effects and, therefore, in the effect of pepsin digestion. If the digestion of at least two-thirds of the *tumor* is acceptable, then these slides will be suitable for hybridizing.
15. The VP2000 should be switched on before to computer to allow the computer to recognize the VP2000.
16. Pretreatment solution contains 8% (w/v) sodium thiocyanate; during each run at 80°C, some water is lost from this solution, and this is replaced by topping up the solution with distilled water. We recommend replacing the solution either every 2 wk or after between 5 and 10 runs.
17. Use protease buffer from the same batch number. The pH of the protease buffer should be checked before use and adjusted if required with 0.1*M* HCl to pH 2.0 ± 0.1. We recommend replacing the solution either every 2 wk or after between 5 and 10 runs.
18. Digestion times on the VP2000 tend to be slightly shorter than those for manual pretreatment, possibly because of greater circulation of buffer within the digestion chamber. However, similar principles apply and a digestion series (*see* **Note 13**) should be produced prior to commencing FISH routinely. We have found sections digested using the automatic protocol to be more reproducibly digested and have a greater success rate, with less requirement for redigestion than those treated manually.
19. A minimum hybridization time of 12–14 h is recommended.
20. Addition of slides to the posthybridization wash will lower the temperature. A maximum of five to six slides per Coplin jar should be added, because the addition of more slides may compromise the stringency of the posthybridization wash. If large batches of slides are to be washed simultaneously, either prepare multiple Coplin jars or use staining dishes.
21. Simply placing the slides in a cupboard will suffice, although use of light-shielded boxes is a useful alternative.
22. Clear nail polish is a useful sealant and can be used to prevent slides from drying out.

23. With experience, it is possible to identify areas for scoring, in most cases, without detailed reference to an adjacent hematoxylin and eosin (H&E) stained slide. However, because of the high rate of amplification observed in ductal carcinoma *in situ* (DCIS), which is currently not clinically relevant in regard to HER2-based therapies, confirmation of the tumor morphology by examination of an H&E-stained section by a trained histopathologist should be regarded as central to the diagnosis of HER2 amplification. For samples where dual scoring is to be performed, note the coordinates either on a New England Finder or using the Vernier scales on the microscope stage.
24. It is essential that only cells with clear nuclear boundaries are scored. Only nuclei with signals for both chromosome 17 and HER2 signals should be included. Our recent data ***(28)*** shows a high rate of aneusomy for chromosome 17 in breast cancer (>55% cases); therefore, the chromosome 17 copy number should be scored in each case.
25. In a small number of cases (1–2%) ***(28)***, heterogeneity of amplification may be observed, scoring cells from three separate areas of the tumor markedly increases the likelihood that such heterogeneity will be correctly observed. In cases where only one or two areas are amplified, we recommend scoring additional cells from these areas and reporting the maximum HER2:chromosome 17 ratio with a note to the effect that the tumor was heterogeneous for HER2 amplification.
26. There are a number of principles embodied in the scoring of FISH signals in tissue sections, many of which are detailed within the Pathvysion protocol document. Dual-observer scoring is a valuable means of ensuring that accurate results are obtained, particularly when new observers are being trained in the interpretation of FISH signals. In our extensive experience, interobserver variation for absolute counts of signals can be routinely controlled below 10% ***(28,30)***. Periodic review of scoring by selective sampling of diagnostic results can be a valuable means of ensuring continued quality control.

References

1. Slamon, D. J., Clark, G. M., and Wong, S. G. (1987) Human breast cancer: correlation of relapse and survival with amplification of the HER-2/neu oncogene. *Science* **235,** 217–227.
2. Coombs, L. M., Pigott, D. A., Sweeney, E., et al. (1991) Amplification and overexpression of c-erbB-2 in transitional cell carcinoma of the urinary bladder. *Br. J. Cancer* **63,** 601–608.
3. Reles, A., Marx, D., Meden, H., et al. (1991) C-erb-b2 oncogene expression in ovarian cancers. *Arch. Gynecol. Obstet.* **250,** 183–184.
4. Tyson, F. L., Boyer, C. M., Kaufman, R., et al. (1991) Expression and amplification of the her-2/neu (c-erb-2) protooncogene in epithelial ovarian-tumors and cell-lines. *Am. J. Obstet. Gynecol.* **165,** 640–646.
5. Albino, A. P., Jaehne, J., Altorki, N., et al. (1995) Amplification of HER-2/neu gene in human gastric adenocarcinomas. *Eur. J. Surg. Oncol.* **21,** 56–60.
6. Underwood, M. A., Bartlett, J., Reeves, J., et al. (1994) C-erbB2 gene amplification as a molecular marker in bladder-cancer. *Cancer Res.* **81,** 1822–1822.

7. Slamon, D. J., Godolphin, W., Jones, L. A., et al. (1989) Studies of the HER-2/neu proto-oncogene in human breast and ovarian cancer. *Science* **244,** 707–712.
8. Revillion, F., Bonneterre, J., and Peyrat, J. P. (1998) ERBB2 oncogene in human breast cancer and its clinical significance. *Eur. J. Cancer* **34,** 808.
9. Ross, J. S. and Fletcher, J. A. (1998) The HER-2/neu oncogene in breast cancer: prognostic factor, predictive factor, and target for therapy. *Stem Cells* **16,** 413–428.
10. Andrulis, I. L., Bull, S. B., Blackstein, M. E., et al. (1998) neu/erbB-2 amplification identifies a poor-prognosis group of women with node-negative breast cancer. Toronto Breast Cancer Study Group. *J. Clin. Oncol.* **16,** 1340–1349.
11. Dalifard, I., Daver, A., Goussard, J., et al. (1998) p185 overexpression in 220 samples of breast cancer undergoing primary surgery: comparison with c-erbB-2 gene amplification. *Bioorg. Med. Chem. Lett.* **1,** 855–861.
12. Press, M. F., Bernstein, L., Thomas, P. A., et al. (1997) HER-2/neu gene amplification characterized by fluorescence *in situ* hybridization: poor prognosis in node-negative breast carcinomas. *J. Clin. Oncol.* **15,** 2894–2904.
13. Piffanelli, A., Dittadi, R., Catozzi, L., et al. (1996) Determination of ErbB2 protein in breast cancer tissues by different methods. Relationships with other biological parameters. *Breast Cancer Res. Treat.* **37,** 267–276.
14. Press, M. F. (1990) Oncogene amplification and expression. Importance of methodologic considerations. *Am. J. Clin. Pathol.* **94,** 240–241.
15. Press, M. F., Hung, G., Godolphin, W., et al. 1994. Sensitivity of HER-2/neu antibodies in archival tissue samples: potential source of error in immunohistochemical studies of oncogene expression. *Cancer Res.* **54,** 2771–2777.
16. Goldenberg, M. M. (1999) Trastuzumab, a recombinant DNA-derived humanized monoclonal antibody, a novel agent for the treatment of metastatic breast cancer. *Clin. Ther.* **21,** 309–318.
17. Bartlett, J. M. S., Mallon, E. A., and Cooke, T. G. (2003) The clinical evaluation of HER2 status, which test to use? *J. Pathol.* **199,** 411–417.
18. Giai, M., Roagna, R., Ponzone, R., et al. (1994) Prognostic and predictive relevance of c-erbB-2 and ras expression in node positive and negative breast cancer. *Anticancer Res.* **14,** 1441–1450.
19. Rosen, P. P., Lesser, M. L., Arroyo, C. D., et al. (1995) Immunohistochemical detection of HER2/neu in patients with axillary lymph node negative breast carcinoma. A study of epidemiologic risk factors, histologic features, and prognosis. *Cancer* **75,** 1320–1326.
20. Carlomagno, C., Perrone, F., Gallo, C., et al. (1996) c-erbB2 overexpression decreases the benefit of adjuvant tamoxifen in early-stage breast cancer without axillary lymph node metastases. *J. Clin. Oncol.* **14,** 2702–2708.
21. Muss, H., Berry, D., and Thor, A. (1999) Lack of interaction of tamoxifen (T) use and ErbB-2/Her-2/Neu (H) expression in CALGB 8541: a randomized adjuvant trial of three different doses of cyclophosphamide, dooxrubicin and fluorouracil (CAF) in node positive primary breast cancer (BC). *Proc. Am. Soc. Clin. Oncol.* **18,** 68A (abstract).

22. Paik, S., Bryant, J., Park, C., et al. (1998) erbB-2 and response to doxorubicin in patients with axillary lymph node-positive, hormone receptor-negative breast cancer. *J. Natl. Cancer Inst.* **90,** 1361–1370.
23. Ravdin, P. M., Green, S., Albain, V., et al. (1998) Initial report of the SWOG biological correlative study of c-erbB-2 expression as a predictor of outcome in a trial comparing adjuvant CAF T with tamoxifen (T) alone. *Proc. Am. Soc. Clin. Oncol.* **17,** 97A (abstract).
24. Thor, A. D., Berry, D. A., Budman, D., et al. (1998) erbB-2, p53, and efficacy of adjuvant therapy in lymph node-positive breast cancer. *J. Natl. Cancer Inst.* **90,** 1346–1360.
25. Arber, D. A. (2000) Molecular diagnostic approach to non-Hodgkin's lymphoma. *J. Mol. Diagn.* **2,** 178–190.
26. Mitchell, M. S. and Press, M. F. (1999) The role of immunohistochemistry and fluorescence in situ hybridization for HER-2/neu in assessing the prognosis of breast cancer. *Semin. Oncol.* **26,** 108–116.
27. Pauletti, G., Godolphin, W., Press, M. F., et al. (1996) Detection and quantitation of HER-2/*neu* gene amplification in human breast cancer archival material using fluorescence *in situ* hybridization. *Oncogene* **13,** 63–72.
28. Bartlett, J. M. S., Reeves, J., Stanton, P., et al. (2001) Evaluating HER2 amplification and overexpression in breast cancer. *J. Pathol.* **195,** 422–428.
29. Ellis, I. O., Dowsett, M., Bartlett, J., et al. (2000) Recommendations for HER2 testing in the UK. *J. Clin. Pathol.* **53(12),** 890–892.
30. Edwards, J., Krishna, N. S., Mukherjee, R., et al. (2001) Amplification of the androgen receptor may not explain the development of androgen-independent prostate cancer. *BJU Int.* **88,** 633–637.

8

Fluorescence *In Situ* Hybridization for BCR-ABL

Mark W. Drummond, Elaine K. Allan, Andrew Pearce, and Tessa L. Holyoake

1. Introduction

The *BCR-ABL* fusion gene arises as a result of a reciprocal translocation between chromosomes 9 and 22, resulting in the so-called Philadelphia (Ph) chromosome (a minute chromosome 22), which is found in 95% of cases of chronic myeloid leukemia (CML) *(1)*. A variable sequence length of the *BCR* gene at 22q11 fuses with *ABL* at 9q34 and encodes the constitutively active BCR-ABL protein tyrosine kinase (reviewed in **refs.** ***2*** and ***3***). Data from animal models have demonstrated that this protein is capable of inducing a CML-like disease in mice, indicating its central importance in the pathogenesis of CML as well as other leukemias (viz. 20% of adult acute lymphoblastic leukemia and the rare chronic neutrophilic leukemia). Detection of the *BCR-ABL* translocation is, therefore, important from both clinical and research perspectives. *BCR-ABL* positive cells do not have a reliable immunophenotypic marker to distinguish them from their normal counterparts; therefore, proof of their clonal origin requires either reverse transcriptase-polymerase chain reaction (RT-PCR), conventional G-banding of metaphase (MP) spreads, or direct visualization of the *BCR-ABL* translocation by fluorescence *in situ* hybridization (FISH). The advantages of FISH over G-banding include applicability to interphase (IP) cells, greater sensitivity (as many more cells can be analyzed), and ability to detect masked translocations. This has led to its use in the clinical setting for monitoring response to therapy, by quantifying the size of the *BCR-ABL* clone on either bone marrow (BM) or peripheral blood (PB) specimens. Equally, it may be applied to research specimens such as individual colonies or selected cell populations to confirm a clonal origin. The initial FISH protocols utilized 5' *BCR* and 3' *ABL* probes, differentially labeled with fluoro-

From: *Methods in Molecular Medicine, vol. 79: Molecular Diagnosis of Cancer*
Edited by: J. E. Roulston and J. M. S. Bartlett © Humana Press Inc., Totowa, NJ

chromes, to generate a single fused signal at the site of the *BCR-ABL* translocation (S-FISH) ***(4,5)***. However, in IP cells, a high false-positive rate can result from random colocalization of the signals, mimicking a fusion signal (reviewed in **ref. *6***). If such problems are taken into account (e.g., by establishing a false-positive threshold on a *BCR-ABL* negative population of similar cells), IP FISH can still provide reliable data in samples where the majority of cells are *BCR-ABL* positive. Using such probes on MP preparations reduces false-positive signals, although this may not be applicable to all samples. Recently, the use of improved probes has reduced these problems significantly. Inclusion of an "extra signal" (ES) in the form of a 5' ABL probe allows simultaneous detection of the derivative chromosome 9 and greatly lowers the likelihood of false-positive signals ***(7)***. Another strategy incorporates extra 5' *ABL* and 3' *BCR* probes, thereby generating fusion signals for both the *BCR-ABL* and *ABL-BCR* translocations, so-called dual fusion (D-FISH) ***(8)***. Such probes also allow detection of the recently described deletions on the derivative chromosome 9, adjacent to the t(9;22) breakpoint ***(9)***. These appear to be of considerable clinical importance: Their occurrence in CML patients at diagnosis (some 15% of patients) appears to be associated with a significantly poorer prognosis ***(10)***. Reliable detection of such deletions is likely to become a prerequisite when considering treatment options at the outset of the disease.

Protocols are presented here for the application of FISH to both research and clinical samples. Preparation of BM, PB, sorted cell populations, and long-term culture initiating cell (LTCIC) colonies for FISH will be discussed prior to a brief summary of the relative merits of the commercially available probes and an outline of a generic FISH protocol. It is clearly impractical to consider all available probes individually, and the manufacturers instructions should be consulted.

2. Materials

All glassware must be cleaned with 0.5% (v/v) Decon and thoroughly rinsed before use. Plasticware and solutions should be sterile.

2.1. Sample Collection

1. Heparin saline, sterile (10,000 units/L).
2. Lithium–heparin blood collection tubes.

2.2. White Cell Count and Sample Preparation

1. Leighton tubes (Nunc).
2. Serological pipets (10 mL).
3. Tissue culture medium: RPMI 1640 (Sigma) with HEPES, supplemented with 20% fetal calf serum (FCS).

2.3. Harvest of BM/PB Cultures

1. Colcemid (KaryoMax; Gibco, 10 μg/μL [w/v] in Hanks' balanced salt solution).
2. Absolute methanol: Glacial acetic acid fixative (3:1, v/v).

2.4. Slide Preparation

1. 0.5% (v/v) Decon 90 solution in distilled water.
2. 70% Ethanol.
3. Frosted microscope slides.
4. 10- or 12-Well Multispot microscope slides (Hendley Ltd., Essex).
5. Poly-L-lysine solution (PLL), 0.1% (w/v) (Sigma-Aldrich, Dorset).
6. Plastic Coplin jars.

2.5. Preparation of IP/MP Nuclei

1. 10X NH_4Cl, 8.3% (w/v).
2. Phosphate-buffered saline (PBS): 0.01*M* phosphate buffer, 0.0027*M* KCl, 0.137*M* NaCl, pH 7.4).
3. 10X Hypotonic solution: 0.75 *M* KCl.
4. Fixative: Methanol:acetic acid 3:1 (must be prepared fresh prior to use).
5. Diamond pencil.
6. Inverted light microscope.
7. Phase-contrast microscope.
8. Glass or plastic Coplin jars (50 mL).

2.6. Generic FISH Procedure

1. 20X Sodium chloride-sodium citrate buffer (SSC) (pH 7.0). Adjust prior to use if necessary with NaOH or HCl) (Sigma).
2. Denaturation solution: 70% Formamide (Sigma) in 2X SSC (*see* **Notes 1** and **2**).
3. 2X SSC, pH 7.0.
4. 0.5X SSC, pH 7.0, for posthybridization wash.
5. Glass Coplin jars (*see* **Note 3**).
6. Microcentrifuge tubes (0.2 or 1.5 mL).
7. NP40 or Tween (Sigma).
8. Ethanol: 70%, 80%, 95%.
9. Glass coverslips (22 × 22, 22 × 50, 26 × 25, or 18 × 18 mm).
10. 4' 6'-diamidino-2-phenylindole (DAPI) (final concentration 0.05–0.1 μg/mL in Antifade or Vectashield [Vector Laboratories Inc., USA]).
11. Rubber cement or cowgum for sealing cover slips.
12. Humidified chamber.
13. 37°C Incubator.
14. Pipets and tips.
15. Water baths at 37°C and 72°C (72°C in fume hood).
16. Commercial probe kit with hybridization buffer (e.g., Vysis LSI *BCR-ABL* Dual Colour Translocation probe; *see* **Note 4** and **Subheading 3.9.**).

17. Epifluorescence microscope (100-W mercury lamp and appropriate filters) with low (×10) and high (×100 oil immersion) objectives.
18. Immersion oil.

3. Methods

3.1. PB and BM Sample Collection

3.1.1. BM

Add 2–5 mL of BM to 15 mL of sterile saline heparin (10,000 U/mL) in a universal container (*see* **Note 5**).

3.1.2. PB

Collect 10 mL of PB into lithium–heparin tube.

3.2. BM (or PB) Preparation and Culture (for MP FISH)

1. A 0.5-mL aliquot of BM/PB is removed with a sterile pipet into a Bijou tube to determine the cell count using either a Coulter analyzer or hemocytometer.
2. Centrifuge the BM/PB at 200*g* for 8 min at room temperature (RT).
3. Remove the plasma with a sterile pipet ensuring that the buffy coat remains intact.
4. Using a 10-mL sterile graduated pipet, add tissue culture medium (RPMI supplemented with 20% FCS) to the remaining cells (buffy coat and red cells) to give a final concentration of 1×10^7 cells/mL (based on the total white cell count).
5. Using a sterile 10-mL graduated pipet, add 4.5 mL of tissue culture medium to a labeled culture tube.
6. Using a sterile graduated pipet, add 0.5 mL of the diluted BM to the culture tube and mix gently by rinsing the pipet with the culture medium (this results in a final concentration of 1×10^6 cells/mL in the culture tube).
7. Place the culture tube in an incubator at 37°C and incubate for 24 h.

3.3. Harvest and Fixation of Cultured BM/PB Cells (for MP FISH)

1. After 24 h incubation at 37°C, add 50 μL of Colcemid to the culture tube.
2. Return the culture to the incubator at 37°C for 1 h.
3. When the incubation is complete, centrifuge the cultures at 200*g* for 8 min. Aspirate the supernatant with a sterile pipet without disturbing the pellet of cells.
4. Gently mix the pellet on a Whirlimix and add 3 mL of hypotonic KCl with a disposable pipet. Mix again.
5. Replace the culture tubes in the incubator at 37°C for 10 min.
6. At the end of this time, centrifuge the tubes at 200*g* for 8 min.
7. Aspirate the supernatant as before using a sterile pipet.
8. Gently mix the pellet using a vortex mixer (to prevent cell clumping), and using a pipet, slowly add 1 mL of methanol:acetic acid.
9. Add a further 2 mL of fixative while mixing on the Whirlimix.
10. Centrifuge at 200*g* for 8 min.

11. Aspirate the supernatant, and using a vortex mixer, resuspend the cells, adding 3 mL of fixative.
12. Repeat **steps 11** and **12** twice, reducing the volume of fixative by 1 mL each time (i.e., 2 mL) and, finally, 1 mL.
13. Store at –20°C until required.

3.4. Fixing PB Mononuclear Cells From Whole Blood for IP FISH

(Prior culture not required.)

1. Prepare 1:10 dilution of 10X NH_4Cl solution with sterile distilled water.
2. Add 1 mL whole blood to 10 mL of 1X NH_4Cl in a sterile 15-mL conical tube to lyse red cells. Incubate at 37°C for 10 min. Invert tube gently during incubation.
3. Centrifuge to pellet cells at 450*g* for 5 min at RT.
4. Decant supernatant.
5. Resuspend cells with PBS to wash.
6. Repeat centrifugation.
7. Resuspend cell pellet with 1 mL PBS and count cells using a hemocytometer.
8. Centrifuge to pellet cells and discard supernatant.
9. Add 10 mL prewarmed (at 37°C) hypotonic solution.
10. Invert gently to mix cells.
11. Incubate at RT for 10–20 min.
12. Add 2 mL freshly prepared fixative and incubate at RT for 5 min.
13. Centrifuge at 450*g* for 5 min.
14. Discard supernatant and resuspend pellet in 10 mL fixative.
15. Leave at RT for 5 min.
16. Centrifuge at 450*g* for 5 min.
17. Repeat **steps 14–17** at least twice.
18. Resuspend cells with fixative to a density of approx 1×10^6 cells/mL and store at –20°C until required.

3.5. Preparation of Slides

Multispot slides, containing 10 or 12 individual wells, are routinely used for fixing samples of low cell numbers because cells are restricted to a considerably smaller surface area than on standard microscope slides to produce a suitable density for FISH. This also permits a more economical use of probes, as lower volumes are used per sample. Also, positive and negative control samples can be analyzed on the same slide as test cells. *Standard microscope slides are also washed and stored in this way.* The latter are used for examination of PB and BM preparations as described. For certain cell types at low numbers (e.g., $CD34^+$ selected cells), slide adhesion should be facilitated by precoating slides with PLL as detailed below. *See* **Subheading 3.7.** for fixing and slide preparation of FACS sorted cells and colonies.

1. Prewash slides by soaking in 0.5% Decon 90 for 1 h.
2. Wash slides for 1–2 h with running tap water with occasional agitation.
3. Dry excess liquid from slides on paper towel.
4. Store slides in 70% ethanol until required.

3.5.1. PLL Coating of Slides

1. Remove slides from 70% ethanol and rinse with cold tap water and dry.
2. Prepare 1:10 dilution of PLL solution, 0.1% (w/v), in sterile distilled water.
3. Coat several slides by placing in 0.01% PLL in a plastic Coplin jar for 5–10 min at RT.
4. Air-dry slides for 1–2 h or overnight.
5. Precoated PLL slides may be stored at RT until required.
6. Proceed to fix cells on slide.

3.6. Preparation of IP/MP Cells From Fixed-Cell Preparations

1. Remove fixed cell pellet from –20°C storage and allow to reach RT.
2. Centrifuge to pellet cells at 200*g* for 5 min.
3. Aspirate supernatant and gently resuspend cell pellet with fresh fixative solution using a Pasteur pipet to required cell density. The volume of the fixative should be sufficiently low so as to confer a slightly milky appearance to the cell suspension.
4. Remove slides from storage in ethanol and thoroughly rinse with slightly cool running tap water.
5. Drain excess water from the microscope slide, leaving a thin film of water.
6. Quickly draw several drops of cell suspension into a Pasteur pipet.
7. Holding the slide upright (frosted end up), rotate the slide slightly away from you. Touch the tip of the pipet to the edge nearest to you, just below the frosted area. Slowly dispense some of the cells away from you, across the slide while turning the slide toward you to allow even distribution of the cells the length and width of the slide.
8. Dry the slide at RT by resting it vertically at a 45° angle.
9. Examine slides for quality and distribution of IP nuclei using phase-contrast microscopy and circle the desired area for FISH analysis using a diamond pencil. Cells should be free from cytoplasm and not in contact with each other (*see* **Note 6**).

3.7. Fixing and Slide Preparation of FACS Sorted Cells for FISH

1. Transfer approx 5000 cells in PBS to a 0.2-mL polymerase chain reaction (PCR) tube and centrifuge at 700*g* for 5 min in a microcentrifuge.
2. Carefully remove the supernatant without disturbing the cell pellet.
3. Resuspend in 50 μL prewarmed (37°C) hypotonic solution.
4. Divide aliquots between duplicate wells of a previously PLL-coated Multispot microscope slide.

5. Incubate for 20 min at RT before removing excess hypotonic solution carefully with a pipet.
6. Check microscopically to ensure that sufficient cells are present in well for FISH (>1000; *see* **Note 7**).
7. Add 20 μL freshly prepared fixative to each well.
8. Incubate at RT for 5 min.
9. Remove excess fixative carefully before the addition of 30 μL fixative for 5–10 min.
10. Repeat **step 9**.
11. Transfer slide to a plastic Coplin jar containing fixative for a further minimum of 5 min (may be left overnight in fixative if desired).
12. Air-dry for several hours or overnight as suitable.
13. Proceed with FISH or wrap in parafilm and store frozen at –20°C until required.

3.8. Fixing and Slide Preparation of LTCIC and CFC Colonies for IP FISH

The LTCIC colonies from CML patients can be plucked directly from methylcellulose medium and fixed on Multispot slides for determination of *BCR-ABL* status by FISH. A number of colonies may be fixed on the one slide along with prefixed positive and negative control cells. Alternatively, if colonies are particularily small, they may be pooled prior to fixing. These steps will remove some of the methylcellulose that can cause problems with subsequent FISH.

3.8.1. Small Colonies

1. Add 25 μL prewarmed (at 37°C) hypotonic solution to one well of a PLL-coated Multispot slide.
2. Locate colonies for plucking using an inverted light microscope. Aspirate individual colonies with a minimum volume of methylcellulose (1–2 μL) using a 20-μL pipet tip.
3. Carefully add plucked colony into 25 μL prewarmed hypotonic solution on slide, taking care to wash all cells out of the pipet tip.
4. Incubate cells on slide for 20 min at RT.
5. Repeat as for sorted cells from **step 5** of **Subheading 3.7**.

3.8.2. Large Colonies

1. Aspirate into 100 μL PBS in a 0.2-mL PCR tube.
2. Wash by centrifugation at 700*g* for 5 min.
3. Resuspend in 25 μL hypotonic solution.
4. Add to Multispot slide.

3.9. FISH Probes

Probes for detection of the *BCR-ABL* fusion gene by FISH are commercially available for several companies and may be used on BM cells, PB cells, and cell lines, either using MP spreads or on IP nuclei. These probes detect fusion genes arising from both major and minor breakpoints regions on chromosome 22.

3.9.1. Choice of Probe

S-FISH probes will detect the *BCR-ABL* fusion signal on the derivative chromosome 22 only. However, because of the random spatial association of probe signals in normal nuclei, these often result in a high incidence of false-positive results ***(6)***. Therefore, these probes are most suitable for analysis of samples with a high percentage of cells possessing this translocation.

ES-FISH probes are a mixture of a *BCR* probe and an *ABL* probe that also spans the *ASS* gene (centromeric of *ABL* on chromosome 9) ***(7)***. In a cell with the t(9:22) translocation, one fusion signal (yellow) is detected plus one normal *BCR* (green) and one *ABL* (red), but, in addition, a further red signal from the derivative chromosome 9 is produced. This will reduce the incidence of false-positive results.

More recently, *D-FISH* probes have become available. These detect the reciprocal translocation *ABL-BCR* on chromosome 9, in addition to the translocation on chromosome 22. Therefore, in a cell possessing the t(9:22) translocation, two yellow fusion signals (or red/green colocalization signals) will be produced in addition to the normal *BCR* and *ABL* single signals, green and red, respectively (depending on probe manufacturer). Consequently, these probes produce a lower incidence of false-positive results and are, therefore, more suitable for analysis of samples with a low percentage of t(9:22) cells, such as for clinical monitoring of therapy or minimal residual disease. These probes will also detect deletions of the derivative 9 chromosome in some CML patient samples, which have been associated with a poor prognosis *(10)*.

3.9.2. Generic FISH Procedure

All FISH procedures using commercial probes should be carried out according to the manufacturer's instructions for optimum results, as these may differ slightly from the methodology detailed below.

1. Remove slides from storage at –20°C and allow to equilibrate to RT.
2. Incubate slides in a glass Coplin jar containing 2X SSC/0.5% NP40 (Igepal, Sigma), pH 7.0 (prewarmed to 37°C), for 30 min (*see* **Note 8**).
3. Remove the slides from the 2X SSC and dehydrate in 70%, 80%, and 95% ethanol for 2 min each at RT.

4. Allow slides to air-dry.
5. Denature slides by immersion in 70% formamide/2X SSC, pH 7.0, at 72 ± 2°C for 2 min. (The pH of the denaturation solution must be 7.0 for optimum results. Verify the temperature is 72°C by placing a clean thermometer directly into the Coplin jar).
6. Repeat **steps 3** and **4** using ice-cold ethanol to stop denaturation rapidly while dehydrating the slides. Leave them in 95% ethanol until required for the next stage.
7. Prewarm vial containing probe at 37°C for 5 min.
8. Aliquot required volume of probe into a foil-covered 0.2 mL microcentrifuge tube (approx 2.5 μL per well of Multispot slide). For standard slides, an 8- to 10-μL probe will be required per sample with a 22 × 22-mm cover slip (smaller cover slips are available that will reduce the volume of probe required).
9. Denature probe by heating at 72 ± 2°C for 5 min.
10. Centrifuge for 2–3 s to collect contents in the bottom of the tube.
11. Incubate probe at 37°C until ready to add to slide.
12. While the probe is denaturing for the final 2 min, remove the slides from the 95% ethanol and transfer to a 45°C hot plate to dry (optional).
13. Apply probe to target area on slide and immediately apply coverslip. For Multispot slides, the size of coverslip used will depend on the number of wells tested. Several wells of a Multispot slide can be covered with a 22 × 50-mm coverslip. It is important to ensure that no air bubbles are trapped under the coverslip, as this will prevent contact of probe with test cells.
14. Seal coverslip with rubber cement.
15. Place slide(s) in a prewarmed humidified box in a 37°C incubator for 16 h.

3.9.3. Washing the Slides

1. Prepare 50 mL of 0.5X SSC from stock 20X SSC. Pour into a glass Coplin jar and heat in a water bath to 72 ± 2°C. Allow at least 30 min to achieve temperature.
2. Pour 50 mL of 2X SSC into another foil-covered Coplin jar at RT.
3. Remove cover slip from slide carefully by peeling back rubber cement sealant using forceps. Gently tap side of slide to dislodge coverslip and carefully remove using forceps. Carefully wipe any excess cement from underside of slide using a piece of tissue.
4. Place slide(s) in 2X SSC for 2 min to rinse prior to posthybridization wash.
5. Remove and quickly place in Coplin jar containing 0.5X SSC at 72 ± 2°C for 5 min without agitation.
6. Transfer slides to Coplin jar containing 2X SSC/0.1% NP40 for 10 min. Again, to minimize light exposure, the Coplin jar can be covered with foil.

3.9.4. Counterstaining of Slides

1. Prepare 0.05 μg/mL DAPI/Antifade (AF) or Vectashield.
2. Add 10 μL DAPI/AF to standard slides and approx 3–5 μL DAPI/AF per well of a Multispot slide.
3. Cover with a 22 × 50-mm glass cover slip and carefully remove any excess counterstain with a paper towel.
4. Store in the dark until ready to evaluate microscopically with an epifluorescence microscope (*see* **Note 9**).

3.10. Analysis of D-FISH Preparations

Slides may be stored for 2–3 wk at 4°C in the dark without total loss of fluorescence signal, although it is better to examine slides as soon as possible after completion of the FISH procedure

Commercial probes such as the Vysis LSI *BCR-ABL* Dual Colour Translocation probe are directly labeled with red and green fluorochromes. Therefore, for optimal visualization of the preparations, an epifluorescence microscope with a 100-W mercury lamp is required, together with one of the following filter arrangements:

- Appropriate single-bandpass filters (including DAPI for the counterstain).
- Appropriate dual-bandpass filter + DAPI filter.
- Appropriate triple-bandpass filter.

1. Initially, the preparation is examined under low magnification (×10 objective). Open the diaphragm from the fluorescence source (if single-bandpass filters or a dual-bandpass filter +DAPI are being used switch to DAPI).
2. Locate the edge of the target area and center the field of view on an appropriate IP/MP cell (i.e., free from surrounding cytoplasm and not in contact with neighboring cells).
3. Place a drop of immersion oil onto the cover slip and switch to the high-magnification (×100) objective.
4. Refocus the microscope on the chosen cell and change to the triple- or dual-bandpass filter. If using single-bandpass filters, select either the red or green.
5. Score the observed signal pattern. If using single-bandpass filters, select the second color (i.e., change from red to green or vice versa) and score the signal pattern.
6. Having scored the first cell, the slide should be examined in an orderly manner. If using single/dual-bandpass + DAPI filters, return to the DAPI filter, keep the high-magnification (×100) objective in place, and scan the slide in overlapping rows so that the entire target area can be covered. Vertical scanning is conventionally preferred (*see* **Fig. 1**).
7. As cells are encountered during the scanning process, assess the suitability for scoring. Try to avoid cells that are in contact with others or surrounded by debris/cytoplasm. If suitable, score the cell.

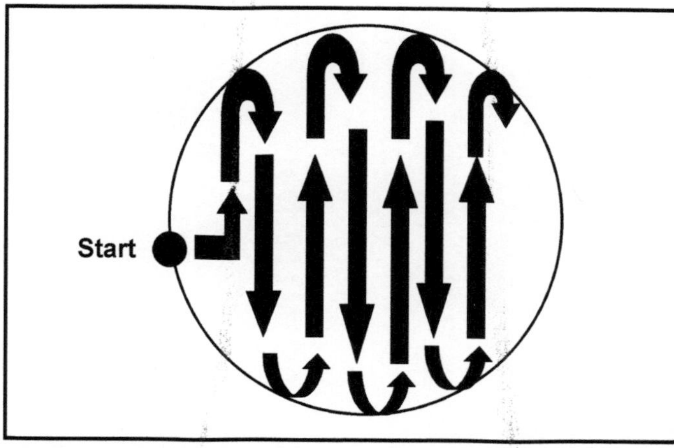

Fig.1. Diagram illustrating the suggested method of slide examination. Rapid horizontal scanning is liable to induce seasickness!

8. Continue with this process until the requisite number of cells have been scored. At first referral and for any subsequent samples, scoring a total of 100 cells is considered to be sufficient to avoid erroneous results through random colocalized signals (*see* **Subheading 3.10.1.**).

3.10.1. Hybridization Patterns

1. The Vysis LSI BCR-ABL Dual Colour Translocation probe displays two red and two green signals where no BCR/ABL rearrangement has occurred (*see* **Fig 2**).
2. The Vysis LSI BCR-ABL Dual Colour Translocation probe displays two fusion signals in addition to single red and green signals for a standard BCR-ABL rearrangement. This largely avoids potential interpretation problems resulting from the random juxtapositioning of red and green signals producing colocalized signals. Fusion signals resulting from a standard BCR-ABL rearrangement will appear as a red and green signal in very close proximity or may be perceived as yellow (*see* **Fig. 3;** *also see* **Note 10**).
3. When single-bandpass filters are used, no fusion signals will be seen; rather, both red and green signals will be observed to occupy the same space when the filters are switched from red to green (and vice versa).

4. Notes

1. Formamide is a mutagen. Always wear gloves when handling substances containing formamide and use in a fume cupboard.
2. Denaturation solution should be prepared fresh prior to use and ensure that pH is 7.0.
3. Glass Coplin jars are preferred for incubation temperatures of over 70°C. Plastic

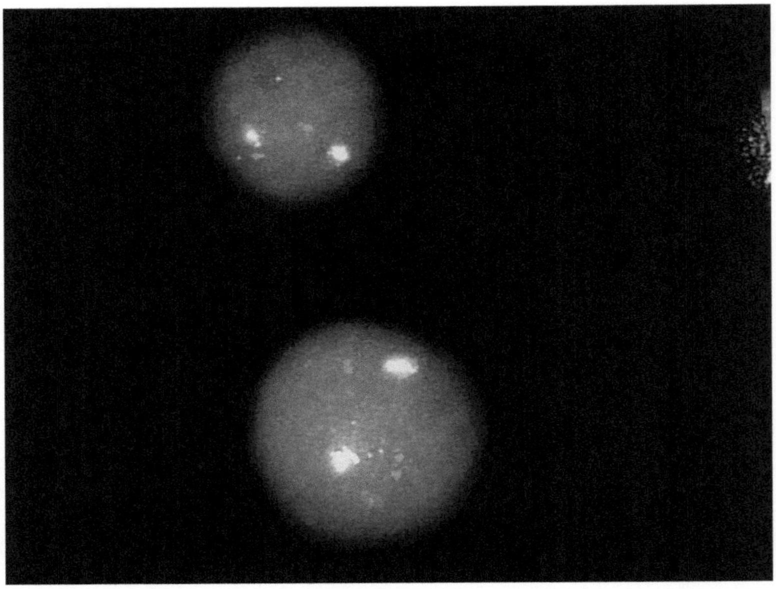

Fig. 2. MP and IP cells from a BM specimen hybridized with the Vysis LSI BCR-ABL Dual Colour Translocation probe. Green signal is the BCR locus on chromosome 22 and red signal is the ABL locus on chromosome 9. No BCR-ABL rearrangement has occurred.

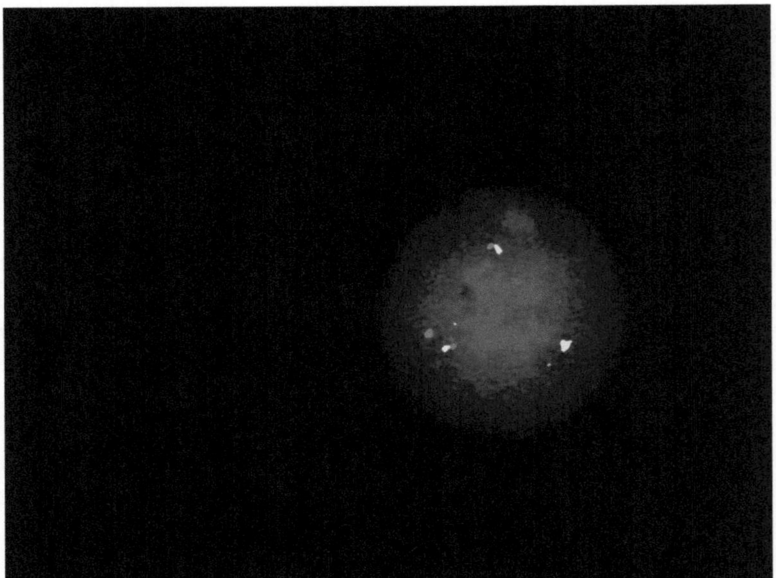

Fig. 3. An IP cell from a BM specimen hybridized with the Vysis LSI BCR-ABL Dual Colour Translocation probe. Green signal is the BCR locus on chromosome 22 and red signal is the ABL locus on chromosome 9. The presence of two fusion signals (here perceived as discrete red and green signals in close proximity) indicates that a standard BCR-ABL rearrangement has occurred.

Coplin jars may not maintain higher temperatures adequately, especially if several slides are processed simultaneously.

4. Probes are light sensitive; therefore, exposure to light should be minimal. Probes are also sensitive to DNases. Therefore, wear gloves at all times and ensure that all pipet tips and plastic and glassware are clean and DNase-free.
5. Bone marrow and PB specimens are potential sources of infection by blood-borne viruses and other agents. When handling unfixed human tissue samples, wear gloves and a laboratory coat. All procedures with open specimen/culture containers should be carried out in a class 2+ biological safety cabinet. To prevent aerosol production, use a centrifuge with sealed buckets.
6. Remember, for successful FISH, the slide quality is extremely important. Visible cytoplasm surrounding nuclei may adversely affect hybridization. For optimum results, FISH should be carried out on the same day as the IP/MP cell preparations are made.
7. It is not recommended to attempt to fix fewer than 1000 cells to the well, as not all of these will adhere, resulting in too low a cell density for later visualization.
8. Alternative methodology uses Tween (instead of NP40 at this stage) during the posthybridization washes (2X SSC + 0.3% Tween and 2X SSC and 0.1% Tween in the first and second Coplin jars, respectively, as described in **Subheading 3.9.3.**).
9. Slides may be stored for 2–3 wk at 4°C in the dark without total loss of fluorescence signal, although it is better to examine slides as soon as possible after completion of the FISH procedure.
10. In approx 15% of Ph+ve CML cases, the derivative chromosome 9 has a deletion adjacent to the translocation breakpoints. On FISH analysis with a dual-fusion probe, this is seen as a variant signal pattern (a single fusion signal in addition to the single red and green signals). It is important to recognize this pattern, as it may be associated with a subset of patients with poor prognosis ***(10)***. Examination of sufficient cells should enable differentiation between those patients with a genuinely deleted derived chromosome 9 and random colocalization of signals in a patient without the BCR-ABL rearrangement.

References

1. Rowley, J. D. (1973) A new consistent chromosomal abnormality in chronic myelogenous leukemia identified by quinacrine fluorescence and Giemsa staining. *Nature* **243,** 290–293.
2. Deininger, M. W. N., Goldman, J. M., and Melo, J. V. (2000) The molecular biology of chronic myeloid leukemia. *Blood* **96,** 3343–3356.
3. Holyoake, T. (2001) Recent advances in the molecular and cellular biology of CML: lessons to be learned from the laboratory. *Br. J. Haematol.* **113,** 11–23.
4. Arnoldus, E. P., Wiegant, J., Noordermeer, I. A., et al. (1999) Detection of the Philadelphia chromosome in interphase nuclei. *Science* **54,** 108–111.
5. Tkachuk, D. C., Westbrook, C. A., Andreefe, M., et al. (1990) Detection of bcr-

abl fusion in chronic myelogeneous leukemia by in situ hybridization. *Science* **250,** 559–562.

6. Chase, A., Grand, F., Zhang, J. G., et al. (1997) Factors influencing the false positive and negative rates of BCR-ABL fluorescence in situ hybridization. *Genes Chromosomes Cancer* **18,** 246–253.
7. Sinclair, P. B., Green, A. R., Grace, C., et al. (1997) Improved sensitivity of BCR-ABL detection: a triple-probe three-color fluorescence *in situ* hybridization system. *Blood* **90,** 1395–1402.
8. Dewald, G. W., Wyatt, W. A., Juneau, A., et al. (1998) Highly sensitive fluorescence in situ hybridisation method to detect double BCR/ABL fusion and monitor response to therapy in chronic myeloid leukemia. *Blood* **91,** 3357–3365.
9. Sinclair, P. B., Leversha, M., Telford, N., et al. (2000) Large deletions at the t(9;22) breakpoint are common and may identify a poor-prognosis subgroup of patients with chronic myeloid leukemia. *Blood* **95,** 738–744.
10. Huntly, B. J., Reid, A. G., Bench, A. J., et al. (2001) Deletions of the derivative chromosome 9 occur at the time of the Philadelphia translocation and provide a powerful and independent prognostic indicator in chronic myeloid leukemia. *Blood* **98,** 1732–1738.

9

UroVysion™ Multiprobe FISH in Urinary Cytology

Lukas Bubendorf and Bruno Grilli

1. Introduction

Urinary cytology is used in combination with cystoscopy for the diagnosis of primary bladder cancer and to monitor the patients for early detection of recurrence after initial transurethral resection. Urinary cytology is highly specific for the detection of poorly differentiated urothelial carcinoma (G3), but notoriously unreliable in case of low-grade urothelial tumors ***(1–3)***. The sensitivity of urinary cytology for the detection of low-grade urothelial tumors is as low as 15–25% ***(1,4)***. Because of a broad cytological overlap between reactive urothelial changes and low-grade urothelial neoplasia, cytologists often have to capitulate by assigning samples to the uncertain and unrewarding category of cellular atypia. Several attempts have been made to improve the detection of neoplastic cells in urinary specimens ***(5–8)***. Common drawbacks of these tests include high false-positive rates resulting from benign conditions and lack of reproducibility if applied in different laboratories. Chromosomal alterations are likely to be more tumor-specific than alterations of protein expression, as they occur frequently in bladder cancer but have only exceptionally been described in non-neoplastic conditions ***(9–11)***. Fluorescence *in situ* hybridization (FISH) allows for visualization of specific DNA sequences and can, therefore, be used for quantitation of chromosomes and genes, including aneusomies, chromosomal deletions, or amplifications ***(12,13)***. Applicability to interphase nuclei makes FISH an ideal tool for chromosomal analyses in cytopathology ***(14)***.

A new commercial assay (UroVysion™, Vysis, Inc., Downers Grove, IL, USA) has recently made the FISH technique available to routine cytology laboratories. This assay is composed of four single-stranded fluorescently labeled nucleic acid probes, including three chromosome enumeration probes (CEP)

From: *Methods in Molecular Medicine, vol. 79: Molecular Diagnosis of Cancer*
Edited by: J. E. Roulston and J. M. S. Bartlett © Humana Press Inc., Totowa, NJ

for the chromosomes 3, 7, and 17, and the single locus-specific identifier (LSI) probe 9p21. The DNA probes are directly labeled with the four different fluorescent dyes SpectrumRed (CEP3), SpectrumGreen (CEP7), SpectrumAqua (CEP17), and SpectrumGold (LSI 9p21). These probes target chromosomal alterations that occur frequently in bladder cancer. This particular probe combination has been selected based on its superior sensitivity for urothelial tumor detection among a set of 10 probes (3, 7, 8, 9, 11, 15, 17, 18, Y, and 9p21) ***(15)***. Chromosomes 3, 7, and 17 are frequently accumulated in urothelial tumors during progression, most likely reflecting general aneuploidy. The 9p21 probe was included to improve coverage of the low-grade, low-stage tumors. Loss of chromosome 9 and 9p21 belongs to the few early chromosomal changes that typically prevail in early, noninvasive tumors (pTa) ***(16–18)***.

Several studies have shown that UroVysion FISH can markedly improve the sensitivity of urinary cytology for the detection of urothelial tumors at a high specificity (>90%) ***(19–23)***. In addition, this test might allow to better predict of the risk of recurrence in individual patients irrespective of cystoscopy and cytology findings ***(21,23,24)***.

2. Materials

A detailed description of the materials required for specimen preparation, hybridization, and scoring is provided in the package insert of the UroVysion assay (Vysis, Inc./Abbott Laboratories). Here, we describe the procedures as used in our laboratory.

2.1. Specimen Selection

1. Standard routine microscope for cytologic evaluation of the specimens.
2. Colored pen to mark the most appropriate specimen or area on a specimen for FISH analysis.
3. Diamond pen for permanent marking of the area for FISH.

2.2. Specimen Pretreatment

Many of the reagents required for the pretreatment are included in the Vysis/Abbott FISH Paraffin Pretreatment Reagent kit (cat. no. 32-801270). Alternatively, the following reagents can be used:

1. Pepsin buffer (0.01*N* HCL).
2. Pepsin (Pepsin A 1:10,000, 25 g; cat. no. 7000, Sigma Chemical Co., St. Louis, MO, USA).
3. Phosphate-buffered saline (PBS).
4. Carnoy's fixative (3:1 methanol:glacial acetic acid).

2.3 Denaturation and Probe Hybridization

1. 4% Neutral-buffered formalin.
2. Immersion oil for appropriate oil immersion objectives. Store at room temperature (15–30°C) (*see* **Note 1**).
3. 100% Ethanol stored at room temperature.
4. Concentrated (2 *N*) HCl.
5. 1*N* NaOH.
6. Purified water, stored at room temperature.
7. Rubber cement (cat. no. 00494; Starkey Inc, IL, USA).
8. Formamide, stored at room temperature.
9. Glass cover slips (Ø 9 mm).
10. Microliter pipettors (1–10 μL and 20–200 μL) and tips.
11. Conical centrifuge tubes (10 and 100 mL).
12. Timer.
13. Magnetic stirrer (e.g., IKA® big-squid, cat. no. 00494; Medos Company, Australia).
14. Vortex mixer (e.g., Vortex Genie 2™; Bender & Hobein AG, Zurich, Switzerland).
15. Microcentrifuge (e.g., EBA 12; Hettich Inc., Bäch, Switzerland).
16. Water baths (37±1°C and 73±1°C).
17. Microwave (e.g., H2800 microwave processor; Energy Beam Sciences Inc, Agawam, MA, USA) (*see* **Note 2**).
18. Humidified hybridization box.
19. Air incubators (37±1°C) (e.g., Memmert Incubator 400; Hettich Inc., Bäch, Switzerland).
20. Forceps.
21. Disposable syringe (5 mL).
22. Coplin jars (10).
23. pH Meter (metrohm 744 pH meter; Metrohm AG; Herisau, Switzerland).
24. Calibrated thermometer.
25. UroVysion Bladder Cancer Recurrence Kit (cat. no. 30-161070, 20 assays; Vysis Inc.).
26. Optional: HYBrite™ Denaturation/Hybridisation system (cat. no. 30-144020; Vysis Inc.).
27. Epifluorescence microscope (e.g., Zeiss Axioplan 2 [Zeiss, Jena, Germany]), equipped with a 100-W mercury lamp and recommended excitation and emission filters (DAPI, yellow, aqua, green, and red single bandpass, or red/green double bandpass) (*see* **Notes 3** and **4**).
28. Optional but highly preferable: digital camera for image documentation (e.g., Zeiss Axiocam [Zeiss, Jena, Germany]); automated stage; appropriate computer and software for microscope, stage, and camera control; relocation software to relocate individual cells or cell groups of interest after hybridization (e.g., "Mark & Find" module of the AxioVision software [Zeiss, Jena, Germany]) (*see* **Note 5**).

2.4. Preparing Working Reagents

1. 100 mL of 1% Buffered formalin: Dilute 25 mL of 4% buffered formalin in 75 mL PBS.
2. 250 mL 20X SSC, pH 5.3: Dissolve 66 g of 20X SSC in 200 mL purified water, adjust pH to 5.3 using concentrated HCl, and bring the total volume to 250 mL with purified water.
3. 1000 mL of Carnoy's fixative: dilute 250 mL glacial acetic acid in 750 mL methanol.
4. Denaturing solution (70% formamide/2X SSC, pH 7.0–8.0) (*Note*: not required for automated assay using HYBrite): Mix 49 mL formamide and 7 mL of 20X SSC and add 14 mL of purified water to a final volume of 70 mL. Verify that pH is 7.0–8.0 using pH meter. This solution can be used for up to 1 wk. Store at 2–8°C in a tightly capped container when not in use (*see* **Note 6**).
5. Ethanol washing dilutions: Prepare dilutions of 70% and 80% using 100% ethanol and purified water, to be used for 1 wk. Store at room temperature in tightly capped Coplin jars to prevent evaporation.
6. 0.4X SSC/0.3% NP40: Add together 20 mL SSC, pH 5.3, 877 mL purified water, and 3 mL NP40 to a final volume of 1000 mL. Discard used solution after 1 d. Unused solution can be stored at room temperature for up to 6 mo.
7. 2X SSC/0.1% NP40: Add together 100 mL of 20X SSC, pH 5.3, 849 mL purified water, and 1 mL NP40 to a final volume of 1000 mL.

3. Methods

In general, the technical part poses no particular problems, as both the FISH protocol and the FISH probes are very robust. In our laboratory, UroVysion FISH gives good or excellent hybridization signals in over 95% of the prospectively collected urinary specimens. Reasons for test failures include severe inflammation, large amounts of bacteria, crystalluria, hematuria, poor preservation of the cells, or poor cellularity (e.g., <50 cells).

3.1. Specimen Collection, Transport, and Processing

1. Add an equal volume of 50% ethanol to the specimen immediately after collection of voided urine or bladder washing to guarantee preservation of the cells during a transport period of 1–2 d at room temperature in a tightly capped plastic container. For longer transports, ice packs are recommended. The specimens remain preserved for up to 7 d when kept refrigerated.
2. Centrifuge the whole volume of urinary fluid at 1425*g* for 10 min.
3. Resuspend the pellet in 10 mL of the supernatant and recentrifuge.
4. Recentrifuge 40–70 μL of the sediment at 71.5*g* using a Cytospin centrifuge. The cell density can easily be adjusted to 100–400 cells per cytospin area by using an appropriate volume for centrifugation based on a visual estimate of the cell density of the sediment.

5. Immediately fix the specimens using a spray fixative (e.g., SprayFix™ [e.g., ethanol and polyethylene glycol; cat. no. 2212.76, Medite, Burgdorf, Germany]) (*see* **Note 7**).
6. Stain the specimens according to Papanicolaou for cytologic evaluation prior to hybridization (*see* **Notes 8** and **9**).
7. Mount a cover slip (24 × 50 mm) using a mounting medium (e.g., Pertex®; cat. no. 41-4010-00, Medite, Burgdorf, Germany).
8. Place the mounted slides in xylene for several hours to remove the coverslip after cytologic evaluation (*see* **Note 10**).
9. Immerse slides in 100% ethanol for 5 min at room temperature. Repeat once.
10. Decolorization of stained specimens is achieved during the process of slide denaturation in the denaturation solution or in a separate decolorization step (*see* **Subheading 3.2.2.**).

3.2. Slide Pretreatment

1. Allow slides to dry at room temperature.
2. Immerse prestained slides in 0.5% HCl for 5–60 min at room temperature (*Note*: this decolorization step is only required for prestained specimens and subsequent use of the automated HYBrite co-denaturation assay).
3. Immerse slides in 2X SSC for 10 min at 37°C.
4. Prepare the protease solution (pepsin 0.5 mg/mL in 0.01 *N* HCl) at 37°C.
5. Immerse slides in protease solution for 13 min (±1 min) at 37°C (*see* **Note 11**).
6. Wash slides in phosphate-buffered saline (PBS) for 5 min at room temperature.
7. Place slides for 5 min in 1% neutral-buffered formalin.
8. Wash slides in PBS for 5 min at room temperature.
9. Wash the slides for 5 min in Carnoy's fixative at room temperature. Repeat twice.
10. Dehydrate slides by immersing in 70% ethanol solution for 5 min at room temperature. Repeat with 80% ethanol, followed by 100% ethanol.
11. Allow slides to dry completely.

3.3. Denaturation and Probe Hybridization (Manual) (see Appendix 1)

When the manual method for the FISH procedure is used, the decolorization of prestained specimens is achieved in the denaturation solution during the denaturation step. Carefully coordinate the timing for denaturing of the specimen DNA (*see* **steps 1–3** and **step 7**) and preparing the probe solution (*see* **steps 5** and **6**).

1. Denature slides in 2X SSC/70% formamide at 73°C (±1°C) for 5 min.
2. Dehydrate slides by immersing in 70% ethanol solution for at least 2 min. Repeat with 80% ethanol, followed by 100% ethanol at room temperature.
3. Remove excess ethanol and let the slides dry for 15 min at room temperature.
4. Remove UroVysion probe from –20°C storage. Allow to warm to room temperature. Vortex to mix. Spin briefly (1–2 s). Gently vortex again to mix.

5. Pipet the appropriate volume of the UroVysion probe solution into a tube (3 μL × the number of specimens).
6. Heat this UroVysion probe solution for 5 min in a 73°C (±1°C) water bath.
7. Put the slides on a 45°C slide warmer for up to 2 min prior to applying the UroVysion probe mixture.
8. Apply 3 μL of UroVysion probe mixture to the target area of the slide.
9. Place a 9-mm round glass coverslip over the probe and seal with rubber cement.
10. Incubate at 37°C overnight in a prehumidified chamber.

3.4. HYBrite Co-Denaturation Assay (Optional)

1. Remove UroVysion probe from –20°C storage. Allow to warm to room temperature. Vortex to mix. Spin briefly (1–2 s). Gently vortex again to mix.
2. Put the slides on a 45°C slide warmer for up to 2 min.
3. Apply 3 μL of UroVysion probe mixture to the target area of the slide.
4. Place a 9-mm round glass cover slip over the probe and seal with rubber cement.
5. Place a moisted paper towel in the channels along the heating surface.
6. Turn on the HYBrite instrument.
7. Set the program for Melt Temp 73°C and Melt Time 5 min (denaturation), and Hybridisation Temperature to 37°C and Hybridisation Time 4–16 h.
8. Place slides on the heating surface of the instrument. Supplement with blank slides.
9. Close HYBrite lid and run program.

3.5. Posthybridization Washes

1. Place a Coplin jar with with 0.4X SSC/0.3% NP40 in a 73°C water bath.
2. Fill two other jars with 2X SSC/0.1% NP40 and place at room temperature.
3. Using forceps, remove the rubber cement and cover slip from the slide.
4. Place slide in the 0.4X SSC/0.3% NP40 immediately after removing the cover slip. Do not wash more than four slides at a time in the same jar. Supplement with blank slides if necessary.
5. Wash for 2 min at 73°C (±1°C) .
6. Wash the slides in the jar containing 2X SSC/0.1% NP40 at room temperature for 2 min. Repeat once.
7. Allow slides to dry in a dark area.
8. Apply 10 μL of DAPI II onto the target area and place a coverslip (18- to 24-mm square is recommended) over the DAPI solution, avoiding air bubbles.

3.6. Scoring and Interpretation

3.6.1. Analysis of Specimen Slides

1. Scan the hybridized area at a magnification of ×400 for morphologically abnormal cells that have increased nuclear size, irregular nuclear contours, patchy DAPI staining of the nuclear chromatin, and/or cells that appear in clusters. If few morphologically abnormal cells are present, select cells with the largest nuclei.

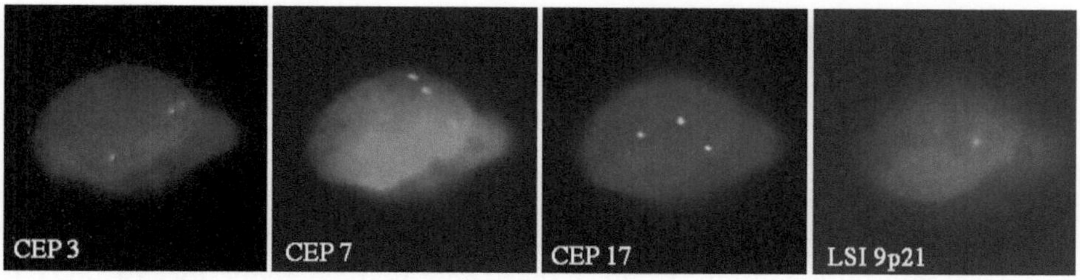

Fig. 1. Identification of bladder cancer cells by FISH in a urinary specimen (gray channel images): cell nucleus showing an abnormally high copy number of the chromosomes 7 and 17 (three copies, each), and heterozygeous loss of 9p21 (only one copy, magnification ×1000).

2. Increase magnification to ×630 to ×1000. Focus up and down to find all of the signals in the nucleus.
3. Determine the number of signals for all four probes by using the four filters. Document the result on an appropriate data sheet (*see* **Appendix 2**).
4. Record the chromosome pattern if there is a gain of two or more of the chromosomes 3 (red), 7 (green), or 17 (aqua) or if there is a loss of both copies of 9p21 (yellow). A scoring template and a worked example are shown in **Appendices 2** and **3**. A representative example of an urothelial cell with multiple chromosomal changes is shown in **Fig. 1**.
5. If you find surrounding cells with abnormal chromosomal patterns, these cells should be recorded, even if they appear morphologically normal.
6. Continue the analysis until at least 25 morphologically abnormal cells have been analyzed.
7. If you do not find at least 4 cells with an abnormal chromosomal pattern as defined in **Subheading 3.6.1., step 4**, screen the whole specimen, including morphologically normal cells.

3.6.2. Cutoff and Interpretation

To avoid false-positive results by artifactual gain of a single probe as a result of signal splitting or technical artifacts, only multiple gains of at least two chromosomes are considered in the guidelines of the manufacturer based on an initial study ***(15)***. Loss of 9p21 is evaluated separately, as bladder tumors can rarely show isolated loss of 9p21. The current scoring guidelines of the manufacturer demand that at least 4 of the 25 cells show multiple chromosomal gains (at least two of the chromosomes 3, 7, and 17) or lack of both copies (homozygeous deletion) of 9p21 in at least 12 of the cells. These criteria appear reasonable, as suggested by the results from previous studies ***(19–21,23–25)***. However, refinements of the scoring criteria may lead to further improvements in the future. For example, the presence of isolated cells with a purely tetraploic chromosomal pattern (four signals of each probe) does not have the same significance as other numerical aberrations. A small population of such cells prevails in up to 30% of benign urinary specimens ***(21)***. Given the reduced diagnostic significance of tetraploic cells, one should be cautious about considering a purely tetraploic pattern as a positive FISH result, unless it is found in a large number of cells. Similarly, results at or near the cutoff level should be interpreted with caution. In our experience, homozygeous loss of 9p21 is less frequent than heterozygeous loss and determines the test result only on very rare occasions. However, there is often a relative loss with a lower number of 9p21 signals than chromosome signals (e.g., two 9p21 signals but four signals of the chromosomes 3, 7, and 1, each). This finding can best be explained by initial heterozygeous 9p21 deletion followed by polyploidization during progression.

3.6.3. Pitfalls in Interpretation

Interpretation of urinary FISH results should always include consideration of the patient's medical history in order to avoid misleading interpretation.

1. A positive urinary FISH test after radiation therapy in the pelvic field for prostate or endometrial cancer should be interpreted with caution. Radiotherapy can lead to persistent chromosomal aberrations in the irradiated field. However, there is no evidence for an increased risk of developing bladder cancer following prostate irradiation ***(26)***.
2. Local or systemic chemotherapy can lead to secondary chromosomal aberrations unrelated to neoplasia ***(27)***.
3. Seminal vesicle cells, which can rarely be found in the urine, may appear strikingly atypical and can be aneuploid ***(28,29)***. The characteristic golden brown and autofluorescent cytoplasmic pigment of seminal vesicle cells is a clue to the correct diagnosis.

4. Notes

1. We recommend oil that has been specifically formulated for use in fluorescence microscopy (e.g., Zeiss fluorescence-free immersion oil: Immersol 518-F oil). The use of fluorescence and standard oil with the same objective leads to diffuse autofluorescence, necessitating careful cleaning of the objective. The cleaning of the objective is best performed using acetone. Oil may form precipitating crystals that can be dissolved by gently warming up in a 37–40°C water bath or microwave.
2. We use a microwave with high-precision heat and time control to heat the fluid reagents in the Coplin jars. Alternatively, one can use a traditional water bath with temperature control.

3. The red and green single-bandpass filters give brighter individual signals than the red/green double-bandpass filter.
4. Regular maintenance of the microscope, including alignment of the mercury lamp, is mandatory to guarantee adequate function.
5. Relocation capability is most helpful, as it allows one to analyze individual cells or cell groups of interest identified in the Papanicolaou staining. Without this automation tool, it is difficult to relocate such individual cells in the DAPI stain after hybridization. Furthermore, automatic relocation facilitates the review of the specimens by a second observer after the initial scoring to confirm the results or to discuss problematic findings. All automated features for FISH analysis are included in high-end microscopic platforms (e.g., Zeiss Axioplan 2 imaging system [Zeiss, Jena, Germany]).
6. The denaturing solution contains formamide, which is toxic and should be handled within a cabinet.
7. Alternative to a spray fixative, one can use other fixatives, including Delaunay solution (equal volumes of absolute ethanol and acetone with 0,5 mL of 1 *M* trichloroacetic acid), acetone, or one can let the specimens air-dry at room temperature using a fan. The type of the fixation type does not recognizably affect the hybridization results. Excellent hybridization results can also be obtained on ThinPrep® slides after fixation in PreservCyt® (Cytyc Corp., Boxborough, MA, USA), which is the preferred method for urinary cytology in some laboratories ***(25)***. In our hands, ThinPreps do not have significant advantages over the less expensive cytospins in routine urinary cytology. The need for higher volumes of probe mixture is a cost-effective disadvantage of ThinPreps, as the target area is larger than on cytospins. As suggested by the manufacturer (Vysis Inc., Downers Grove, IL), one can also use sedimentation preparations, where the specimens are concentrated on small areas on a 16-well slide. However, this method is more expensive and markedly more time-consuming than the preparation of cytospins.
8. We prefer the standard cytological staining according to Papanicolaou for morphological evaluation of the cytologic specimens prior to FISH analysis. Alternatively, one can use May–Grünwald–Giemsa (MGG) and hematoxylin–eosin without adversely affecting the result of a subsequent FISH analysis. The morphologic analysis of the stained slides prior to FISH analysis allows one to better control for suitability and representativity of the slides before hybridization. For example, a FISH analysis is of little or no value in nonrepresentative specimens with an insufficient number of urothelial cells (e.g., <50 cells) or heavy contamination with normal vaginal cells. Similarly, FISH analysis is hampered in specimens with acute granulocytic inflammation, crystalluria, or hematuria because of signal overlay or background autofluorescence.
9. Preparing two or more specimens per urinary sample retains at least one stained specimen to be archived. One cytospin specimen is considered as representative of the whole urinary sample because of the random mixture of urothelial cells in the fluid ***(30)***. We keep the pellet for 1 wk at 4°C in case additional analyses are required.

10. For retrospective applications, one needs to consider that the removal of the mounting medium of the cover slip in xylene may take up to several days, depending on the length of the preceding archival period.
11. In archived cytologic specimens, hybridization efficiency decreases with time of storage, requiring adjustments of the pretreatment conditions. Increasing the protease concentration or the exposure time of the slides to protease are the most appropriate means to improve the hybridization result. This variability may be a concern in retrospective studies, but does not affect diagnostic applications of UroVysion FISH. Usually, diagnostic UroVysion FISH tests are not performed later than 1 or 2 wk after the cytological assessment.

Acknowledgments

We are grateful to Michelle Herzog and Audrey Barascud for their helpful suggestions and their contributions in further developing the FISH technology in diagnostic cytology. We also thank the whole staff of the Cytology Division of the Institute for Pathology, University of Basel, for their support.

References

1. Koss, L.G., Deitch, D., Ramanathan, R., et al. (1985) Diagnostic value of cytology of voided urine. *Acta Cytol.* **29,** 810–816.
2. Renshaw, A. A. (2000) Compassionate conservatism in urinary cytology. *Diagn. Cytopathol.* **22,** 137–138.
3. Renshaw, A. A. (2000) Subclassifying atypical urinary cytology specimens. *Cancer* **90,** 222–229.
4. Bastacky, S., Ibrahim, S., Wilczynski, S. P., et al. (1999) The accuracy of urinary cytology in daily practice. *Cancer* **87,** 118–128.
5. Ross, J. S. and Cohen, M. B. (2000) Ancillary methods for the detection of recurrent urothelial neoplasia. *Cancer* **90,** 75–86.
6. Konety, B. R. and Getzenberg, R. H. (2001) Urine based markers of urological malignancy. *J. Urol.* **165,** 600–611.
7. Saad, A., Hanbury, D. C., McNicholas, T. A., et al. (2001) The early detection and diagnosis of bladder cancer: a critical review of the options. *Eur. Urol.* **39,** 619–633.
8. van der Poel, H. G. and Debruyne, F. M. (2001) Can biological markers replace cystoscopy? An update. *Curr. Opin. Urol.* **11,** 503–509.
9. Richter, J., Jiang, F., Gorog, J. P., et al. (1997) Marked genetic differences between stage pTa and stage pT1 papillary bladder cancer detected by comparative genomic hybridization. *Cancer Res.* **57,** 2860–2864.
10. Richter, J., Beffa, L., Wagner, U., et al. (1998) Patterns of chromosomal imbalances in advanced urinary bladder cancer detected by comparative genomic hybridization. *Am. J. Pathol.* **153,** 1615–1621.
11. Sauter, G., Moch, H., Wagner, U., et al. (1995) Y chromosome loss detected by FISH in bladder cancer. *Cancer Genet. Cytogenet.* **82,** 163–169.
12. Hopman, A. H., Poddighe, P. J., Smeets, A. W., et al. (1989) Detection of numeri-

cal chromosome aberrations in bladder cancer by *in situ* hybridization. *Am. J. Pathol.* **135,** 1105–1117.

13. Werner, M., Wilkens, L., Aubele, M., et al. (1997) Interphase cytogenetics in pathology: principles, methods, and applications of fluorescence *in situ* hybridization (FISH). *Histochem. Cell. Biol.* **108,** 381–390.
14. Jiang, F. and Katz, R. L. (2002) Use of interphase fluorescence *in situ* hybridization as a powerful diagnostic tool in cytology. *Diagn. Mol. Pathol.* **11,** 47–57.
15. Sokolova, I., Halling, K. C., Jenkins, R. B., et al. (2000) The development of a multitarget, multicolor fluoroescence *in situ* hybridization assay for the detection of urothelial carcinoma in urine. *J. Mol. Diagn.* **2,** 116–123.
16. Hopman, A. H., Moesker, O., Smeets, A. W., et al. (1991) Numerical chromosome 1, 7, 9, and 11 aberrations in bladder cancer detected by *in situ* hybridization. *Cancer Res.* **51,** 644–651.
17. Zhao, J., Richter, J., Wagner, U., et al. (1999) Chromosomal imbalances in noninvasive papillary bladder neoplasms (pTa). *Cancer Res.* **59,** 4658–4661.
18. Eleuteri, P., Grollino, M. G., Pomponi, D., et al. (2001) Chromosome 9 aberrations by fluorescence *in situ* hybridisation in bladder transitional cell carcinoma. *Eur. J. Cancer* **37,** 1496–1503.
19. Halling, K. C., King, W., Sokolova, I. A., et al. (2000) A comparison of cytology and fluorescence *in situ* hybridization for the detection of urothelial carcinoma. *J. Urol.* **164,** 1768–1775.
20. Halling, K. C., King, W., Sokolova, I. A., et al. (2002) A comparison of BTA stat, hemoglobin dipstick, telomerase and Vysis UroVysion assays for the detection of urothelial carcinoma in urine. *J. Urol.* **167,** 2001–2006.
21. Bubendorf, L., Grilli, B., Sauter, G., et al. (2001) Multiprobe FISH for enhanced detection of bladder cancer in voided urine specimens and bladder washings. *Am. J. Clin. Pathol.* **116,** 79–86.
22. Placer, J., Espinet, B., Salido, M., et al. (2002) Clinical utility of a Multiprobe FISH assay in voided urine specimens for the detection of bladder cancer and its recurrences, compared with urinary cytology. *Eur. Urol.* **42,** 547–552.
23. Sarosdy, M. F., Schellhammer, P., Bokinsky, G., et al. (2002) Clinical evaluation of a multi-target fluorescent *in situ* hybridization assay for detection of bladder cancer. *J. Urol.* **168,** 1950–1954.
24. Takahashi, T., Lohse, C. M., Pankratz, S., et al. (2002) Predicting urothelial carcinoma recurrence with fluorescence *in situ* hyridization analysis of urine. *J. Urol.* **167(Suppl.)** p. 62 (abstract 651).
25. Skacel, M., Pettay, J. D., Tsiftsakis, E. K., et al. (2001) Validation of a multicolor interphase fluorescence *in situ* hybridization assay for detection of transitional cell carcinoma on fresh and archival thin-layer, liquid-based cytology slides. *Anal. Quant. Cytol. Histol.* **23,** 381–387.
26. Movsas, B., Hanlon, A. L., Pinover, W., et al. (1998) Is there an increased risk of second primaries following prostate irradiation? *Int. J. Radiat. Oncol. Biol. Phys.* **41,** 251–255.
27. Lopez de Mesa, R., Sierrasesumaga, L., Calasanz, M. J., et al. (2000) Nonclonal

chromosomal aberrations induced by anti-tumoral regimens in childhood cancer: relationship with cancer-related genes and fragile sites. *Cancer Genet. Cytogenet.* **121,** 78–85.
28. Arber, D. A. and Speights, V. O. (1991) Aneuploidy in benign seminal vesicle epithelium: an example of the paradox of ploidy studies. *Mod. Pathol.* **4,** 687–689.
29. Wojcik, E. M., Bassler, T. J., Jr., and Orozco, R. (1999) DNA ploidy in seminal vesicle cells. A potential diagnostic pitfall in urine cytology. *Anal. Quant. Cytol. Histol.* **21,** 29–34.
30. Burton, J. L., Goepel, J. R., and Lee, J. A. (2000) Demand management in urine cytology: a single cytospin slide is sufficient. *J. Clin. Pathol.* **53,** 718–719.

Appendix 1

DAY 1		UroVysion air-dried unstained specimens	UroVysion prestained specimens[1]
preparing steps	unfreeze 30' at RT	yes	no
	2X 5' in xylene	no	yes
	2X 5' in absolute ethanol	no	yes
	let dry for 15'	no	yes
pretreatment	2XSSC 10' at 37 °c in microwave	yes	yes
	pepsin 0.5mg/ml in 0.01N HCL 13' at 37 °c in microwave	yes	yes
	5' PBS at RT	yes	yes
	5' in 1% neutral buffered formalin	yes	yes
	5' PBS at RT	yes	yes
	3X 5' in Carnoy's fixative[2]	yes	yes
	5' ethanol 70 % at RT	yes	yes
	5' ethanol 80 % at RT	yes	yes
	5' ethanol 100% at RT	yes	yes
	let dry 15'	yes	yes
denaturation	slide denaturation	no	5' at 73 °c in denaturing solution[3]
	2' ethanol 70% at 4°c (on ice)	no	yes
	2' ethanol 80% at 4°c (on ice)	no	yes
	2' ethanol 100% at RT	no	yes
	let dry 15'	no	yes
	probe denaturation	no	5' at 73 °c in denaturing solution[3]
	slide 2' on heat plate at 45°c	yes	yes
	probe volume	3 µl	3 µl
	round coverslip, Ø9mm	yes	yes
	seal coverslip with rubber cement	yes	yes
	co-denaturation slide & probe	HYBbrite, 5' at 73 °c	no
hybridization	hybridization overnight	HYBrite at 37°c	humified hybridization chamber at 37°c
DAY 2			
washing	wash 2' in 0.4XSSC/0.3%NP40 at 73°c	yes	yes
	wash 2' in 2XSSC/0.1%NP40 at RT	yes	yes
	wash 2' in 2XSSC/0.1%NP40 at RT	yes	yes
	let dry in the dark	yes	yes
cover	10 µl DAPI, coverslip (21x26mm)	yes	yes

[1]Papanicolaou, May-Grünwald-Giemsa, or Hematoxylin-Eosin

[2]Carnoy's fixative: 3:1 methanol/glacial acetic acid

[3]Denaturing solution: 49 mL formamide, 7 mL 20X SSC, 14 mL $H_2$0 nanopure, pH=7.0-8.0 with 2*N* HCL (Store ar 4°C, 1 w)

Appendix 2
Scoring Template for UroVysion FISH

UROVYSION

Date hybridization: **Pat.ID:** **voided urine** ☐ **bladder wash** ☐

other:

	not optimal	good	excellent
material			
signal intensity			
background			
overall quality			
evaluation	not evaluable		evaluable

cells	blue CEP17	red CEP3	green CEP7	gold 9p21	positive cells
1					
2					
3					
4					
5					
6					
7					
8					
9					
10					
11					
12					
13					
14					
15					
16					
17					
18					
19					
20					
21					
22					
23					
24					
25					
total					

comments: Date: signature:

Appendix 3
Scoring Sheet from a Worked Example

UROVYSION

Date hybridization: **Pat.ID:** **voided urine** ☐ **bladder wash** ☐

other:

	not optimal	good	excellent
material		x	
signal intensity		x	
background			x
overall quality		x	
evaluation	not evaluable		evaluable (circled)

cells	blue CEP17	red CEP3	green CEP7	gold 9p21	positive cells
1	2	4	4	0	X
2	3	4	2	1	X
3	2	2	2	1	
4	4	5	5	1	X
5	4	4	4	1	X
6	2	4	4	1	X
7	3	4	4	1	X
8	4	4	5	1	X
9	4	3	2	1	X
10	4	4	2	2	X
11	3	4	2	1	X
12	5	4	2	2	X
13	2	3	2	2	X
14	3	4	2	2	X
15	2	2	2	1	
16	4	4	5	1	X
17	4	3	2	1	X
18	4	5	4	1	X
19	4	5	5	2	X
20	4	4	3	1	X
21	3	4	3	0	X
22	3	4	4	1	X
23	4	5	3	0	X
24	5	4	4	1	X
25	5	4	4	2	X
total					23/25

comments: Date: signature:

10

Chromogenic *In Situ* Hybridization in Tumor Pathology

Jorma Isola and Minna Tanner

1. Introduction

Ever since the correlation was found between the pathogenesis of diseases and genomic alterations, molecular cytogenetic techniques have found a place in molecular medicine. These techniques are used in tracing gene and genomic abnormalities that are underlying in the development of cancer and genetic diseases. In 1969, Gall and Pardue introduced a technique known as "*in situ* hybridization" (ISH) to localize nucleic acids in individual cells *(1)*. At that time, the capabilities of ISH were limited to highly repetitive sequences using radioactively labeled probes that were subsequences visualized by autoradiography. The use of radioisotopes has many disadvantages and has been replaced in DNA ISH by nonradioactive detection methods. The most commonly used reporter molecules are haptens, such as biotin and digoxigenin, which can be incorporated easily in the probe DNA. The tagged probes are then detected with labeled antibodies against the specific tag or, as in the case of biotin, with a labeled avidin molecule. Since the first report of fluorescent *in situ* hybridization (FISH) *(2)*, the principle of FISH has remained essentially the same, with the exception that biotin and digoxigenin have partly been replaced by directly fluorochrome-conjugated nucleotides, which simplifies the laboratory protocol.

Fluorescent *in situ* hybridization is currently a standard tool in cytogenetics laboratories in the diagnostics of hereditary disorders, chromosomal aberrations, and hematologic cancer markers. The application of FISH became feasible for pathology laboratories along with the development of modifications of FISH, which make it possible to analyze formalin-fixed and paraffin-embedded tissue samples. The main obstacle for widespread use is fluorescense microscopy, which is rarely used in pathology laboratories. Although chromo-

From: *Methods in Molecular Medicine, vol. 79: Molecular Diagnosis of Cancer*
Edited by: J. E. Roulston and J. M. S. Bartlett © Humana Press Inc., Totowa, NJ

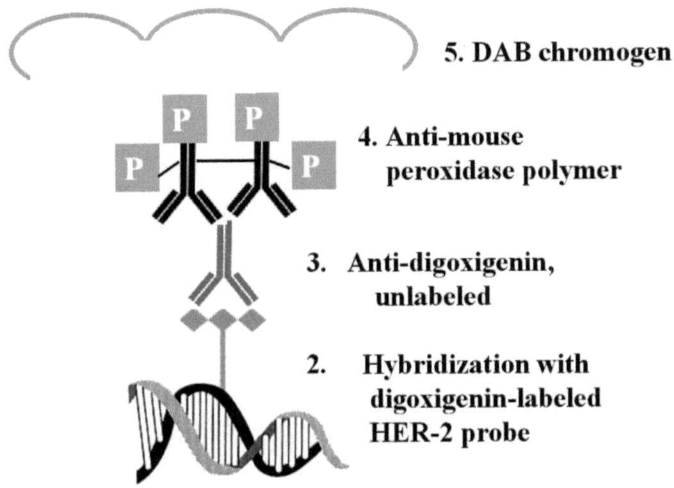

Fig. 1. Principle of CISH.

some copy enumeration with centromere probes has been made with chromogenic detection methods since the early 1990s (reviewed in **ref. *3***), the chromogenic detection of unique sequences (like the HER-2 oncogene) was first published in 2000 ***(4)***. The present review focuses on chromogenic *in situ* hybridization (CISH) technology as a new alternative to FISH in cancer diagnostics. The principle of CISH is illustrated in **Fig. 1.**

1.1. Methodological Aspects of CISH

1.1.1. Probes and Probe Labeling in CISH

The requirements of probes used in CISH and FISH are largely the same. The DNA probes specific to the cancer genes can be selected from P1, PAC, and BAC libraries, which all have successfully been used to prepare probes for FISH and CISH. The probe DNA can be labeled by nick translation, polymerase chain reaction (PCR), random priming, or chemical conjugation. Biotin and digoxigenin can use labels, which are incorporated into probe DNA as dUTP conjugates. As in FISH, the probe labeling is a critical factor for signal intensity, and the important issues are discussed in detail in Chapter 8. The repetitive DNA sequences are blocked either with Cot-1 DNA or they are removed from the probe DNA as described in **ref. *5***. The different probes used so far in CISH are listed in **Table 1**.

1.1.2. CISH Hybridization and Microscopy

The reagents needed and the workflow of CISH hybridization is described in detail in **Subheadings 2.** and **3.** and the explanatory notes. The hybridiza-

Table 1
Probes Used in CISH (as of November 2002)

Probe/gene	Application
Chromosome centromere probes	Chromosome enumeration
Human papilloma virus (HPV)	High-risk HPV detection
HER-2	Prognostication and Herceptin eligibility
Topoisomerase IIα	Therapy response prediction
EGFR	Brain tumor research
C-MYC	Breast cancer research
Cyclin D1	Breast cancer research
EWS, bcr/abl	Translocations in hematologic malignancies and sarcomas

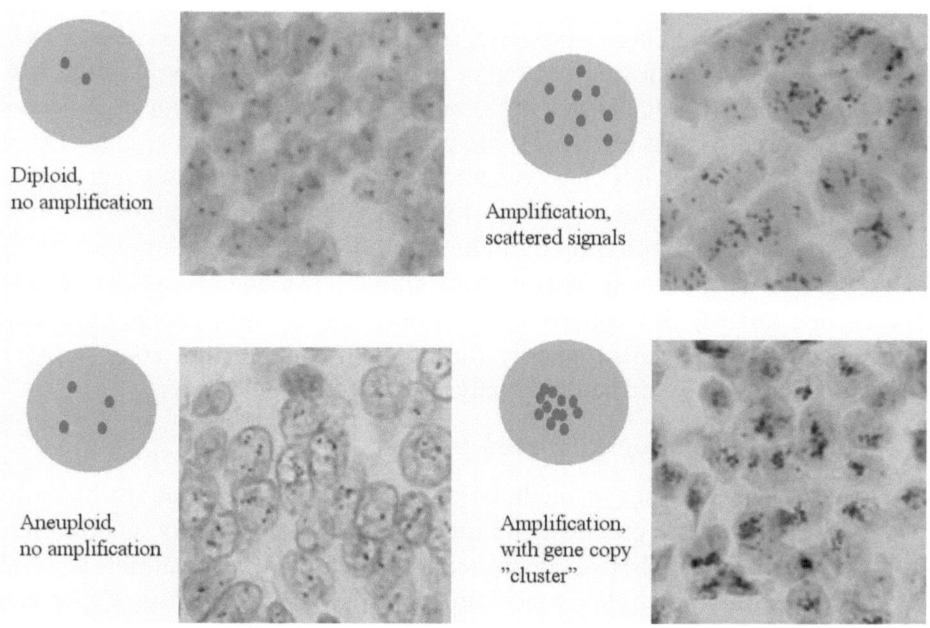

Fig. 2. Microscopic evaluation of oncogene copy number status by CISH.

tion signals (dots) of CISH can easily be visualized with ×40 objective. Because oil immersion objectives are not needed, it is easy to change magnification from low magnification (useful in histopathological orientation) to high magnification, which is needed in copy number evaluation (×40 objective). Verification of histopathology can be done easily, because CISH slides are counterstained with hematoxylin. A schematic illustration and examples of CISH are shown in **Fig. 2**.

Unlike in the well-established two-color FISH, the currently used version of CISH is based on colorimetric detection of one probe only. After careful optimization, we have adopted a cutoff of six or more copies as a definition for amplification of HER-2 oncogene. Tumors with no HER-2 amplification show one to two signals per cell, or in chromosomally aneuploid cases, three to five copies per cell. Because of DNA replication during the S- and G2/M-phases of the cell cycle, a small proportion (up to 10–30%) of aneuploid cancer cells may contain five to eight signals per nucleus (often as signal doublets). This should also be regarded as a negative finding (no HER-2 amplification). If CISH shows no hybridization signals, the hybridization had failed because of technical reasons ***(6)***.

A typical gene amplification by CISH is a peroxidase-positive cluster of multiple gene copies, which is easy to identify in the microscope with 40× objective magnification. The exact enumeration of gene copies is not possible, but in clinical HER-2 diagnostics, enumeration of gene copies exceeding 10 is not needed. The most difficult category in CISH is the "low level" amplification (6–10 gene copies/cell), in which enumeration of the gene copies is necessary. In these cases, it is often useful to perform a chromosome 17 centromere CISH on an adjacent slide and compare the copy numbers. However, in the case of the HER-2 oncogene, tumors with a borderline copy number seem to comprise only a small minority of all breast tumors. Based on our experience, pathologists who have experience from immunohistochemistry learn CISH microscopy quickly. Interobserver variation is small, in the range of 1–2%. The discordant cases are typically the ones with borderline copy number counts, which are also difficult to analyze with FISH.

1.2. Future Methodological Developments

There are several lines of methodological developments that are likely to make CISH even more practical and user-friendly for pathology laboratories. In terms of making CISH easier to perform in clinical laboratories, several companies are developing immunostaining robots that can perform CISH in a fully automated manner. In line with this development, it would also be practical if the hybridization reaction could be shortened to allow CISH to be performed in 1 d.

Because CISH has been criticized because of the lack of reference probe, two-color CISH has recently been developed (*see* **Fig. 2**). In this system, a biotin-labeled centromere probe is hybridized together with HER-2 and detected simultaneously with HER-2 using a rabbit antibiotin antibody and an anti-rabbit alkaline phosphatase polymer (Powervision™). The HER-2 gene copies show up deep red, which is distinguishable from the typical brown color of the DAB precipitate (*see* **Fig. 3**). This technology may have wide applica-

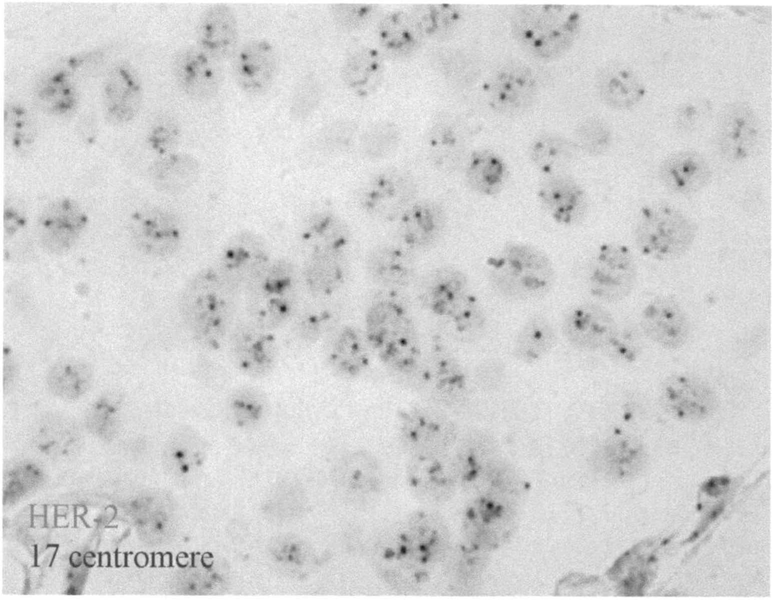

Fig. 3. Example of one-color CISH and its new two-color version (A and B, respectively). The chromosome 17 centromere is visualized with alkaline phosphatase and Fast Red chromogen, whereas the HER-2 oncogene is shown with peroxidase and DAB.

tions also in the detection of diagnostically important chromosome translocations. A related ongoing development aims at combining HER-2 CISH with simultaneous HER-2 protein immunohistochemistry. This method would allow a complete HER assessment (gene amplification and protein overexpression) on one slide.

1.3. Applications of CISH

Although the potential advantages of chromogenic detection over fluorescence detection in DNA ISH have been recognized for many years, the low sensitivity of the chromogenic detection has restricted its use with centromere probes *(3)*. These probes target tens or hundreds of repetitive α-satellite sequences, thereby decreasing the sensitivity requirements of the detection system. Unfortunately, chromosome copy number assessment with centromere probes CISH has limited applicability in diagnostic pathology and has never become a standard diagnostic practice.

The need for CISH increased with the assays of HER-2 oncogene, the amplification of which is strongly associated with clinical outcome and response to the anti-HER-2 therapy with Herceptin™ *(7,8)*. HER-2 diagnostics with protein immunohistochemistry is now widely spread, but it is well known

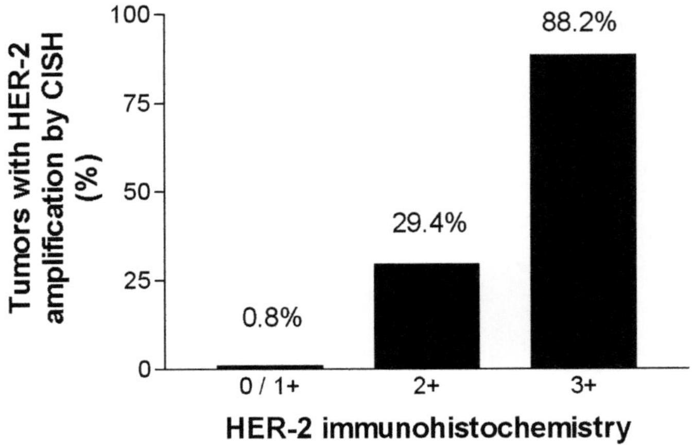

Fig. 4. Amplification of HER-2 by CISH versus immunohistochemistry in standard clinical practice in Finland in 2001 to November 2002. Immunohistochemistry was done in 14 local pathology laboratories and CISH in the author's reference laboratory. In total, there were 122 tumors immunostaining score 0 or 1+, 394 tumors with 2+, and 373 tumors with 3+ HER-2 score.

that for the moderately HER-2 overexpressing (2+) tumors, this method is not very accurate ***(9)***. Because FISH is carried out mainly in reference laboratories, CISH has been recognized as a promising alternative for ordinary pathology laboratories. There are an increasing number of studies reporting positive experiences of CISH in breast cancer ***(4,6,10–17)***. Although definitive interlaboratory validation of CISH (vs FISH) is still underway, the positive scientific evidence makes it possible to already recommend CISH as an additional test to confirm positive immunohistochemical HER-2 results. Probably the largest experience of CISH comes from Finland, where CISH was selected as the immunostaining positivity confirmation test in a nationwide adjuvant Herceptin therapy trial. During 2001–2002, over 2000 diagnostic CISH tests have been made in two reference laboratories. Based on the overview of the results, less than 1% of IHC 0 or 1+, 29.4% of the 2+, and 88.2% of the 3+ tumors showed HER-2 amplification by CISH (*see* **Fig. 4**). Thus, a significant number of noneligible patients would have been treated with Herceptin, and, conversely, many patients with amplification would not have received Herceptin if immunohistochemistry were used as the only HER-2 test.

Chromogenic *in situ* hybridization of HER-2 may have applicability in other tumor types as well. To our knowledge, CISH has already been applied in ovarian, gastric, and prostatic tumors, as well as extramammary Paget's disease, which all have previously been recognized as HER-2-positive tumor entities. In addition to HER-2, other cancer genes can be studied with CISH equally

Table 2
Comparison of FISH and CISH for the Detection of HER-2 Oncogene Amplification

CISH	FISH
First study published November 2000 (Tanner et al.)	First study published in 1992 (Kallioniemi et al., 1992)
Reagent kits since November 1999	Reagent kits since 1995
Approximately 10 original articles published (by November 2002)	Ten published studies
Single color (reference probe on another slide)	Two color (HER-2 and 17 centromere with different colors)
Uses standard microscopes (×40 dry objective most suitable)	Requires expensive epifluorescence microscopes (63×–100× oil objectives)
Microscopy is straightforward for pathologists	Microscopy is laborious and difficult
Allows one to evaluate histology	Proper evaluation of histology not possible; only few pathologists have experience in FISH microscopy
CISH slides are permanent (can be archived)	FISH slides are not permanent (cannot be archived)

well. CISH has been used to study Topoisomerase IIα, which is often coamplified with HER-2; it is an interesting new cancer gene because of its possible relationship with response to doxorubicin therapy ***(6)***. Similarly, CISH of c-*myc* has been published ***(13)***, and studies of epithelial growth factor receptor (EGFR), androgen receptor, and cyclin D1 are underway (*see* **Table 1**). CISH may find important applications also in tumors containing diagnostic chromosome translocations. For example, CISH reagents to detect bcr/abl and EWS translocations have recently become commercially available (by Zymed Inc.).

1.4. Comparison of CISH and FISH

At present, FISH can be regarded as the gold standard test (in HER-2/neu diagnostics). CISH was originally developed for clinical diagnostics of the HER-2 oncogene to overcome the difficulties of FISH microscopy. The main features of CISH and FISH are compared in **Table 2**.

The main advantage of CISH over FISH is the simple laboratory methodology and the ability to perform oncogene analysis in the proper histologic context. The use of 60× or 100× oil immersion objectives, which are necessary to see the hybridization signals in FISH, makes it laborious to screen the tissue section to find the most representative cancerous areas and to evaluate tumor histopathology. In CISH, histologic evaluation of a tissue section is straightforward because of the hematoxylin counterstain. Switching from low magnification to copy number evaluation using a 40× objective is easy because oil immersion objectives are not needed. Time-consuming enumeration of the gene copies is necessary in a minority of samples because the HER-2 amplicon usually presents as a typical and pathogenomic peroxidase-positive gene copy "cluster." The large size and irregular shape of the cluster allows one to distinguish amplification from individual nonamplified gene copies. Of significant help in evaluation are the nonmalignant cells, which show the pattern and size of nonamplified copies of HER-2. Because most pathologists are familiar with peroxidase-based immunostainings, the time and effort needed to learn CISH microscopy is shorter than that needed for FISH.

Because of these practical advantages, CISH is a promising new alternative to FISH in clinical diagnostics as a more user-friendly technique that allows morphological identification of the target cells. Studies aiming to validate CISH directly with the response to trastuzumab therapy are currently underway.

2. Materials

1. Silanized or SuperFrost Plus microscope slides.
2. Xylene and ethyl alcohol to remove wax.
3. Reveal target unmasking solution (Biocare Inc., Walnut Creek, CA).
4. A desktop autoclave, a pressure cooker, or a microwave oven for heat pretreatment.
5. A ready-to-use pepsin solution (Digest-All III; Zymed Inc.).
6. Graded ethanols (70–99.5%).
7. A ready-to-use probe mixture for the gene or centromere to be studied (Spot-Light probe series; Zymed Inc, South San Francisco, CA).
8. CISH-UnderCover Slips (Zymed Inc.).
9. Thermal plate set at 94°C.
10. Incubator (oven) set at 37°C.
11. Water bath set at 75°C (needed in the posthybridization wash on d 2).
12. Phosphate buffered saline (PBS) and Tris-buffered saline (TBS) buffers (pH 7.0).
13. 0.5X SSC: Dissolve 175.3 g NaCl and 88.2 g sodium citrate in 800 mL distilled water, pH to 7.0 with 10 *M* NaOH; make up to 1 L with distilled water and autoclave. Dilute 1:40 with distilled water for 0.5X SSC).
14. Coplin jars.
15. Mouse anti-digoxigenin antibody (Roche Biochemicals).
16. Powervision+ detection kit (ImmunoVision Inc., Daly City, CA).

17. Hematoxylin solution for counterstaining.
18. Permanent mounting medium, coverslips.

3. Methods

1. Cut 5-μm tissue sections onto silanized slides (*see* **Note 1**) and bake at 56–60°C for 2–4 h. Store at room temperature until required.
2. Immerse slides in xylene for 5 min.
3. Repeat **step 2**.
4. Immerse slides in 70% ethanol for 5 min.
5. Repeat **step 4**.
6. Air-dry slides.
7. Place slides in the pressure cooker in Coplin jars filled with Reveal solution. Boil 2 min at 120°C (*see* **Note 1**).
8. Allow slides to cool down to room temperature.
9. Wash slides in distilled water for 5 min.
10. Wash slides in PBS for 5 min.
11. Apply dropwise Digest-All III solution onto slides. Incubate 3–5 min at room temperature (*see* **Note 1**).
12. Wash 5 min in PBS.
13. Dehydrate slides in graded ethanols (70–99.5%, 2 min each) and air-dry.
14. Apply 10- to 15-μL probe solution (Zymed Spot-Light series) and seal the slides under UnderCover Slips (*see* **Note 2**).
15. Denature probe and target DNA by placing slides on a thermal plate, 94°C for 3 min (*see* **Note 3**).
16. Hybridize overnight at 37°C.
17. Remove UnderCover Slips and wash with 0.5X SSC buffer for 5 min at 75°C.
18. Wash with TBS buffer, 5 min at room temperature.
19. Apply mouse antidigoxigenin antibody (diluted 1:300 in the Powervision+ blocking solution). Incubate for 20–30 min at room temperature (*see* **Note 4**).
20. Wash for 5 min with TBS.
21. Apply Powervision+ postantibody blocking solution, incubate 10–20 min at room temperature (*see* **Note 4**).
22. Wash 5 min with TBS.
23. Apply Powervision+ poly-HRP-goat-x-mouse polymer. Incubate 20–30 min at room temperature (*see* **Note 4**).
24. Wash 5 min with TBS.
25. Prepare the Powervision+ DAB solution: 1000 μL distilled water + 50 μL DAB reagent A + 50 μL DAB reagent B. Apply onto slides and incubate 5 min at room temperature.
26. Wash 1 min with H_2O.
27. Perform counterstaining with standard hematoxylin. Incubate for 5–10 s at room temperature.
28. Wash slides with H_2O.

Table 3
Probe Detection in CISH

	Steps in probe detection			
Probe label	1st layer	2nd layer	Chromogen	Sensitivity
Digoxigenin	Anti-digoxigenin–HRP	None	DAB	+/–
Digoxigenin	Mouse anti-digoxigenin	Anti-mouse HRP[a] polymer	DAB	+++
Digoxigenin	Mouse anti-digoxigenin	Anti-mouse AP polymer	Fast Red	+++
Digoxigenin	Anti-digoxigenin FITC	Anti-FITC–HRP	DAB	+/++
Biotin	Mouse anti-biotin	Anti-mouse HRP polymer	DAB	+++
Biotin	Streptavidin–HRP	None	DAB	+/–

[a] Using PicTure (Zymed); EnVision+ (Dako); Powervision+ (ImmunoVision).
[b]Powervision (ImmunoVision).

29. Dehydrate slides with graded ethanols and xylene (or xylene substitute) and mount with any permanent mounting medium.

4. Notes

1. Formalin and embedding in paraffin require one to use specific pretreatments to uncover the DNA sequences. Common to all pretreatment methods is enzymatic digestion to dissolve DNA protein crosslinks and high-temperature incubation to restore DNA in hybridizable configuration. The most efficient heat treatment is boiling in an autoclave or pressure cooker in various buffer solutions. The success rate in CISH using the described protocol is over 95%.
2. The Zymed probes work well in CISH. The repetitive DNA sequences have been removed from the clone DNA by subtractive hybridization *(5)*. CISH can be successfully performed with conventional repeat-containing DNA probes as well. The different probes used so far in CISH are listed in **Table 1**.
3. For practical reasons, the probe and the target DNA denaturation is carried out simultaneously after applying the probe on the slide.
4. The most critical step in CISH is the probe detection, which must be highly sensitive to produce clearly visible signals. Early experiments with simple one-layer protocols (anti-digoxigenin–peroxidase or streptavidin–peroxidase) were unsuccessful. To increase the detection sensitivity, a two-layer antibody approach was introduced and successfully used in CISH of clinical tumor samples *(4)* (*see* **Table 3**). A major improvement in detection sensitivity was incorporation of the antibody–HRP-containing polymers (trade names Powervision™, PicTure™, EnVision™). The choice of the reporter enzyme (HRP or alkaline phosphatase) seem to result in similar signal brightness. A CISH modification using tyramide-

based probe detection has recently been published *(16)*. The different detection schemes and their relative sensitivity are compared in **Table 2**.

References

1. Gall, J. G. and Pardue, M. L. (1969) Formation and detection of RNA–DNA hybrid molecules in cytological specimens. *PNAS* **63,** 378–383.
2. Pinkel, D., Straume, T., and Gray, J. (1986) Cytogenetic analysis using quantitative high sensitivity fluorecense hybridization. *PNAS* **83,** 2934–2938.
3. Hopman, A. H., Claessen, S., and Speel, E. J. (1997) Multi-colour brightfield *in situ* hybridisation on tissue sections. *Histochem. Cell. Biol.* **108,** 291–298.
4. Tanner, M., Gancberg, D., Di Leo, A., et al. (2000) Chromogenic *in situ* hybridization (CISH): a practical new alternative for FISH in detection of HER-2/neu oncogene amplification. *Am. J. Pathol.* **157,** 1467–1472.
5. Davison, J. M., Morgan, T. W., Hsi, B. L., et al. (1998) Subtracted, unique-sequence, *in situ* hybridization: experimental and diagnostic applications. *Am. J. Pathol.* **153,** 1401–1409.
6. Tanner, M., Järvinen, P., and Isola, J. (2001) Amplification of HER-2/neu and topoisomerase IIα in primary and metastatic breast cancer. *Cancer Res.* **61,** 5345–5348.
7. Pauletti, G., Godolphin, W., Press, M. F., et al. (1996) Detection and quantitation of HER-2/neu gene amplification in human breast cancer archival material using fluorescence *in situ* hybridization. *Oncogene* **13,** 63–72.
8. Press, M. F., Bernstein, L., Thomas, P. A., et al. (1997) HER-2/neu gene amplification characterized by fluorescence *in situ* hybridization: poor prognosis in node-negative breast carcinomas. *J. Clin. Oncol.* **15,** 2894–2904.
9. Ross, J. S. and Fletcher, J. A. (1999) HER-2/neu (c-erb-B2) gene and protein in breast cancer. *Am. J. Clin. Pathol.* **112,** S53–S67.
10. Dandachi, N., Dietze, O., and Hauser-Kronberger, C. (2002) Chromogenic *in situ* hybridization: a novel approach to a practical and sensitive method for the detection of HER2 oncogene in archival human breast carcinoma. *Lab. Invest.* **82(8),** 1007–1014.
11. Isola, J., Tanner, M., Salminen, T., et al. HER-2/neu oncogene status by chromogenic *in situ* hybridization and immunohistochemistry: a study on 1,728 breast cancer patients. (Submitted.)
12. Kumamoto, H., Sasano, H., Taniguchi, T., et al. (2001) Chromogenic *in situ* hybridization analysis of HER-2/neu status in breast carcinoma: application in screening of patients for trastuzumab (Herceptin) therapy. *Pathol. Int.* **51(8),** 579–584
13. Rummukainen, J., Salminen, T., Lundin, J., et al. (2001) Comparison of c-myc oncogene amplification by chromogenic *in situ* hybridization (CISH) and FISH in archival breast cancer tissue array samples. *Lab. Invest.* **81,** 1545–1552.
14. Savinainen, K., Linja, M., Saramäki, O., et al. (2002) Expression and gene copy number analysis of ERBB2 oncogene in prostate cancer. *Am. J. Pathol.* **160,** 339–345.

15. Tanskanen, M., Jahkola, T., Asko-Seljavaara, S., et al. (2003) HER-2 oncogene amplification in extramammary Paget's disease. *Histopathology,* in press.
16. Tubbs, R., Pettay, J., Skacel, M., et al. (2002) Gold-facilitated *in situ* hybridization: a bright-field autometallographic alternative to fluorescence *in situ* hybridization for detection of Her-2/neu gene amplification. *Am. J. Pathol.* **160(5),** 1589–1595.
17. Zhao, J., Wu, R., Au, A., et al. (2002) Determination of HER2 gene amplification by chromogenic *in situ* hybridization (CISH) in archival breast carcinoma. *Mod. Pathol.* **15(6),** 657–665.

11

Comparative Genomic Hybridization and Fluorescence *In Situ* Hybridization in Chronic Lymphocytic Leukemia

Marie Jarosova

1. Introduction

The first reported recurring chromosome aberrations in B-cell chronic lymphocytic leukemia (B-CLL) were published in the early 1980s. Over the past 10 yr, a number of studies ***(1–4)*** as well as data from the International Workshop on Chromosomes in CLL ***(5)*** confirmed that the chromosomal changes in B-cells are frequent and, using modern molecular cytogenetic techniques, genomic aberrations can be diagnosed in approx 80% of CLL patients ***(6,7)***. The genomic regions recurrently affected by chromosomal deletions, trisomies, and, less frequently, translocations probably contain tumor suppressor genes and oncogenes. The identification of these changes is important for the understanding of the pathogenesis of the disease and has prognostic information, which is independent from that obtained by the conventional clinical markers.

The methodological aspects of genetic analysis in CLL have shown that conventional chromosomal banding analysis showed a normal karyotype because of its limits caused by the low in vitro mitotic activity of clonal B-cells. Using solely conventional cytogenetics, clonal abnormalities were detected in only 40–50% of patients ***(6)***.

The introduction of new molecular cytogenetic methods, such as fluorescence *in situ* hybridization (FISH) and comparative genomic hybridization (CGH), has greatly improved our ability to detect chromosomal changes in tumor cells.

1.1. Fluorescence In Situ *Hybridization in CLL*

Fluoresence *in situ* hybridization (FISH) is a molecular cytogenetic technique enabling determination of specific nucleotide sequences in chromo-

From: *Methods in Molecular Medicine, vol. 79: Molecular Diagnosis of Cancer*
Edited by: J. E. Roulston and J. M. S. Bartlett © Humana Press Inc., Totowa, NJ

somes, cells, and tissues. The principle of this technique is based on the ability of single-stranded DNA, called probe, to hybridize to target DNA and complete double-stranded DNA according to the complementarity of bases.

One of the greatest advances in cytogenetic analysis facilitated by FISH has been the ability to examine nondividing cells as targets. This enables the screening of large numbers of cells and provides access to a variety of sources of hemopoietic cells. The main advantage is to examine hematological malignancies characterized by low proliferative and mitotic activity. Such an example is CLL.

Data published by Döhner et al. *(6)* show that genomic aberrations can be detected in 82% of the cases analyzed. Based on the conventional cytogenetics, trisomy of chromosome 12 was the first abnormality reported to be associated with shorter survival *(5)*. Other aberrations associated with inferior prognosis are 17p and 11q deletions *(2,3,5–9)*. In contrast, patients with aberrations of chromosome 13, mostly deletion of 13q, and patients with normal karyotype seemed to have a favorable prognosis *(7)*. The most frequent aberrations detected in CLL patients are 13q deletion (55%), followed by 11q deletion (18%), 12q trisomy (16%), and 17p deletion (7%) *(6,10,11)*. Multivariate analysis identified six significant prognostic factors: 17p deletion, 11q deletion, age, Binet stage, serum lactate dehydrogenase level, and white blood cell count. As genomic aberrations represent important independent prognostic factors for the progression of the disease as well as for the survival, the determination of these changes have to be part of diagnostic and follow-up laboratory examinations. The routine diagnostic assessment for the determination of frequent chromosomal changes in CLL is FISH.

1.2. Comparative Genomic Hybridization in CLL

Because most aberrations detected in CLL patients are unbalanced changes, CGH is a useful method for the detection of such aberrations, too *(9,10)*. The CGH method was introduced to detect regions in the genome of tumor cells undergoing quantitative changes—gain and losses of copy number. Two different green and red probes prepared from normal (reference) and tumor (tested) DNA are mixed in equal amounts and hybridized to normal metaphase chromosomes mounted on glass slides *(11–13)*.

The advantage of CGH is that it requires only genomic DNA from tumor and normal tissue. CGH has its limitations: It cannot detect balanced chromosomal translocations, inversion, point mutation, and aberrations present in low frequency, such as in multiclonal tumors. The detection limit is 2–10 megabases (Mb).

The method involves the following work procedure. Reference DNA from healthy donors and tumor DNA from fresh, cryopreserved, or paraffin-embedded tumor samples are isolated using standard molecular genetic methods ***(14)***. The tumor (test) DNA is usually labeled using the nick-translation method with green fluorescence, whereas the normal (reference) one is then labeled with red fluorescence. After nick translation, the probes are prepared for hybridization and are then cohybridized for 48–72 h to normal metaphase chromosome on a slide with the presence of Cot-1 DNA to block repetitive sequences. After finishing the hybridization by washing the slides in wash solution to remove unhybridized probes, the result of the hybridization is evaluated in a fluorescence microscope using an appropriate software program.

2. Materials

2.1. FISH

1. SuperFrost microscope slides (e.g., Menzel-Glaser, Germany).
2. Coverslips.
3. Water bath (capable of heating to 100°C).
4. 37°C Incubator.
5. Fluorescence microscope with an appropriate set of filters.

2.1.1. Preparation of Slides for FISH, Pretreatment, and Denaturation

1. 3:1 (v/v) Absolute methanol:glacial acetic acid fixative, freshly prepared and refrigerated before use.
2. Coplin jars containing 100%, 85%, and 70% ethanol (EtOH) at ambient temperature.
3. RNAse: Mix 25 mg RNAse (Cambio Ltd., UK) and 5 mL Tris-HCl, and allow to boil in water bath for 15 min. Add 2X SSC solution to bring it up to 250 mL.
4. 20X SSC: Dissolve 132 g of 20X SSC (Vysis Inc., USA) in 500 mL of purified H_2O and adjust pH to 5.3 with HCl.
5. 2X SSC: Prepare 500 mL of 2X SSC by adding 50 mL of 20X SSC and 450 mL of distilled water. Verify the solution is pH 5.3 before use.
6. Denaturation solution (*see* **Note 1**): Mix thoroughly 49 mL of formamide, 7 mL of 20X SSC (pH 5.3), and 14 mL purified H_2O. Verify pH, which is to be 7.0–7.8. Place the Coplin jars with formamide in a 73±1°C water bath about half an hour before the denaturation in order to bring the solution to the required temperature.

2.1.2. Preparation of the FISH Probe Mix

1. Centromeric probe chromosome 12 (CEP 12; Vysis Inc., USA).
2. LSI p53 probe (Vysis Inc., USA).
3. Dual-color LSI RB1 probe (Vysis Inc., USA).
4. Dual-color LSI MLL probe (Vysis Inc., USA).
5. LSI hybridization buffer and/or CEP hybridization buffer (Vysis Inc., USA).
6. Purified H_2O.

2.1.3. FISH Posthybridization Washes, Detection, and Evaluation of Hybridization

1. 0.4X SSC/0.3% NP40: Prepare 0.4X SSC/0.3% NP40 by adding: 20 mL of 20X SSC (pH 5.3), 950 mL purified water, 3 mL NP40. Mix thoroughly and add H_2O to bring the solution up to the total volume of 1 L.
2. 2X SSC/0.1% NP40: Prepare 2X SSC/0.1% NP40 by adding: 100 mL of 20X SSC (pH 5.3), 1 mL of NP40. Add H_2O to bring it up to the total volume of 1 L and adjust pH to 7.0. Use this wash solution at ambient temperature.
3. DAPI II: 125 mg DAPI/mL in antifade mounting solution (Vysis Inc., USA).

2.2. CGH Materials

1. Water bath.
2. 37°C incubator.
3. Slide warmer.

2.2.1. Isolation of Tumor (Test) DNA

DNA isolation kit (Gentra Inc., USA).

2.2.2. Labeling of DNA Using Nick Translation

1. SpectrumRed™ normal female total human genomic DNA, 100 ng/μL (Vysis Inc., USA).
2. SpectrumRed™ normal male total human genomic DNA, 100 ng/μL (Vysis Inc., USA).
3. CGH nick translation kit (Vysis Inc., USA) includes nick translation enzyme, 10X nick translation buffer, dTTP, dCTP, dATP, dGTP, nuclease-free water, CGH hybridization buffer.
4. 0.2 m*M* SpectrumGreen dUTP: Add 10 μL of 1 mM dUTP to 40 μL of nuclease-free water.
5. 0.1 m*M* dTTP: Add 10 μL of 0.3 m*M* dTTP to 20 μL of nuclease-free water.
6. 0.1 m*M* dNTP mix: Mix together 10 μL each of 0.3 m*M* dCTP, dGTP, and dATP.

2.2.3. Denaturation of CGH Target Slide

1. CGH metaphase target slides (Vysis Inc., USA).
2. Denaturation solution: 49 mL deionized formamide, 7 mL of 20X SSC (pH 5.3), 14 mL purified H_2O; mix and verify that pH is 7.0–7.5 at ambient temperature.
3. 70%, 80%, and 100% Ethanol: Dilute 100% ethanol (v/v) with purified H_2O to prepare 70%, 80%, and 100% ethanol (EtOH).
4. 20X SSC (pH 5.3): Dissolve 66 g of 20X SSC (Vysis Inc., USA) in 200 mL purified water, fill to 250 mL, and adjust to pH 5.3 using concentrated HCl.

2.2.4. Preparation and Denaturation of CGH Probe

1. Human Cot-1® DNA (Gibco-BRL, USA).

2. 3*M* Sodium acetate (NaAc) (pH 5.5).
3. 100% EtOH.

2.2.5. CGH Hybridization and Posthybridization Washing

1. Rubber cement.
2. NP40.
3. 0.4X SSC/0.3 NP40 wash solution: Mix 20 mL of 20X SSC with 950 mL purified H_2O and add 3 mL NP40. Mix to dissolve NP40.
4. 2X SSC/0.1% NP40 wash solution: Mix 100 mL 20X SSC with 850 mL purified H_2O and add 1 mL of NP40. Mix and add purified H_2O to bring it up to the total volume to 1 L. Adjust pH to 7.0–7.5 using NaOH.
5. Counterstaining: DAPI II (4, 6-diamidino-2-phenylindole) (Vysis Inc., USA).

2.2.6. Evaluation of CGH Results

1. Fluorescence microscope with appropriate set of fluorescence filters.
2. Cooled CCD camera.
3. CGH software program based on an image analysis (e.g., MetaSystems, Germany).

3. Methods

3.1. FISH Method

The cells prepared for FISH analysis are treated to facilitate disruption of the cell membrane. This procedure is important for successful FISH. Undisrupted cell membranes prevent the probe from penetrating into cell nuclei. Cell nuclei and chromosomes are applied to slides, which are then allowed to dry at room temperature. Heating of the slides is not recommended for *in situ* hybridization. The preparation is pretreated using RNAse, dehydrated, and allowed to dry at ambient temperature. The slides are denatured and hybridized using the denatured probe mix. After the hybridization, excess unhybridized probe is removed using series of washes. All probes used are directly labeled. Visualization is made in fluorescence microscope with the appropriate set of fluorescence filters.

3.1.1. Preparation of Specimen Target and Pretreatment

1. Cell suspension prepared by a conventional cytogenetic procedure (peripheral blood, bone marrow, or lymph node), wash by adding fresh 3:1 fixative and drop the cells without baking onto SuperFrost slides.
2. Check the area under the microscope to evaluate cell density and mark area to be hybridized with a diamond-tipped pen.
3. Allow the slide to dry at room temperature.
4. Immerse the dried and marked specimen slide in RNAse for 1 h at 37°C.

5. Dehydrate the slide for 1 min in 70% EtOH, followed by 1 min in 85% EtOH, and 1 min in 100% EtOH.
6. Allow the slide to dry at room temperature.

3.1.2. Denaturation of Specimen Target

1. Ensure that the temperature of the denaturation solution is 73±1°C.
2. Immerse the slides in the denaturation solution for 5 min.
3. Immediately dehydrate the slides for 1 min in 70%, 80%, and, finally, in 100% EtOH at room temperature.
4. Allow the slide to dry at room temperature.

3.1.3. Preparation of the Probe Mix

1. Add the following components to a microcentrifuge tube at room temperature (per slide):
   7 µL LSI hybridization buffer and/or CEP hybridization buffer
   1 µL LSI probe or CEP probe
   2 µL purified H_2O.
2. Vortex gently and centrifuge the tube for 1–3 s.
3. Vortex and then centrifuge again.
4. Place the tube in a 73±1°C water bath for 5 min.
5. Remove the tube from the water bath.
6. Immediately apply the probe to the slide.

3.1.4. Hybridization

1. Prepare humidified box and prewarm in 37°C incubator.
2. Apply 10 µL of the probe mixture to the target area on the slide and cover this area by a coverslip immediately.
3. Seal the coverslip using rubber cement, place the slide in the humidified box, and allow it to hybridize in 37°C incubator for 16–20 h.

3.1.5. Posthybridization Washes and Detection

1. Fill one Coplin jar with the 0.4X SSC/0.3% NP40 and place in 73±1°C water bath at least 30 min before using.
2. Carefully remove the rubber cement and cover slip using forceps and immediately transfer the slide to a Coplin jar containing 0.4X SSC/0.3% NP40. Agitate the slide for 20 s and then let it stand for 2 min.
3. Immerse the slide in 2X SSC/0.1% NP40. Agitate the slide for 20 s and then let it stand for 1 min.
4. Dry the slides by resting the lower edge of the slide on a blotter and then let them dry in darkness.
5. Apply 10 µL of counterstaining DAPI II (Vysis Inc., USA) and cover with cover slip.

3.1.6. Evaluation of the Results

In order to evaluate the results of hybridization, a fluorescence microscope with an appropriate set of filters is used. In the hybridized area, at least 300–500 interphase cells are evaluated. Because positive signals (e.g., for the deletion of RB1 gene can be detected in only a proportion of the potential targets), a cutoff level must be developed.

For each rank of probe, the determination of cutoff level is based on the data specified in the protocol supplied with the probe as well as on the results of control hybridizations with normal cells from a healthy donor. In order to minimize false-positive or false-negative results, the probes are combined. For example, hybridization with probe p53 (labeled with SpectrumRed) is combined with the centromere for chromosome 12 (labeled with SpectrumGreen), or the probe for the centromere of chromosome 12 is hybridized with RB1 probe. Both combined probes are always labeled with different fluorochromes. Currently, for visualization and evaluation of fluorescent signals, the different imaging systems are used. These systems allow the use of high-performance cooled charge-coupled device (CCD) camera analysis of even the weakest signals and digital archiving of the results of FISH.

3.2. CGH Methods

3.2.1. Extraction of DNA

The DNA for CGH should be of a high quality. It is possible to use a number of commercially available kits (Gibco or Gentra, USA) or use an in-house extraction procedure. High-quality DNA is obtained using standard phenol:chloroform extraction ***(14)***.

The quality and quantity of DNA is measured using spectrophotometers. Approximately 500 ng to 1 μg of DNA is recommended for CGH hybridization for a patient. It is important to remember that some volume of DNA is lost during the whole procedure. Therefore, at least 1.7 μg of DNA is required for the analysis.

3.2.2. Nick-Translation Procedure

The nick-translation labeling kit efficiently incorporates fluorescent-labeled dUTP into genomic DNA by nick translation. The optimal size of labeled DNA for CGH is 300–3000 bp (*see* **Fig. 1**). In CGH analysis, the test (tumor) DNA is labeled with SpectrumGreen, whereas the normal (reference) DNA is labeled with SpectrumRed (commercially available from Vysis Inc., USA).

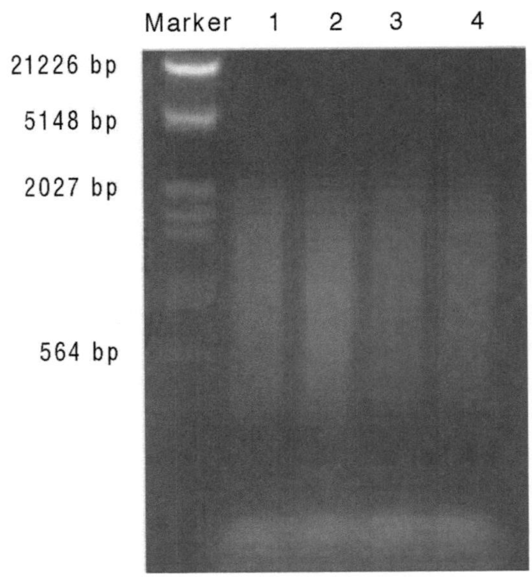

Fig. 1. The result of nick translation after agarose gel electrophoresis. Line 1 represents Lambda DNA/*Eco*RI+*Hin*dIII marker and in lines 2–4 are different test DNAs after nick translation in the range of 300–3000 bp.

1. Place a microtube (500 µL) on ice and allow the tube to cool.
2. Add the following components to the tube in the order listed:

   (17.5–x) µL nuclease-free water
   x µL for 1.7 µg of extracted genomic DNA
   2.5 µL of 0.2 m*M* SpectrumGreen dUTP
   5 µL of 0.1 m*M* dTTP
   10 µL of dNTP mix
   5 µL of 10X nick-translation buffer
   10 µL of nick-translation enzyme

   ---

   350 µL total volume

3. Vortex the tube briefly.
4. Incubate for 1–3 h at 15°C.
5. Check the size of DNA probe on the gel.
6. Allow the probe to stand on ice in the dark until reaction ceases.
7. After checking the results on gel, stop the reaction by heating in a 70°C water bath for 10 min.
8. Chill on ice.

3.2.3. Determination of Probe Size

Determination of the probe size is an essential part of the CGH procedure. This is provided on gel (for detailed instructions for preparing and running an agarose gel, see original Nick Translation Kit protocol from Vysis Inc., USA).

1. Prepare 1% agarose gel by adding 1 g agarose to 100 mL of TBE or TAE buffer ***(14)***. Heat the solution in the microwave to melt agarose.
2. Cool agarose solution to 55°C and add 10 µL of EtBr (ethidium bromide in final concentration of 0.01% [v/v]).
3. Pour the agarose into a gel-running apparatus with comb and allow agarose to cool until solid.
4. Pour enough TBE buffer into gel-running apparatus to cover the gel by approx 5 mm.
5. Remove 7 µL of the reaction mix containing the nick-translated DNA and add 1 µL of gel-loading buffer.
6. Run the samples in one lane, and as in the first lane, a sample of the DNA size marker to size the probe.
7. Run the gel at 10 V/cm until the gel-loading buffer is 2–3 cm from the end of the gel.
8. Check the results of nick translation by finding DNA smear in the 300- to 3000-bp range (*see* **Fig. 1**).
9. To produce smaller probe fragments, you can increase the amount of the enzyme or lengthen the time of nick translation.

3.2.4. Preparation of the Probe Mix

1. Combine the following components in a microcentrifuge tube:
   a. 20 µL (400 ng) of SpectrumGreen-labeled tumor (tested) DNA
   b. 1 µL (100 ng) of SpectrumRed total genomic reference DNA (Vysis Inc., USA)
   c. 10 µL (10 µg) of human Cot-1 DNA
   d. Mix gently and add 3.1 µL (0.1 volume) of sodium acetate, then add 77.5 µL (2.5 vol) of 100% ethanol to precipitate the DNA. Vortex briefly and place on dry ice or at –70°C for 30 min.
2. Centrifuge at 3000*g* for 30 min at 4°C to pellet DNA.
3. Discard the supernatant and let the pellet dry for 10 min in a vacuum drier.
4. Prepare the probe mix by resuspending the pellet in 3 µL of purified water and 7 µL of CGH hybridization buffer (Vysis Inc., USA). Mix gently, centrifuge, and let stand at 4°C overnight so that DNA dissolves well.

3.2.5. Denaturation of the Target Metaphase

1. Mark the hybridization area on the slide using a diamond-tipped pen.
2. Heat the denaturation solution to 73±1°C. Immerse the slide containing normal metaphase spread into the solution for 5 min.

3. Dehydrate the slides in 70%, 80%, and 100% EtOH, for 1 min each.
4. Dry the slide by resting the bottom edge on a blotter and place the slide in a slide warmer at 40°C to allow the remaining EtOH to evaporate. Allow to stand in slide warmer until used.

3.2.6. Denaturation of the Probe and Hybridization of the Probe to the Target Metaphase

1. On the following day, continue by denaturating the probe mix by heating it for 5 min in a 73±1°C water bath.
2. Immediately apply 10 μL of denatured probe mix to the slide.
3. Immediately apply the coverslip and seal with rubber cement.
4. Place the slide a in sealed, humidified box and place it in a 39°C incubator for 48–72 h for hybridization.

3.2.7. Washing the Slide

1. Place the Coplin jar containing 0.4X SSC/0.3% NP40 wash solution in a 74±1°C water bath for at least 30 min before using.
2. Remove the rubber cement seal and the cover slip and immediately place the slide into the 0.4X SSC/0.3% NP40 wash solution at 74±1°C. Agitate the slides for 10–20 s and then allow to stand for 2 min. (Repeat this step for each slide but do not wash more than four slides at once.)
3. Remove the slide in the 2X SSC/0,1% NP40 wash solution at room temperature. Agitate the slide for 10–20 s and then allow to stand for 1 min.
4. Dry the slide by resting the bottom edge on a blotter and place the slide in darkness to dry at ambient temperature.

3.2.8. Visualizing of Hybridization

1. Apply 10 μL of DAPI II counterstain (Vysis Inc., USA) and cover with coverslip.
2. View the results of hybridization in the fluorescence microscope using recommended set of fluorescence filters (Vysis Inc., USA).

3.2.9. Evaluation and Interpretation of the Results

Evaluation is based on an appropriate software program developed on the basis of image analysis. Software is used to acquire the metaphase image and to determine the ratio profile of the fluorescence intensities and a statistical analysis of the ratio. Chromosomes are counterstained with DAPI, resulting in a Q bandinglike pattern that is used for chromosome identification. After karyotyping each metaphase, the software program then calculates the intensity profiles of the SpectrumGreen and SpectrumRed images of the tumor and control DNA for each chromosome. Ratio profiles of each individual chromosome is calculated using a dedicated software. For each case, the mean ratio profiles from at least 10 metaphase cells are computed. Thresholds for the identifica-

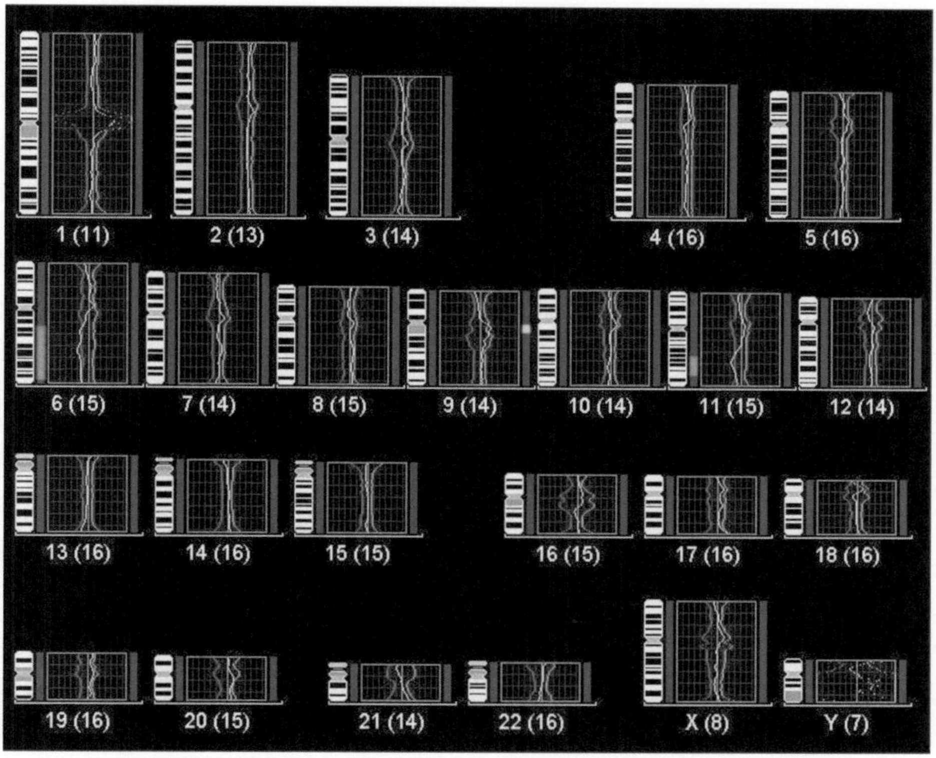

Fig. 2. The average ratio profile in patient suffering from CLL shows deletion of chromosome 6q and deletion of chromosome 11q.

tion of imbalances are defined as 0.75 (lower threshold) and 1.25 (upper threshold). These are the theoretical values that identify in diploid tumor cell population monosomy and trisomy present in 50% of the test cells. The chromosomes and chromosomal regions with a ratio outside of this thresholds are considered to be underrepresented or overrepresented (*see* **Fig. 2**) The value 1 is used to indicate that no change in copy number has occurred.

A CGH analysis results in the determination of relative DNA sequence copy number and diploid tumors cannot be distinguished from tetraploid tumors because there is no difference in the green and red ratio across the chromosomes. Other limitations include the cautious evaluation of changes in the profile ratio in the chromosome telomere regions and/or in the heterochromatic pericentromeric regions on chromosomes 1, 9, 16, and Y. Labeling artifacts that lead to a spurious profile ratio in the CG-rich regions on chromosomes 1pter, 19, and 22 are also common. Several factors influencing the results of CGH analysis were recognized and it is therefore recommended to verify the results using control hybridization with total genomic DNA with known unbalanced changes (e.g., SpectrumGreen MPE 600 DNA extracted from female breast cancer cell line; Vysis Inc., USA).

To date, CGH has been an important laboratory tool improving cytogenetic analysis of many tumors, including CLL *(9,10,15)*. As a routine method, it is a rapid strategy for the screening of chromosomal imbalances and their chromosomal locations.

4. Notes

1. The denaturation solutions contain formamide, a teratogen. Swallowing, inhalation, and absorption through the skin should be avoided. Any work must be performed with safety glasses, pipets, and gloves.

References

1. Gahrton, G., Robért, K. H., Friberg, K., et al. (1980) Nonrandom chromosomal aberrations in chronic lymphocytic leukemia revealed by polyclonal B-cell-mitogen stimulation. *Blood* **56,** 640–647.
2. Bird, M. L.,Ueshima, Y., Rowley, J. D., et al. (1989) Chromosome abnormalities in B cell chronic lymphocytic leukemia and their clinical correlations. *Leukemia* **3,** 182–191.
3. Döhner, H., Stilgenbauer, S., Fischer, K., et al. (1997) Cytogenetic and molecular cytogenetic analysis of B cell chronic lymphocytic leukemia: specific chromosome aberrations identify prognostic subgroups of patients and point to loci of candidate genes. *Leukemia* **11,** S19–S24.
4. Matutes, E., Oscier, D., Garcia-Marco, J., et al. (1996) Trisomy 12 defined a group of CLL with atypical morphology: correlation between cytogenetic, clinical and laboratory features in 544 patients. *Br. J. Haematol.* **92,** 382–388.
5. Juliusson, G., Oscier, D., Gahrton, G., for the International Working Party on Chromosomes in CLL (IWCCLL). (1991) Cytogenetic findings and survival in B-cell chronic lymphocytic leukemia. Second IWCCLL compilation of data on 662 patients. *Leuk. Lymphoma* **5,** 21–25.
6. Döhner, H., Stilgenbauer, S., Benner A., et al. (2000) Genomic aberrations and survival in chronic lymphocytic leukemia. *N. Engl. J. Med.* **343,** 1910–1916.
7. Juliusson, G., Oscier, D., Fitchett, M., et al. (1990) Prognostic subgroups in B-cell chronic lymphocytic leukaemia defined by specific chromosomal abnormalities. *N. Engl. J. Med.* **323,** 720–724.
8. Döhner, H., Fisher, K., Benz, M., et al. (1995) p53 gene deletion predict for poor survival and non-response to therapy with purine analogs in chronic B-cell leukemias. *Blood* **85,** 1580.
9. Jarosová, M., Jedlicková, K., Holzerová, M., et al. (2001) Contribution of comparative genomic hybridization and fluorescence *in situ* hybridization to the detection of chromosomal abnormalities in B-cell chronic lymphocytic leukemia. *Onkologie* **24,** 60–65.

10. Bentz, M., Huck, K., du Manoir, S., et al. (1995) Comparative genomic hybridization in chronic B-cell leukemias shows a high incidence of chromosomal gains and losses. *Blood* **85,** 3610–3618.
11. Kallioniemi, A., Kallioniemi, O. P., Sidar, D., et al. (1992) Comparative genomic hybridization for molecular cytogenetic analysis of solid tumors. *Science* **258,** 818–821.
12. Du Manoir, S., Schröck, E., Benz, M., et al. (1995) Quantitative analysis of comparative genomic hybridization. *Cytometry* **19,** 27–41.
13. Lichter, P., Joos, S., Bentz, M., et al. (2000) Comparative genomic hybridization: use and limitation. *Semin. Hematol.* **37,** 348–357.
14. Maniatis, T., Fritsch, E. F., and Sambrook, J. (1982) in *Molecular Cloning. A Laboratory Manual, 9th ed.,* Cold Spring Harbor Laboratory Press, New York, NY.
15. Werner, C. A., Döhner, H., Joos, S., et al. (1991) High-level DNA amplifications are common genetic aberrations in B-cell neoplasms. *Am. J. Pathol.* **51,** 335–342.

12

Molecular Characterization of Human Papillomaviruses by PCR and *In Situ* Hybridization

Suzanne D. Vernon and Elizabeth R. Unger

1. Introduction

The goal of early detection and screening is the diagnosis and treatment of cancer before it spreads beyond the organ of origin, perhaps even in its preinvasive state. Unfortunately, available early detection and screening techniques pick up many tumors at a relatively late stage in their natural history. As a result, decrements in mortality even with the best available detection modalities are likely to be modest. On the other hand, some early detection and screening techniques identify changes with a low probability of progression to life-threatening cancer, thereby resulting in unnecessary diagnosis and overtreatment. New technologies coming from the field of molecular and cellular biology are able to identify genetic as well as antigenic changes during the early stages of malignant progression. Some of these changes show promise as biomarkers for preneoplastic development or for malignant transformation.

Early detection technologies are rapidly evolving while existing technologies are undergoing progressive refinement in their sensitivity, specificity, and throughput. Improved analytic tools have allowed more detailed examination of the molecular basis of carcinogenesis and provided the ability to identify the molecular and cellular signatures of cancer and explore gene–environment interaction relevant to early detection. To fully explore the application of molecular profiles for earlier detection, it is essential to understand the molecular pathogenesis of cancer (i.e., the natural history of tumor progression at the molecular level), so that the biological behavior of an evolving lesion (e.g., dysplasia or field change) can be predicted with greater accuracy. Cur-

From: *Methods in Molecular Medicine, vol. 79: Molecular Diagnosis of Cancer*
Edited by: J. E. Roulston and J. M. S. Bartlett © Humana Press Inc., Totowa, NJ

rent observations indicate that cancers usually evolve through many complex cellular processes, pathways, and networks. A better understanding of the circuits in these pathways is critical if we are to successfully apply these molecular-based technologies to earlier detection.

Cervical cancer is a malignancy whose preinvasive lesions are well described as a result of the relative accessibility of the affected organ and because of over 50 yr experience with cytologic and histologic correlations with biologic behavior. Progressive reduction in the incidence and mortality of cervical cancer in the United States occurred at the same time that widespread cervical cytology screening (Pap smear) was being introduced. This led to the optimistic belief that cervical cancer could be eliminated with improved screening practices and outreach to high-risk populations. Although impressive reductions in cervical cancer mortality have been achieved, cervical cancer remains a significant public health problem. The American Cancer Society has estimated that in 1999 there were 12,800 new cases in the United States, resulting in 4800 deaths *(1)*.

It is now known that of the more than 100 closely related human papillomavirus (HPV) types, at least 30 can be found in the genital tract *(2)*. The types found in cancers or those having phylogenetic similarity to those found in cancers are referred to as "high-risk" types. There are numerous epidemiologic studies indicating the central role of HPV infection in cervical neoplasia *(3–6)*, plausible molecular mechanisms for viral oncogenesis have been described *(7–10)*, and the immortalizing and transforming capacity of HPV has been demonstrated using in vitro and model systems *(11–16)*.

Although much remains to be understood about HPV interactions with the host, the general course of infection is known. The virus is small and the outside of the virus particle is made up of two capsid proteins called L1 and L2. Inside the virus particle is a double-strand DNA molecular that is the viral genome encoding eight known viral genes (*see* **Fig. 1**). The L1 capsid gene is a highly conserved among papillomaviruses, and because of this sequence conservation, it is used as a target for consensus primer generation and amplification that will be discussed in this chapter. HPV infection is initiated in the basal layer of epithelium with the virus maintained as an episome. In common with other papillomaviruses, HPV is epitheliotropic. Viral replication and transcription are dependent on cellular enzymes, and both are linked to epithelial differentiation. Both cellular and viral proteins influence transcription by binding to the regulatory region located upstream of the major promoter. Accumulation of high copy numbers of viral DNA and RNA is restricted to the mature upper layers of the epithelium *(17)*.

Methods for diagnosing HPV are all dependent on detection of viral DNA. This is because the agent cannot be cultivated in routine tissue culture and

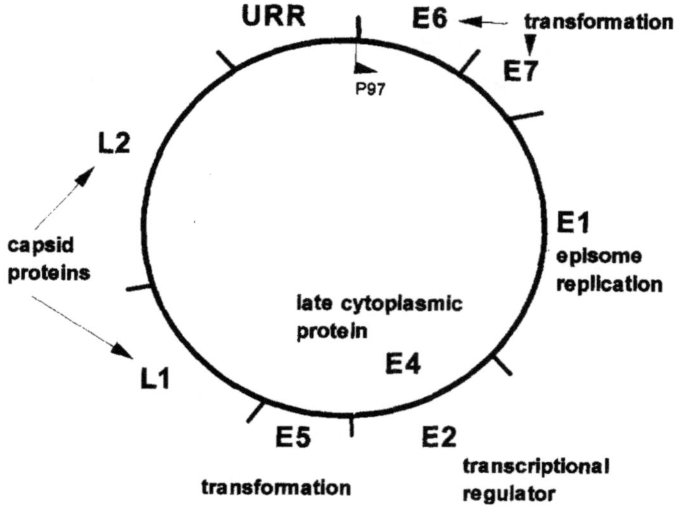

Fig. 1. The organization of the human papillomavirus genome. The double stranded viral DNA has eight open reading frames that code for eight proteins. The L1 gene is highly conserved among papillomaviruses and therefore is an ideal target for consensus PCR.

antibody methods lack sensitivity. Detection of HPV DNA therefore requires analysis of cellular material from the viral lesion. The assay format and sampling method influences how often HPV will be detected. In this chapter, we discuss several HPV consensus polymerase chain reaction (PCR) assays and present the method for a sensitive colorimetric *in situ* hybridization (ISH) assay. Both PCR and ISH assays can be used for DNA analysis in formalin-fixed archival tissues. Both assay formats require small amounts of tissue and thus conserve material essential for clinical management. In addition, both formats tolerate some degradation of target nucleic acids and can utilize nonradioactive detection methods ***(18)***.

2. PCR and the Sample

Similar to most viral infections, many more people are infected with HPVs than will ever experience disease. The significance of these subclinical HPV infections is not well understood, but there is evidence suggesting that persistence of HPV in a subclinical state increases the risk of cervical neoplasia ***(19)***. For this reason, any sample for use in HPV detection that is intended for screening or patient management should be representative of the disease process. In the case of cervical cancer, screening by cytology has been so effective because the sample is derived directly from the cervix. Yet, for HPV detection and typing, many different approaches have been used for sampling the cervix, ranging from self-sampling with a Dacron swab to cervical lavage. A recent study found only a 50% concordance between the HPV types detected in a self-collected sample compared to a physician-collected cervical sample ***(20)***. It is likely that automated, liquid-based cervical screening devices that use thin-layer cytology and HPV DNA testing will become the standard for routine primary screening for cervical cancer and its precursors. For this reason, it is critical that cervical sampling, cervical cytology, and cervical HPV testing become standardized and integrated.

Much has been done to standardize and integrate the cervical sampling approach for use in liquid-based cytology and HPV testing. Cervical sampling devices and collection jars with preservation media are sold as kits by several companies, such as Wellcerv LTD (Bridgewater, UK), CYTYC Corporation (Boxborough, MA, USA), and TriPath Imaging Inc. (Burlington, NC, USA). The preservation media in the collection vial fixes and disperses the cervical cells in preparation for thin-layer cytology. In addition to preserving cell morphology, the nucleic acid can be readily extracted from the preserved cells for HPV detection by PCR ***(21)***. Several commercially available DNA extraction kits are effective for obtaining ample DNA for HPV testing. For example, by extending the proteinase K digestion step of the QIAmp DNA Mini Kit (Qiagen Inc., Valencia, CA, USA) to overnight at 56°C rather than 1 h, a 250-μL aliquot of the 20-mL cervical cytology sample often yields several micrograms of DNA. Following isolation of the DNA, PCR inhibitors can be removed and the DNA concentrated using a centrifugal filter device such as a Centricon Centrifugal Filter Device YM-100 (Millipore Corp., Bedford, MA, USA). The small amount of preserved sample required for DNA extraction and HPV testing by PCR leaves sufficient sample for cytology and, if desired, ISH. Thus, from one cervical sample, there is integration of cytology and HPV testing, making this approach ideally suited for cervical cancer screening and patient management.

3. Technical Considerations for PCR

Once the DNA has been extracted from the cervical cytology sample, it is ready for HPV detection by PCR. PCR is an incredibly sensitive method capable of detecting a single molecule in a cell. For this reason, great care has to be taken when collecting and preparing the sample for HPV testing by PCR and an excellent technique is required when setting up the PCR to avoid contamination and the possibility of false-positive results. At least three distinct sites within the laboratory should be used for the different steps of routine PCR. All surfaces should be thoroughly cleaned with a DNA-contaminant-removal solution. The initial PCR preparation, including reagent master mixes, is completed in the first location. Test samples are added to the master mix in a second location. Amplified samples are handled and analyzed in the third location. Each location should have a dedicated set of micropipettors, and sterile, disposable, aerosol block tips should be used. A set of positive, negative, and contamination controls should be included for every 12 samples. For the HPV consensus PCR, an HPV-containing cell line such as SiHa or CaSki (both containing HPV 16) are good positive controls. Avoid the use of cloned HPV DNA unless used at a very high dilution, as the high copy number easily results in cross-contamination of samples. Human placental DNA is used as the negative control. A tube that contains all of the reagents, with water in place of the test sample, serves as the contamination control. Another important control performed on all samples in parallel with the HPV consensus PCR is amplification of a housekeeping gene such as β-globin. These reactions test for inhibitors or insufficient quantity of the test sample. Finally, it is very useful to run a water sample through the DNA extraction procedure along with the actual cervical samples. This water extraction sample should also go through the same HPV PCR and typing procedures and is an excellent way to monitor the source of any contamination that may occur during sample processing and extraction.

4. HPV Consensus PCR

There are several methods for amplifying HPV DNA in cervical cytology samples, but the fundamentals are similar for each: sample collection and processing, amplification, and characterization of the amplified product. Amplification of HPV DNA will occur in the presence of the target molecule (in this case, HPV), HPV sequence-specific primers, *Taq* polymerase, nucleotides, and buffers. Other than the sample and primers, the reagents necessary for PCR are commercially available. One highly effective amplification strategy is to target conserved sequences among the family of organisms of interest. Such broad-range PCR strategies have been effective in identifying and characterizing several HPVs *(22)*. Consensus primers designed to amplify the highly conserved L1 region of the HPV genome have become the most widely used in clinical and epidemiological studies and will be the focus of this section. **Table 1** lists primer sets that will be described in this section and the primary reference where the primer sequences and amplification conditions can be found.

One of the most widely used and successful consensus primer sets are called MY09 and MY11 *(23)*. These primers were designed to have several degenerate nucleotide positions, thus enabling the amplification of a 450-bp region of L1 of at least 25 different anogenital HPV types. However, it was noted that the amplification efficiency with this primer set was affected by the presence a

Table 1
Consensus Primer Sets for Amplification of the HPV L1 Region

Primers	Product size (bp)	Primary ref.	Commercially available
MY09/11	450	*23*	http://home.appliedbiosystems.com/
PGMY09/11	450	*24*	No
GP5+GP6+	150	*25*	No
SPF1/2	65	*26*	No

multiple HPV types *(27)* and, indeed, genital infection with multiple HPV types is common *(28)*. Inefficient amplification of several HPV types occurred because of sequence mismatch between the target HPV and the MY09 and MY11 primers, despite degenerate base sites. The MY09 and MY11 primers were redesigned to increase amplification efficiency of the genital HPV types by using the same primer-binding regions in the L1 open reading frame and creating a sequence-specific primer cocktail mix called PGMY09 and PGMY11 *(24)*. Now, rather than having degenerate sites in the primer sequence, HPV sequence heterogeneity is accommodated by having multiple primer sequences in an upstream cocktail of 5 oligonucleotides (PGMY11) and a downstream cocktail of 13 oligonucleotides (PGMY09). The PGMY primer set has proven to be more efficient in amplifying the 30 most commonly detected genital HPV types *(29)* and will likely replace the use of the MY09/11 primers.

Another widely used L1 consensus amplification approach uses the general primers GP5+GP6+ *(25)*. The GP5+-GP6+ primers are a mixture of fixed nucleotide oligonucleotides that amplify a 150-bp region of L1 of a wide range of HPV types by lowering the annealing temperature during PCR. The 150-bp sequence amplified by these general primers has sufficient internal heterogeneity for generation of HPV-type-specific probes for the amplified products. HPV types amplified using the GP primers can be characterized using a high- and low-risk probe cocktail *(30)* or a more recently developed reverse line blot assay *(31)*.

A novel PCR primer set that amplifies a short fragment of the L1 region was developed. This short PCR fragment approach for HPV amplification is called SPF PCR *(26)*. The SPF PCR amplifies a 65-bp region of the L1 gene. There is a 22-bp region between the SPF primers that allow for discrimination of most of the genital HPV types using a reverse hybridization line probe assay *(32)*.

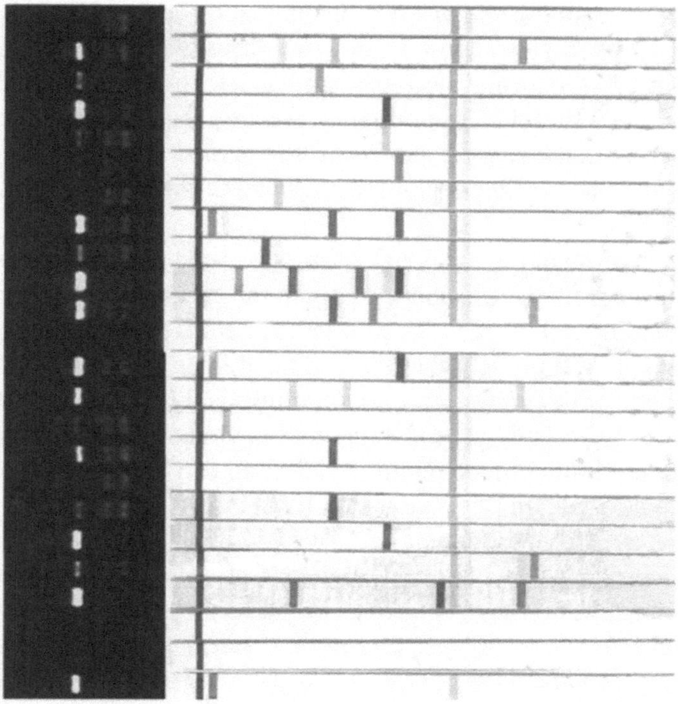

Fig. 2. A photograph of an ethidium bromide (EB) stained agarose gel following electrophoresis of PCR products amplified using the PGMY primter set (left portion of figure). The PCR products are denatured and hybridized to nylon strips in a reverse line blot assay (right portion of the gel). PCR products that hybridize to the probes on the nylon strip are detected and appear as blue stripes. The center blue stripe present on most shows hybridization of the globin PCR product. There are 23 HPV specific probes boun to the nylon that can hybridize to the type(s) amplified by the consensus primers. Note that one PCR product can have multiple HPV types present.

5. Typing Methods of PCR Products

The advantage of HPV consensus PCR is that if 1 or more of the 30 anogenital HPV types are present in the sample, the consensus primers will amplify those types, yielding a positive result. Thus, one reaction is used to determine if a sample has HPV DNA. However, further testing is required to characterize the HPV type(s) in the sample. There are several different approaches for typing the amplified product, ranging from hybridization with HPV-type-specific probes to direct sequencing of the amplified product. The most rapid and efficient method is a reverse hybridization, where the HPV-type-specific probe immobilized to a solid support and the sample is denatured and subsequently allowed to hybridize to the probe(s) (*see* **Fig. 2**). The conventional solid support is either nylon strips decorated with HPV-type-specific probes or microwell plates, with each well coated with a different HPV-type-specific probe. Either format permits sensitive detection of multiple HPV types present in a single sample. The limitation is that a separate hybridization must be performed for each sample. However, the reverse hybridization method is likely to be the most efficient and most adaptable for high-throughput typing of samples.

A reverse hybridization assay has been developed for all three widely used HPV consensus primers sets and the details for each method are described in the corresponding references. The PGMY primers are biotinylated to produce a biotin-labeled PCR product that is hybridized to an array of 27 immobilized HPV oligonucleotide probes representing high- and low-risk HPV types *(33)*. In addition to the 27 HPV probes, high- and low-concentration β-globin-positive controls are immobilized on this nylon strip that allows for assessment of sample adequacy and amplification efficiency. Because each sample requires an individual strip, it is useful to assess by agarose gel electrophoresis whether each sample produced an amplified product. Only samples with an HPV product that is visualized on the gel need to be characterized by reverse hybridization. We have shown excellent correlation between visualization of an HPV product on a gel and positive hybridization *(28)*. Positive HPV products that do not hybridize likely represent HPV types that are not represented by HPV probes on the nylon strip. This reverse line blot assay was developed by Roche Molecular Systems Inc. (Alameda, CA, USA) and is not yet commercially available. However, the probe sequences and reverse line blot production and assay procedure have been published *(33)*.

The INNO-LiPA HPV assay is a reverse line blot designed for typing HPV amplified with the SPF 10 primer set but can also detect and type HPV amplified with the MY09/11 primer set *(32)*. The 25 HPV probes immobilized on this nylon strip can discriminate among HPV types 6, 11, 16, 18, 31, 33, 34, 35, 39, 40, 42, 43, 44, 45, 51, 52, 53, 54, 56, 58, 59, 66, 68, 70, and 74. Both the PGMY reverse line blot assay and the INNO-LiPA HPV assay give comparable HPV detection and typing results *(34)*.

Recently, a reverse line blot assay was developed that types up to 37 distinct HPV types amplified with the GP5+GP6+ primers *(31)*. This system has been miniaturized and takes advantage of multichannel pipettors so that multiple amplified products can be applied to the membrane strips, making this one of the most high-throughput assays available. The method is comparable to both the PGMY and SPF 10 reverse line blots, but it has some advantages in that more type-specific probes are represented on the blot, and because of the size of the GP5+GP6+ amplified product, the HPV probes are highly specific with little cross-hybridization among HPV types. Because of these attributes, this assay should be conducive to and of value for epidemiology studies when large numbers of samples need to be characterized.

6. *In Situ* Hybridization of HPV

In situ hybridization (ISH) is the demonstration of specific genetic information within a morphologic context. Success requires working familiarity with the disparate disciplines of molecular biology and histology: molecular biology for probe design and hybridization and histology for tissue preparation and interpretation of results. Although originally developed with radioactive probes and autoradiographic detection methods, nonradioactive methods, including colorimetric, fluorescent, and chemiluminescent, have made ISH possible in a diagnostic setting. Methods of colorimetric detection and interpretation are the same as those used for immunohistochemistry, making ISH the molecular technique with the greatest potential for ready incorporation into diagnostic histopathology laboratories.

There are many different ISH formats and applications, even restricting consideration to HPV detection and diagnosis. Here, we will focus on colorimetric ISH for detection of HPV DNA in routinely processed formalin-fixed, paraffin-embedded material as found in anatomic pathology archives and describe the strengths and limitations of ISH. A step-by-step ISH protocol can be found at the end of the chapter.

7. The Sample for ISH

In situ hybridization is a specialized version of a solid-support hybridization assay. The microscopic slide is the solid support and the affixed tissue with preserved morphology is the sample. It is the nature of the sample that differentiates ISH from other hybridization assays. The requirement for morphologic preservation means that the nucleic acid must remain at least partially associated with membranes, proteins, and other cellular components that provide the framework recognized as cell and tissue structure by light microscopy. This limits the ability of the sample nucleic acids to interact with the probe. All ISH assays strike a balance between accessibility of the probe to target and preservation of morphology. This compromise is central to understanding both the strengths and limitations of ISH.

In situ hybridization is conceptually straightforward. Although there is a bewildering array of published techniques, all share several basic steps: tissue processing and pretreatment, denaturation of probe and tissue nucleic acids, hybridization, washes, and detection. Even using similar methods, results can vary widely depending on the experience of the laboratory and quality control of each step of the process.

Optimal results will be achieved only with carefully fixed and processed tissue samples. Formalin, a crosslinking fixative, can be quite effective in preserving and retaining nucleic acids in tissues, as well in preserving morphology. To achieve ideal results, tissues must be rapidly placed in an adequate volume of fresh formalin and be cut thin enough to allow rapid and even penetration of the fixative. In addition, the time and temperature of fixation should be standardized, and processing to the paraffin block should use fresh reagents. Routine tissue processing in many clinical histology laboratories does not meet this standard. There are unavoidable variations in tissue handling before fixation, as well as variable conditions of time and temperature during fixation. Reagents in automated tissue processors vary in potency, depending on the numbers of cases processed and the frequency of reagent replacement. These variables are all well tolerated for histologic analysis but contribute to differences in nucleic acid preservation. Techniques developed for archival formalin-fixed, paraffin-embedded starting material must include controls that will detect and adjust for variations in tissue crosslinking and nucleic acid preservation.

The importance of good histologic sectioning is often overlooked. Sections must be without folds or tears. The thickness must be uniform from section to section to allow for even and reproducible penetration of reagents. Tissue adherence to glass is also crucial. Conditions for the hybridization assay are drastic and loss of tissue may occur during the assay if steps are not taken to ensure tissue adherence. Treatment of the glass slides with 3-aminopropyltriethoxysilane has largely replaced other techniques, such as coating glass with poly-L-lysine or glue. When tissue sections are cut and floated in a protein-free tap water bath, the silane-treated glass will form a covalent bond with the tissue section.

Once fixed to glass, tissue preparation for ISH includes removal of paraffin and steps to permeabilize the tissues to reagents. Usually, some form of protein digestion is used to make the target nucleic acids more accessible to the probe. Acid conditions also contribute to protein removal and permeabilization. Pretreatment conditions are empirically determined and will vary depending on the degree of crosslinking.

8. The Probe for ISH

Genetically complex probes increase the amount of label that can be localized to the target, but the final size of the probe after labeling must be less than 300 bases to allow for effective tissue penetration. Sizing of the probe can be achieved during enzymatic incorporation of an affinity label, such as biotin- or digoxigenin-tagged dUTP in a nick-translation reaction. Quality control of probe labeling requires verification of label incorporation as well as determination of the final size of the labeled product. Because the affinity labels are large bulky side groups that are indirectly detected by other even larger multimeric complexes (i.e., avidin–enzyme conjugates or antibody–enzyme conjugates), increasing the specific activity of the affinity label does not directly increase the sensitivity of detection, a difference from direct labeling methods such as radioactivity or fluorescence. Too many affinity labels may actually decrease sensitivity because of steric hindrance of the side chains to the formation of a stable helical structure.

Short oligonucleotide probes are convenient because of the ease of chemical synthesis. Label can be incorporated during synthesis or by a tailing reaction. However, because of the small area of the target that will specifically hybridize to the short probe, sensitivity is limited. Some investigators have attempted to overcome this limitation by using a mixture of oligonucleotides to expand the final target size and increase sensitivity.

For HPV, the entire genome can be propagated in bacterial plasmids. These genomic probes can be used with or without purification from the vector sequences. Although inclusion of the whole HPV genome in the probe results in good sensitivity, the genetic similarity between HPV types means that cross-hybridization between HPV types can be anticipated, particularly for high-copy-number infections. Most colorimetric ISH reactions use simultaneous denaturation of probe and tissue nucleic acids. This seems to favor probe penetration and minimize reannealing of target that limits probe–target interaction. The time and temperature of denaturation are empirically determined and influenced by the extent of crosslinking as well as the extent of protease digestion. The hybridization cocktail as well as time and temperature of the hybridization and final stringency washes determine the degree of cross-hybridization that the assay will tolerate.

9. *ISH* and Detection

The final sensitivity of the reaction is greatly influenced by the colorimetric detection reagents as well as the enzyme–substrate combination. Low background is essential for optimal results. For tissues with high levels of endogenous biotin such as liver or kidney, most investigators recommend using an affinity label other than biotin because background can be hard to control. Although affinity labels result in some signal increase during the detection process, further increases are achieved with recently described signal amplification methods termed "catalyzed reporter deposition" or "tyramide signal amplification" ***(35)***. In these methods, the first steps of detection are the same. The affinity label is used to localize horseradish peroxidase. Instead of using a histochemical substrate in the next step, the peroxidase enzyme activity acts on an affinity-tagged substrate, such as biotinylated tyramide, to yield short-lived affinity-tagged intermediates that deposit at the site of enzyme activity. The newly localized and greatly amplified affinity tags are then detected by another round of enzyme histochemistry. These methods have been successfully used for detection of HPV *(36–38)*, and reagents are commercially available.

With so many facets of the ISH assay being empirically determined, it is clear that laboratories must carefully control and monitor the results of each test. Interpretation of a precipitated product as evidence of an identified segment of nucleic acid requires that all other explanations be eliminated. With each assay, a sample known to contain the target must be run to demonstrate that all components of the assay are working. This positive tissue control should be fixed and processed identically to test tissues and should be run as an additional sample in each assay. Cervical cancer cell lines with well-defined characteristics and known copy numbers of HPV are often used as dependable and consistent controls for many HPV assays. When prepared as formalin-fixed, paraffin-embedded cell blocks, they form very effective tissue controls for monitoring the sensitivity of the ISH reaction. Suggested lines include the following: CaSki, 400–600 copies HPV 16/cell; HeLa, 10–50 copies of HPV 18/cell; SiHa, 1–2 copies of HPV 16/cell; HTB-31, HPV negative. The HPV 16 in SiHa cells is near the limits of detection of the colorimetric ISH assay currently in use in our lab *(39)* and results on this cell block clearly demonstrate when any component of the assay is failing. This allows for small variations between runs to be noticed and corrected.

Because of unavoidable variations in tissue fixation and processing, the use of an endogenous positive control probe on each sample is absolutely essential. This probe is selected to be positive on all tissues if the target nucleic acid has been adequately preserved and made available. This probe should be labeled and used at the same concentration as the test probe. If the positive control probe does not give positive results on a tissue, a negative result for the test probe cannot be interpreted. Adjustment of digestion conditions will often allow positive results to be obtained, but, at times, preservation is poor or tissues are so overfixed that the assay must be termed unsatisfactory. Human placental DNA is a simple and effective endogenous positive control probe for patient samples.

The negative control probe is selected to evaluate the specificity of probe target interaction. It should be of similar size and basepair composition as the test probe but should not hybridize in the absence of the specific organism. For recombinant DNA probes, unmodified plasmid sequences are commonly used as the negative control. The negative control probe is labeled and used at the same concentration as the test probe. A negative result with the negative control probe does not prove specificity of the test probe interaction but is, at least, a guide to monitoring that specificity. The negative control probe also monitors nonspecific interaction of detection reagents and tissue. If the negative control probe yields positive results, use of a cocktail-only reaction (no probe) will demonstrate if the problem is attributable to detection reagents. Therefore, for each patient sample, a minimum of three slides is required to validate assay results for one target. Desired results are illustrated in **Figure 3**. The tissue should even yield signal with the positive control probe (*see* **Fig. 3A**) and negative results with the negative control probe (*see* **Fig. 3B**). If these two conditions are met and if the positive control tissue (run as an additional sample in the same assay) is positive with the test probe, then the results with the test probe on the patient sample can be interpreted (*see* **Fig. 3C**). If more than one test probe is used on each sample in the same run of the assay (e.g., if ISH is being performed for HPV 16 and HPV 18), one set of positive and negative slides suffice per block.

The control blocks Caski and HeLa should be positive with HPV 16/18 and negative with the other probe groups. SiHa cells are at the limit of sensitivity of the assay and should be weakly positive with HPV 16/18. Assays in which CaSki or HeLa controls do not give appropriate results must be repeated. A negative result with SiHa is acceptable but indicates that one or more components of the assay could be failing. The positive control probe (human placental DNA; HG) demonstrates whether the assay conditions allow for hybridization of DNA in the test tissue. Tissues hybridized with the HG probe should have an even dark blue-black signal over every nucleus. Hybridization with the negative control probe (pBR322) should result in no detectable signal. If these two conditions are met, the hybridization with the HPV probes may be interpreted. Signal with the HPV probe is seen as a blue-black color primarily over the nuclei of infected cells containing the target DNA. Some samples may demonstrate reaction with more than one group of HPV probes. This is most often the result of cross-hybridization between the probe groups, and the sample should be typed as the group giving the strongest signal. In some instances, the intensity of multiple probe groups is identical, indicating the presence of more than one HPV type. The assay may be repeated with more stringent washes if HPV-type questions occur.

This assay must be interpreted within the context of the histologic lesion and the clinical setting. It is not intended to replace routine histopathological diagnosis but to provide additional information in a manner analogous to immunohistochemical assays. Interpretation must be made by a pathologist. The hematoxylin and eosin (H&E) slide of the original lesion must be reviewed by the pathologist to verify that the recut sections assayed by ISH are representative of the lesion.

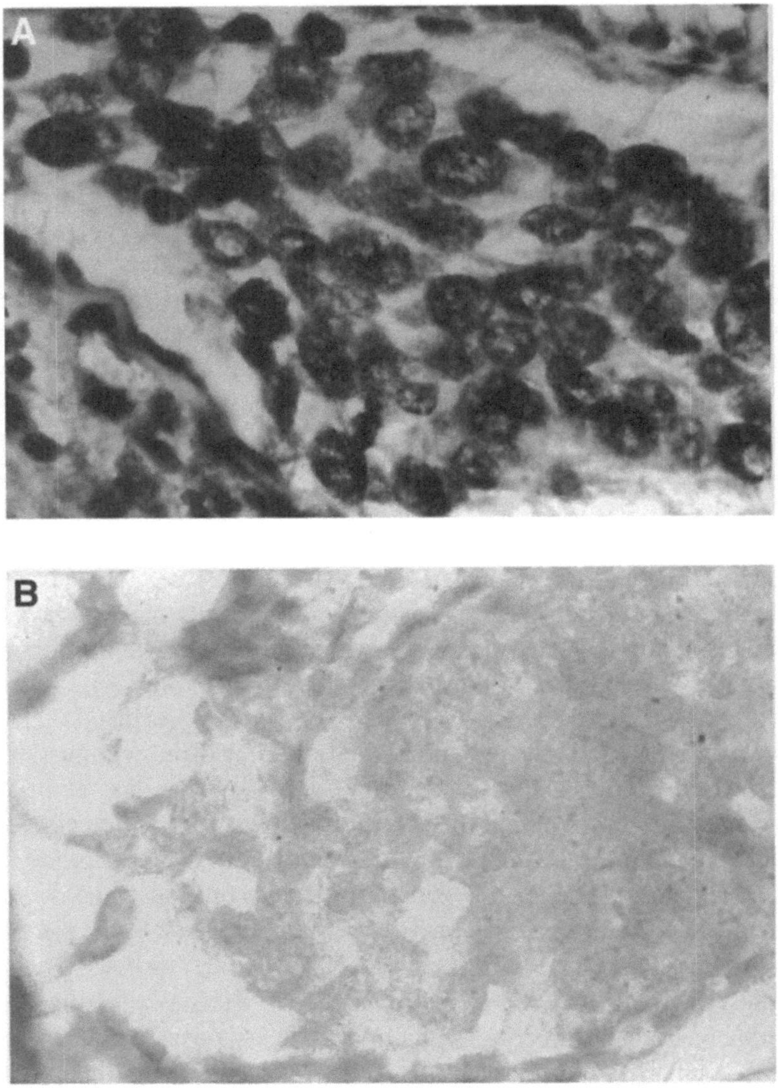

Fig. 3. Appropriate use of controls for ISH. Original magnification ×400. Nuclear fast red counterstain, 5-bromo-4-chloro-3indoyl phosphate/nitroblue tetrazolium chromogen. **(A)** Human placental DNA used as positive control probe. All nuclei show a dark even signal indicating adequate preservation and availability of tissue DNA. **(B)** Plasmid without insert (pBR322) used as negative control probe. No signal is observed, indicating no apparent problems with nonspecific reactions of probe and detection reagent.

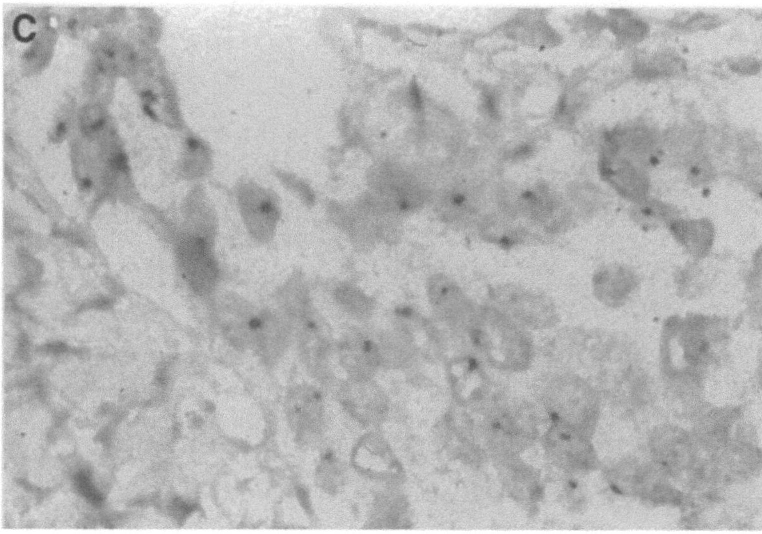

Fig. 3. *(continued)* **(C)** HPV 16 plasmid used as test probe. Signal can be interpreted as specific detection of HPV 16.

10. Strengths and Limitations of HPV ISH

The real strength of ISH lies in the high-resolution detection of HPV sequences within a specific tissue. Spatial localization of HPV genetic information within tissues provides important insights into pathogenesis. Both ISH and PCR can be used effectively on archival tissues, and we have found the results to yield complementary information ***(18)***. The ability to use diagnostic material is a significant advantage for both methods. Histopathology allows the optimal block to be selected for testing, so that representative well-preserved tissues are analyzed. In addition, both ISH and PCR are very conservative of patient material. This allows results of molecular testing to be incorporated into the diagnostic setting without compromising patient care. It also allows molecular epidemiologic studies to be performed on clinically well-characterized material available in pathology archives, minimizing the danger of depleting a valuable resource for future diagnostic and research efforts.

In situ hybridization allows for spatial localization of targets within tissues. Determination of which cell or tissue areas contains the HPV can have implications for pathogenesis. For example, we identified an unusual cervical carcinoma that had HPV 16 in both the malignant epithelium and the benign reactive stroma ***(40)***. This exception to the epitheliotropic nature of HPV, illustrated in **Figure 4**, would not have been noted if the tissue had only been tested by PCR. In another study, several anal condylomas in human immunodeficiency patients

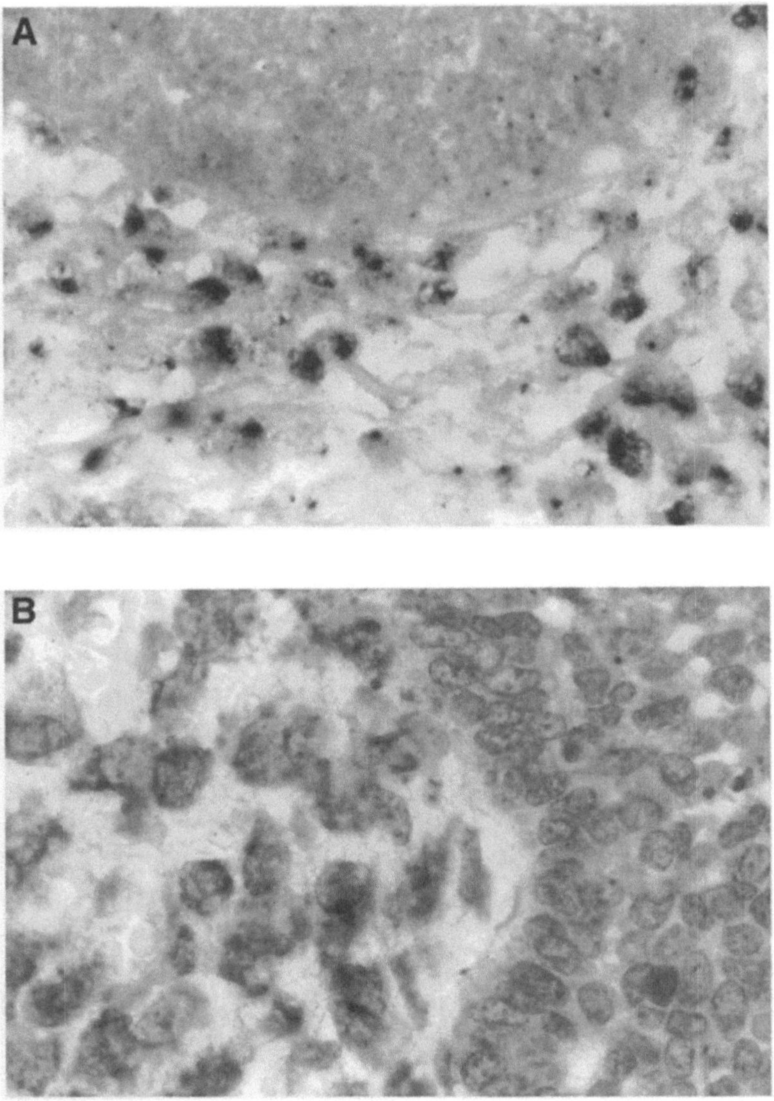

Fig. 4. Localization of HPV 16 DNA to stroma and epitehlium of unusual cervical carcinoma. Original magnification ×400. **(A)** Immunohistochemical detection of vimentin, highlighting stromal elements (i.e., hematoxylin counterstain, diaminobenzidine chromogen). **(B)** *In situ* hybridization localization of HPV 16 DNA to both epithelium and stroma. Strong patchy nuclear signal is present in the stromal nuclei and fine dot-like signal in epithelial nuclei. (Nuclear fast fed counterstain 5-bromo-4-chloro-3indoyl phosphate/nitroblue tetrazolium chromogen.)

were positive for both high- and low-risk HPV types. ISH was able to localize the two different HPV types to morphologically distinct areas of the tissue *(41)*. This differential spatial localization is really only the way to clearly identify multiple HPV types within lesions. The number of multiply-infected lesions is probably underdetected.

Probably, the most important reason to test lesions for HPV by ISH is to determine the integration status of the virus. HPV exists as an episome in condylomas and most dysplasias, whereas in most carcinomas, HPV is integrated into the host chromosome. Integration has been postulated to be an important step in oncogenesis. For stage Ib cervical cancer, we found integration to be a marker of decreased disease-free survival *(42)*. Examples of the patterns of HPV detection within invasive carcinomas are illustrated in **Figure 5**. The pattern associated with the integrated state is shown in **Figure 5A**, whereas that associated with episomal status is shown in **Figure 5B**. The long-term clinical implication of HPV of any type is not clear, and the clinical utility of HPV testing is still under investigation. Other methods that determine integration status (Southern blot hybridization and two-dimensional gel electrophoresis) require relatively large amounts of fresh starting material. The ability to determine the physical state of HPV in archival tissues makes it possible to study HPV integration in many stages of disease evolution, including small precursor lesions.

One of the biggest concerns about ISH is that sensitivity is limited, particularly with nonradioactive methods of detection. ISH sensitivity will vary greatly depending on quality control procedures and experience with the technique. Each laboratory should determine their own sensitivity and specificity rather than relying on literature or manufacturer's results. When optimized, colorimetric ISH can detect one to two copies of integrated HPV in formalin-fixed, paraffin-embedded tissues *(26)*.

Side-by-side comparison of HPV results using ISH and PCR is an ideal way to understand the strengths and limitations of each method. We compared results of colorimetric ISH to L1 consensus PCR for the detection and typing of HPV in 180 blocks of archival tissues (up to 9 yr in storage) from cervical cancer patients *(18)*. Fifteen samples could not be amplified by PCR, but assays were concordant in 75.1% (124/165) of samples that could be analyzed by both methods. Similar numbers of ISH+/PCR– *(23)* and ISH–/PCR+ *(18)* cases were found. Eight of the 18 ISH–/PCR+ cases were attributable to PCR detection of HPV types not included in the ISH assay. Clearly, ISH and PCR assays for HPV yield complementary results. Under the conditions we used, the probability of a sample being positive by either method was not statistically different. In addition, ISH did yield a result on 15 cases (8.3%) that failed to yield amplifiable material for PCR.

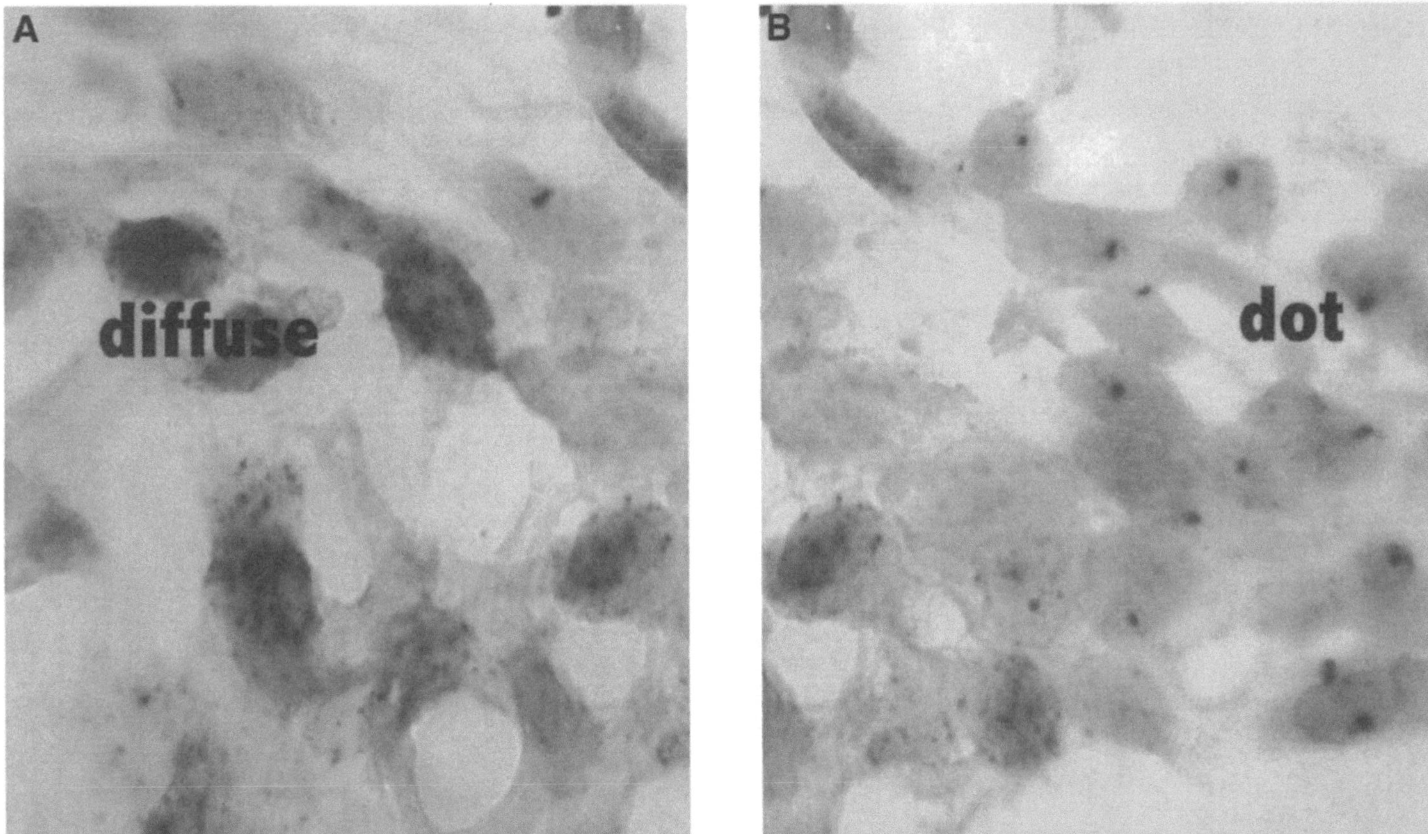

Fig. 5. Localization of the HPV DNA by *in situ* reveals physical state of viral genome. **(A)** A punctuate, dot-like hybridization pattern represents HPV DNA that has integrated into the host genomic DNA. **(B)** A patchy, diffuse hybridization pattern represents HPV DNA that is episomal to the host genomic DNA.

It must be emphasized that these results were not obtained by simply doing the same assay on each block. Considerable effort was spent in determining the optimal conditions for each tissue block. For ISH, digestion conditions varied between 0.5 and 6 mg pepsin/mL of 0.01 *N* HCl. The conditions were selected to yield the strongest signal with the endogenous positive control probe (human placental DNA). In addition, the ISH sensitivity was monitored by including a low positive tissue control in each assay (SiHa cells) to ensure that the probe and detection reagents performed at maximal efficiency. Similarly, we closely monitored the PCR assay by adjusting the template concentrations to yield positive results for the β-globin amplification.

Genomic HPV probes are susceptible to cross-hybridization between closely related types. The ISH PCR comparison described here did detect some type-discordant cases. Limited type specificity of the ISH assay has been described by others ***(43)***. Increasing the stringency of the ISH assay, either through the hybridization itself or during the final washes, may help differentiate between closely related types that yield signal in the same tissue. However, in tissues with very high copy numbers of virus, as in low-grade cervical dysplasias or warts, accurate typing may not be possible. The use of HPV consensus PCR is recommended to confirm HPV type.

The large number of HPV types that are found in clinical lesions presents significant challenges for the ISH format. For optimal sensitivity, the HPV probe includes one to three different types. That means that if all types were to be investigated, as many as 30 sections would have to be processed. The technical difficulty of handling that many tissues as well as the limit in preparing that many different probes means that, in practice, only a few HPV types are tested by ISH, usually those most prevalent in the population. The cross-hybridization of HPV probes can actually be an advantage, allowing assays to detect types not included in the probe mixture. As noted earlier, consensus PCR readily detects most types and use of both techniques allows the most information to be gathered from the tissue.

References

1. American Cancer Society. (1999) *Cancer Facts & Figures—1999,* American Cancer Society, Washington, DC.
2. Munger, K. (2002) The role of human papillomaviruses in human cancers. *Front. Biosci.* **7,** d641–d649
3. Reeves, W. C., Rawls, W. E., and Brinton, L. A. (1989) Epidemiology of genital papillomaviruses and cervical cancer. *Rev. Infect. Dis.* **11,** 426–439.
4. Muñoz, N., Bosch, F. X., de Sanjosé, S., et al. (1992) The causal link between human papillomavirus and invasive cervical cancer: a population-based case-control study in Columbia and Spain. *Int. J. Cancer* **52,** 743–749.

5. Schiffman, M. H., Bauer, H. M., Hoover, R. N., et al. (1993) Epidemiologic evidence showing that human papillomavirus infection causes most cervical intraepithelial neoplasia. *J. Natl. Cancer Inst.* **85,** 958–964.
6. Eluf-Neto, J., Booth, M., Muñoz, N., et al. (1994) Human papillomavirus and invasive cervical cancer in Brazil. *Br. J. Cancer* **69,** 114–119.
7. Dyson, N., Howley, P. M., Münger, K., et al. (1989) The human papillomavirus-16 E7 oncoprotein is able to bind to the retinoblastoma gene product. *Science* **243,** 934–947.
8. Scheffner, M., Werness, B. A., Huibregtse, J. M., et al. (1990) The E6 oncoprotein encoded by human papillomavirus types 16 and 18 promotes the degradation of p53. *Cell* **63,** 1129–1136.
9. Werness, B. A., Levine, A. J., and Howley, P. M. (1990) Association of human papillomavirus types 16 and 18 E6 proteins with p53. *Science* **248,** 76–79.
10. Gao, Q., Srinivasan, S., Boyer, S. N., et al. (1999) The E6 oncoproteins of high-risk papillomaviruses bind to a novel putative GAP protein, E6TP1, and target for degradation. *Mol. Cell. Biol.* **19,** 733–744.
11. Pirisi, L., Creek, K. E., Doniger, J., et al. (1988) Continuous cell lines with altered growth and differentiation properties originate after transfection of human keratinocytes with human papillomavirus type 16 DNA. *Carcinogenesis* **9,** 1573–1579.
12. Woodworth, C. D., Bowden, P. E., Doniger, J., et al. (1988) Characterization of normal human exocervical cell immortalized in vitro by papillomavirus types 16 and 18 DNA. *Cancer Res.* **48,** 4620–4628.
13. Halbert, C. L., Demers, G. W., and Galloway, D. A. (1991) The E7 gene of human papillomavirus type 16 is sufficient for immortalization of human epithelial cells. *J. Virol.* **65,** 473–478.
14. Griep, A. E., Herber, R., Jeon, S., et al. (1993) Tumorigenicity by human papillomavirus type 16 E6 and E7 in transgenic mice correlates with alterations in epithelial cell growth and differentiation. *J. Virol.* **67,** 1373–1384.
15. Arbeit, J. M., Munger, K., Howley, P. M., et al. (1994) Progressive squamous epithelial neoplasia in K14-human papillomavirus type 16 transgenic mice. *J. Virol.* **68,** 4358–4368.
16. Herber, R., Liem, A., Pitot, H., et al. (1996) Squamous epithelial hyperplasia and carcinoma in mice transgenic for the human papillomavirus type 16 E7 oncogene. *J. Virol.* **70,** 1873–1881.
17. Stoler, M. H., Rhodes, C. R., Whitbeck, A., et al. (1992) Human papillomavirus type 16 and 18 gene expression in cervical neoplasia. *Hum. Pathol.* **23,** 117–128.
18. Unger, E. R., Vernon, S. D., Lee, D. R., et al. (1998) Detection of human papillomavirus in archival tissues: comparison of in situ hybridization and polymerase chain reaction. *J. Histochem. Cytochem.* **46,** 535.
19. Ferenczy, A. and Franco, E. (2002) Persistent human papillomavirus infection and cervical neoplasia [review]. *Lancet Oncol.* **3,** 11–16.
20. Lorenzato, F. R., Singer, A., Ho, L., et al. (2002) Human papillomavirus detection for cervical cancer prevention with polymerase chain reaction in self-collected samples. *Am. J. Obstet. Gynecol.* **186,** 962–968.

21. Dimulescu, I., Unger, E. R., Lee, D. R., et al. (1998) Characterization of RNA in cytologic samples preserved in a methanol based collection medium. *Mol. Diagn.* **3,** 1–7.
22. Xi, L. F., Carter, J. J., Galloway, D. A., et al. (2002) Acquisition and natural history of human papillomavirus type 16 variant infection among a cohort of female university students. *Cancer Epidemiol. Biomarkers Prev.* **11,** 343–351.
23. Ting, Y. and Manos M. (1990) Detection and typing of genital human papillomaviruses, in *PCR Protocols: A Guide to Methods and Applications* (Innis, M. A., Gelfand, D. H., Sninsky, J. J., and White, T. J., eds.), Academic, New York, pp. 356–367.
24. Gravitt, P. E., Peyton, C. L., Alessi, T. Q., et al. (2000) Improved amplification of genital human papillomaviruses. *J. Clin. Microbiol.* **38,** 357–361.
25. de Roda Husman, A. M., Walboomers, J. M., Meijer, C. J., et al. (1994) Analysis of cytomorphologically abnormal cervical scrapes for the presence of 27 mucosotropic human papillomavirus genotypes, using polymerase chain reaction. *Int. J. Cancer* **56,** 802–806.
26. Kleter, B., van Doorn, L. J., ter Schegget, J., et al. (1998) A novel short-fragment PCR assay for highly sensitive broad-spectrum detection of anogenital human papillomaviruses. *Am. J. Pathol.* **153,** 1731–1739.
27. Tucker, R. A., Johnson, P. R., Reeves, W. C., et al. (1993) Using the polymerase chain reaction to genotype human papillomavirus DNAs in samples containing multiple HPVs may produce inaccurate results. *J. Virol. Methods* **43,** 321–333.
28. Vernon, S. D., Unger, E. R., and Williams, D. (2000) Comparison of human papillomavirus detection and typing by cycle sequencing, line blot and hybrid capture. *J. Clin. Microbiol.* **38,** 651–655.
29. Coutlee, F., Gravitt, P., Kornegay, J., et al. (2002) Use of PGMY primers in L1 consensus PCR improves detection of human papillomavirus DNA in genital samples. *J. Clin. Microbiol.* **40,** 902–907.
30. Jacobs, M. V., de Roda Husman, A. M., van den Brule, A. J., et al. (1995) Group-specific differentiation between high- and low-risk human papillomavirus genotypes by general primer-mediated PCR and two cocktails of oligonucleotide probes. *J. Clin. Microbiol.* **33,** 901–905.
31. van den Brule, A. J., Pol, R., Fransen-Daalmeijer, N., et al. (2002) GP5+/6+ PCR followed by reverse line blot analysis enables rapid and high-throughput identification of human papillomavirus genotypes. *J. Clin. Microbiol.* **40,** 779–787.
32. Kleter, B., van Doorn, L. J., Schrauwen, L., et al. (1999) Development and clinical evaluation of a highly sensitive PCR–reverse hybridization line probe assay for detection and identification of anogenital human papillomavirus. *J. Clin. Microbiol.* **37,** 2508–2517.
33. Gravitt, P. E., Peyton, C. L., Apple, R. J., et al. (1998) Genotyping of 27 human papillomavirus types by using L1 consensus PCR products by a single-hybridization, reverse line blot detection method. *J. Clin. Microbiol.* **36,** 3020–3027.
34. van Doorn, L. J., Quint, W., Kleter, B., et al. (2002) Genotyping of human papillomavirus in liquid cytology cervical specimens by the PGMY line blot assay and the SPF(10) line probe assay. *J. Clin. Microbiol.* **40,** 979–983.

35. Kerstens, H. M. J., Poddighe, P. J., and Hanselaar, A. G. J. M. (1995) A novel *in situ* hybridization method based on the deposition of biotinylated tyramide. *J. Histochem. Cytochem.* **43,** 347.
36. Plummer, T. B., Sperry, A. C., Xu, H. S., et al. (1998) *In situ* hybridization detection of low copy nucleic acid sequences using catalyzed reporter deposition and its usefulness in clinical human papillomavirus typing. *Diagn. Mol. Pathol.* **7,** 76.
37. Sano, T., Hikino, T., Niwa, Y., et al. (1998) *In situ* hybridization with biotinylated tyramide amplification: detection of human papillomavirus DNA in cervical neoplastic lesions. *Mod. Pathol.* **11,** 19.
38. Cheung, A. L. M., Graf, A.-H., Hauser-Kronberger, et al. (1999) Detection of human papillomavirus in cervical carcinoma: comparison of peroxidase, nanogold, and catalyzed reported deposition (CARD)-nanogold *in situ* hybridization. *Mod. Pathol.* **12,** 689.
39. Unger, E. R., Hammer, M. L., and Chenggis, M. L. (1991) Comparison of ^{35}S and biotin as labels for *in situ* hybridization: use of an HPV model system. *J. Histochem. Cytochem.* **39,** 145.
40. Unger, E. R., Vernon, S. D., Hewan-Lowe, K. O., et al. (1999) An unusual cervical carcinoma showing exception to epitheliotropism of human papillomavirus. *Hum. Pathol.* **30,** 483.
41. Unger, E. R., Vernon, S. D., Lee, D. R., et al. (1997) Human papillomavirus type in anal epithelial lesions is influenced by human immunodeficiency virus. *Arch. Pathol. Lab. Med.* **121,** 820.
42. Unger, E. R., Vernon, S. D., Thoms, W. W., et al. (1995) Human papillomavirus and disease-free survival in FIGO stage Ib cervical cancer. *J. Infect. Dis.* **172,** 1184–1190.
43. Southern, S. A., Graham, D. A., and Herrington, C. S. (1998) Discrimination of human papillomavirus types in low and high grade cervical squamous neoplasia. *Diagn. Mol. Pathol.* **7,** 114.

13

A Nested RT-PCR Assay to Detect BCR/*abl*

Linda M. Wasserman

1. Introduction

Chronic myelogenous leukemia (CML), a clonal myeloproliferative disorder in adults, and some pediatric and adult acute lymphoblastic eukemias (ALLs) are characterized by the presence of a Philadelphia chromosome, t(9;22)(q34;q11) *(1)*. In this chromosomal translocation, exons from a major breakpoint cluster region (M-bcr), located on chromosome 22q11, are joined to the c-*abl* protooncogene, located on chromosome 9q34. When this chromosomal translocation occurs in a hematopoietic stem cell, the resulting BCR/*abl* fusion protein has increased tyrosine kinase activity and a transforming capacity that is critical to the pathogenesis of these leukemic disorders.

The Philadelphia chromosome can be detected in 95% of adults with CML, and 23–50% of adult ALL, and 11% of childhood ALL *(2)*. In the M-bcr, most translocations occur within intronic sequences between the second and fourth exons. Most translocations in c-*abl* occur across a large region 5' to c-*abl* exon II. Although breakpoints in the M-bcr and c-*abl* can be widely distributed along their respective chromosomes, mRNA processing of the fusion transcript consistently links either M-bcr exons b1–b3 or exons b1 and b2 to c-*abl* exon II, or occasionally to c-*abl* exon Ia (*see* **Fig. 1**). Because of the consistent processing of the fusion transcript, reverse transcriptase-polymer chain reaction (RT-PCR) assays, which use mRNA as a starting material, can readily detect almost all Philadelphia chromosome translocations despite the variability in the location of chromosomal breakpoints.

Detection of the BCR/*abl* fusion transcript by RT-PCR is used clinically either to confirm a CML or ALL diagnosis or to detect and monitor the presence of minimal residual disease in leukemic patients following treatment *(3)*. The sensitivity of an RT-PCR assay, particularly if it is a nested two-step PCR,

From: *Methods in Molecular Medicine, vol. 97: Molecular Diagnosis of Cancer*
Edited by: J. E. Roulston and J. M. S. Bartlett © Humana Press Inc., Totowa, NJ

Table 1
BCR/*abl* and β-Catenin Primer Sequences

BCR/*abl*	
Oligo A: 5'-ggA gCT gCA gAT gCT gAC CAA C-3'	(Genset HG099)
Oligo B: 5'-CTg Agg CTC AAA gTC AgA Tg-3'	(Genset HG101)
Oligo C: 5'-gCT TCT CCC TgA CAT CCg Tg-3'	(Genset HG098)
Oligo D: 5'-CgA gCg gCT TCA CTC AgA CC-3'	(Genset HG100)
β-Catenin	
Sense 4: 5'-TTC CAC gAC TAg TTC AgT TgC-3'	
Antisense 4: 5'-CTA CAg gCC AAT CAC AAT gC-3'	
Antisense 3: 5'-AAC AgC AgC TgC ATA TgT Cg-3'	

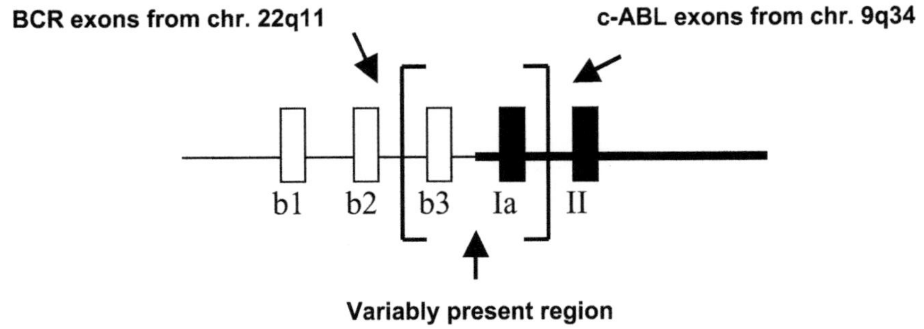

Fig. 1. BCR/abl translocation.

typically enables the detection of one positive cell within a background of 10^5–10^7 normal cells. In the multiplexed, nested RT-PCR assay described here, RNA is extracted either from peripheral blood leukocytes or from bone marrow hematopoietic cells. The RNA is first reverse-transcribed and then subjected to two rounds of PCR. The final PCR product is electrophoresed through an ethidium bromide-stained agarose gel and detected by fluorescence under ultraviolet light.

The multiplexed PCR reactions described in this chapter contain primers for the BCR/*abl* translocation ***(4)*** as well as a set of control primers for the β-catenin gene ***(5)*** to confirm the quality and amplifiability of the cDNA's being tested. The positive control β-catenin primers ensure that the cDNA in each specimen is intact and that the RNA extraction and reverse-transcription procedures were successful. A BCR/*abl* cDNA containing M-Bcr exons b1–b3 generates a 194-bp second-round PCR product, whereas a BCR/*abl* cDNA containing only M-Bcr exons b1 and b2 generates a 119-bp second-round PCR product. Presence of the second-round β-catenin PCR amplicon is detected by the presence of a 372-bp product. The round 1 and round 2 PCR primer sequences for both BCR/*abl* and β-catenin are given in **Table 1**. In the round 2 PCR, an aliquot of the PCR product from round 1 is amplified using BCR/*abl* primers, which are both internal to the round 1 primers and β-catenin primers, which are internal to the round 1 antisense primer.

2. Materials

2.1. Positive Control Cell Line

The K562 cell line is available from ATCC (cat. no. CCL 243) (http://www.atcc.org) and contains a BCR/*abl* translocation containing M-bcr exons b1–b3.

2.2. RNA Extraction

1. 1.5-mL sterile plastic microcentrifuge tubes.
2. Presterilized aerosol-resistant pipet tips.
3. Purescript RNA Isolation Kit (cat. no. R-5000; Gentra Systems, Inc., Minneapolis, MN).
4. Sterile, double-deionized water treated with diethyl pyrocarbonate (DEPC) and autoclaved.
5. Glycogen, 20 mg/mL (Boehringer Mannheim, cat. no. 901 393).
6. 100% Isopropanol, dedicated to RNA extraction use only, stored at 4°C.
7. 70% Ethanol, dedicated to RNA extraction use only, stored at 4°C.
8. Agarose DNA grade (Fisher BP164-100).
9. Ethidium bromide, 10 mg/mL.
10. 1X TBE prepared with DEPC-treated water.
11. 80% Glycerol/BPB loading buffer.

2.3. Reverse Transcription

1. GeneAmp RNA PCR Core Kit (Perkin-Elmer, cat. no. N808-0143).
2. 200 μL Sterile microcentrifuge tubes.
3. Presterilized aerosol-resistant pipet tips.
4. RNA extracted from the K562 cell line.
5. RNA extracted from a "normal" subject (i.e., an individual with no evidence of leukemia to use as a negative control).
6. RNA extracted from patient sample(s).

2.4. PCR Rounds 1 and 2

1. GeneAmp RNA PCR Core Kit (Perkin-Elmer, cat. no. N808-0143), that includes dNTPs, *Taq*, PCR buffer II, and 25 m*M* $MgCl_2$).
2. 200 μL Sterile microcentrifuge tubes.
3. Presterilized aerosol-resistant pipet tips.
4. Patient and control cDNAs.
5. Sterile double-deionized water.

2.5. Gel Electrophoresis

1. NuSieve 3:1 agarose (FMC BioProducts, cat. no. 50090).
2. 1X TBE.
3. Ethidium bromide, 10 mg/mL.
4. 80% Glycerol/BPB loading buffer.
5. DNA size standards: either pBR322/*Hae*III (Sigma, cat. no. D 9655) or ϕ X174 DNA/*Hae*III (Sigma, cat. no. D 0672).

3. Method

3.1. RNA Extraction

1. Note that RNA is more labile than DNA and degrades relatively quickly. Thus, RNA should be extracted from blood or bone marrow specimens as soon as possible after the specimen is received and accessioned in your laboratory. The specimen should be stored at 4°C from the time it is received in the laboratory until the RNA is extracted (*see* **Notes 1** and **2**).
2. The following method uses components of the the Purescript RNA Isolation Kit and includes some modifications of the original protocol found useful in our laboratory to increase RNA yield.
3. For best results, use at least 3 mL of peripheral blood or bone marrow. If the patient's specimen is less than 3 mL, use the entire specimen (*see* **Note 3**).
4. Use pipetmen dedicated to nucleic acid extraction, ideally, dedicated to RNA extraction. Do not use these pipetmen when assembling the master mixes for the reverse transcription and PCR steps.
5. For each milliliter of peripheral blood or bone marrow, add 3 mL of RBC lysis solution, using a Corning 15-mL centrifuge. Cap tube and invert once to mix. Incubate at room temperature for 10 min, inverting the tube once more in the middle of the incubation.
6. Centrifuge at high speed in a desktop centrifuge for 1 min to pellet the white cells.
7. Aspirate off the supernatant and vortex the pellet to loosen it from the bottom of the tube.
8. Add 300 μL of cell lysis solution and pipet up and down no more than three times to lyse the white cells. Place the cell lysate in a microcentrifuge tube.
9. Add 175 μL of protein precipitation solution, cap the tube, and invert it gently 10 times to mix. Place the microcentrifuge tube on ice for 5 min.
10. Centrifuge at highest speed for 3 min (*see* **Note 4**).
11. Carefully remove the supernatant with a pipetman and place in a new microcentrifuge tube. With your pipetman, measure the approximate volume of the supernatant.
12. Add an equivalent volume of 100% isopropanol and 1 μL of glycogen (20 mg/mL). Cap the tube and invert gently 50 times.
13. Centrifuge at highest speed for 5 min.
14. Carefully pour off isopropanol and drain tube on clean paper towels or absorbent paper.

15. Carefully pipet 300 µL of 70% ethanol into the microcentrifuge, directing the stream of fluid along the side of the tube rather than directly onto the pellet in order to avoid dislodging it. Centrifuge at highest speed for 1 min.
16. Either carefully pour off the 70% ethanol without dislodging the pellet or remove most of it with a pipetman and allow the remainder of the ethanol to drain out of the microcentrifuge tube onto paper towels.
17. When no drops of ethanol remain on the sides of the microcentrifuge tube, rehydrate the pellet with 20–40 µL RNA hydration solution (*see* **Note 5**).
18. Quantifying your RNA yield
    a. There are two methods of quantifying your RNA yield: by spectroscopic analysis of the optical density (OD) 260/280 and by visual inspection on an agarose gel. Taking the OD 260/280 provides the concentration (in micrograms per microliter) of nucleic acid in your preparation but can include DNA as well as RNA. Analysis of an aliquot of RNA on ethidium bromide-stained agarose demonstrates the 18S and 28S bands of RNA and is a visual check that you have obtained high-molecular-weight RNA.
    b. OD 260/280: Dilute 6 µL RNA into 600 µL DEPC-treated sterile double-deionized water (ddH$_2$O). The RNA concentration (in micrograms per milliliter) is obtained by multiplying the OD 260 by 400. The OD 260/280 should be greater than or equal to 1.8
    c. 1% Agarose gel: Make a 1% agarose gel using 1X TBE prepared with DEPC-treated ddH$_2$O. For a small gel, add 0.4 g agarose to 40 mL TBE and melt in a microwave oven. Add 10 mg/mL of 4 µL ethidium bromide, to the molten agarose prior to pouring the gel. When the gel sets, cover with 1X TBE and remove the comb. Mix 3 µL RNA with 3 µL of 80% glycerol/BPB loading buffer and load into the gel. Run at 80 V until the dye front is two-thirds of the way down the gel. Photograph the gel under ultraviolet (UV) light. 18S RNA migrates at 1.9 kb; 28S RNA migrates at 4.7 kb.
19. RNA can either be frozen at –80°C indefinitely until needed for reverse transcription or can go immediately into the reverse-transcription step. If the RNA is frozen prior to reverse transcription, it should be thawed on ice.

3.2. Reverse Transcription

1. Prepare a master mix for reverse transcription according to the kit directions, calculating the total volume needed based on the number of patient and control reactions needed. Volumes of ingredients per reaction are as follows:
    4 µL of 25 m*M* MgCl$_2$.
    2 µL of 10X PCR buffer II.
    2 µL of each dNTP, at 10 m*M* initial concentration.
    1 µL RNAsin (20 U/µL).
    1 µL MULV reverse transcriptase (50 U/µL).
    1 µL either random hexamers (50 µ*M*) or oligo dT (50 µ*M*).
2. Set up the reactions in a biosafety hood, if available, or in the space in your

laboratory dedicated to assembling PCR ingredients. Use pipetmen dedicated to setting up PCR reactions.

3. Make duplicate reverse-transcription reactions for each patient sample, one positive control reaction each for a BCR/*abl* exon b1–b3 translocation (i.e., K562), a BCR/*abl* exon b1 and b2 translocation, if available, and one reaction for the negative RNA control (i.e., an RNA known *not* to contain a BCR/*abl* translocation).
4. Pipet 17 μL master mix into each 200 = μL microcentrifuge tube. Each tube should be capped and remain capped after the addition of the master mix and should be opened only when pipetting in the appropriate RNA aliquot.
5. Add 3 μL RNA to each patient positive and negative control tubes, recapping each tube. Allow tubes to sit at room temperature for 10 min to enhance binding of the random hexamer or oligo dT primer to the RNA.
6. Place tubes in a thermocycler. Program the thermocycler for one cycle of 42°C for 60 min, followed by one cycle of 90°C for 5 min to inactivate the reverse transcriptase.
7. Either use the cDNA immediately for the first PCR round or store at –20°C until needed.

3.3. PCR Round 1

1. Prepare the first-round PCR master mix with dedicated PCR reagents, pipetmen, and consumable supplies in the location within your laboratory dedicated to preparing PCR reactions. Include duplicate tubes for each patient specimen, single tubes for the positive and negative control reactions, and a single tube for a water-only control. Prepare the round 1 PCR master mix according to the following reaction volumes:

Sterile ddH_2O	23.5 μL
25 m*M* $MgCl_2$	3.0 μL (1.5 m*M* final concentration)
10X PCR buffer II	5.0 μL (1X final concentration)
10 m*M* dATP	1.0 μL (200 μ*M* final concentration)
10 m*M* dGTP	1.0 μL (200 μ*M* final concentration)
10 m*M* dCTP	1.0 μL (200 μ*M* final concentration)
10 m*M* dTTP	1.0 μL (200 μ*M* final concentration)
10 μ*M* β-catenin Sense 4 primer	1.0 μL (200 μ*M* final concentration)
10 μ*M* β-catenin Antisense 4 primer	1.0 μL (200 μ*M* final concentration)
25 μ*M* Oligo C	1.0 μL (500 μ*M* final concentration)
25 μ*M* Oligo D	1.0 μL (500 μ*M* final concentration)
Taq (5 U/μL)	0.5 μL (2.5 U/reaction)
	40.0 μL

2. Aliquot 40 μL master mix into each reaction tube. Cap the tubes and carry them to the area in your laboratory dedicated to the addition of DNA, cDNA, or PCR products to PCR reactions (*see* **Notes 6–8**).

3. Using pipetmen dedicated to the addition of DNA, cDNA, or PCR reaction products and aerosol-resistant pipet tips, add 10 µL of the appropriate cDNA to each PCR tube or 10 µL sterile ddH_2O to the water-only control, uncapping each tube only to add the appropriate cDNA or sterile water and then recapping each tube prior to uncapping the next tube.
4. Vortex or pulse spin the tubes and place in your thermocycler.
5. Use the following PCR cycle conditions:
   Step 1: 94°C for 10 min for one cycle;
   Step 2: 94°C for 1 min, 50°C for 1 min, 72°C for 1 min;
   Step 3: 72°C for 10 min for one cycle.
6. Repeat the second step for 40 cycles for PCR round 1.
7. Allow tubes to cool to room temperature. Store at 4°C until ready to assemble PCR round 2.

3.4. PCR Round 2

1. PCR round 2 is the nested PCR reaction and uses an aliquot of the PCR round 1 product. Prepare the PCR round 2 master mix in your laboratory's PCR setup area using dedicated reagents, pipetmen, and aerosol-resistant pipet tips according to the following reaction volumes:

Sterile ddH_2O	29.5 µL
25 m*M* $MgCl_2$	3.0 µL (1.5 m*M* final concentration)
10X PCR buffer II	5.0 µL (1X final concentration)
10 m*M* dATP	1.0 µL (200 µ*M* final concentration)
10 m*M* dGTP	1.0 µL (200 µ*M* final concentration)
10 m*M* dCTP	1.0 µL (200 µ*M* final concentration)
10 m*M* dTTP	1.0 µL (200 µ*M* final concentration)
10 µ*M* β-catenin Sense 4 primer	1.0 µL (200 µ*M* final concentration)
10 µ*M* β-catenin Antisense 3 primer	1.0 µL (200 µ*M* final concentration)
25 µ*M* Oligo A	1.0 µL (500 µ*M* final concentration)
25 µ*M* Oligo B	1.0 µL (500 µ*M* final concentration)
Taq (5 U/µL)	0.5 µL (2.5 U/reaction)
	46.0 µL

2. Aliquot 46 µL into each reaction tube. Cap each tube and carry to the area in your laboratory dedicated to the addition of DNA or PCR products. Using dedicated pipetmen and aerosol-resistant pipet tips, add 4 µL of PCR round 1 product to each tube, recapping each tube immediately afterward.
3. Vortex or pulse spin each tube and carry to thermocycler.
4. Use the same PCR cycling conditions as round 1 except repeat the second step of **step 5** for 30 cycles.
5. Allow tubes to come to room temperature and store at 4°C until ready for gel electrophoresis.

3.5. Gel Electrophoresis

1. For 100 mL of molten agarose, add 9 g NuSieve 3:1 to 100 mL of 1X TBE and melt in a microwave oven to make a 3% gel. Add 10 μL ethidium bromide (10 mg/mL) and pour into a gel apparatus, using a wide-tooth comb.
2. When the gel is set, add enough 1X TBE to just cover the agarose and carefully remove the comb.
3. Mix 20 μL of each PCR round 2 product with 4 μL of 80% glycerol/BPB loading buffer and load into gel.
4. Use either pBR322/*Hae*III, 1 μg/μL (Sigma, cat. no. D 9655) or φ X174 DNA/*Hae*III, 1 μg/μL (Sigma, cat. no. D 0672) as DNA size markers.

4. Notes

1. All buffers and consumable plastics needed for this assay should be kept dedicated to work with RNA. They should be kept separate from similar laboratory supplies used for work with DNA and should be labeled "FOR RNA USE ONLY."
2. All glassware used to measure reagents or to contain buffers and any sterile ddH_2O used to work with RNA should first be treated with 0.1% DEPC to inactivate RNases. One milliliter of DEPC is added to each liter of sterile ddH_2O, allowed to sit for at least 12 h at room temperature and then autoclaved for 15 min on the liquid cycle. Glassware can be filled to the brim with sterile ddH_2O and an appropriate amount of DEPC added and allowed to sit in the vessel for 12 h at room temperature. The DEPC–H_2O is removed from the glassware prior to autoclaving. DEPC is unstable in the presence of Tris buffers and breaks down to ethanol and carbon dioxide. Thus, when preparing the 5X TBE buffer, which will be used to check the quality of the RNA on an agarose gel prior to the reverse-transcriptase step, prepare the buffer in DEPC-treated glassware, using DEPC-treated ddH_2O rather than adding DEPC directly to the 5X TBE.
3. If you have never extracted RNA before, it is wise to practice on specimens of peripheral blood prior to extracting a patient's sample in order to acquaint yourself with the extraction protocol you are using and to become familiar with manipulating the RNA pellet following isopropanol precipitation and ethanol wash and rehydrating the RNA pellet following the ethanol wash. The RNA extraction step is critical to the success of the assay because it is the starting material on which the remainder of the assay depends.

   There are many RNA extraction kits available and you may want to try several to determine which kit or extraction method gives the best results in your laboratory. No matter which kit or RNA extraction protocol you use, it is wise to keep your white RNA cell pellet on ice, to complete the extraction protocol without interruption once you start it, and, when precipitating the RNA, to use equal volumes of supernatant to isopropanol.
4. After completing the protein–DNA precipitation step using the Purescript reagents, the red-brown pellet, consisting of residual red cell debris, protein, and DNA, should be tight and well compacted at the bottom of the microcentrifuge

tube. If the pellet is rather loose and not well compacted, adding additional protein precipitation reagent may be beneficial. When the pellet is loose and has a mucuslike appearance, it can be difficult to remove the supernatant and the volume of supernatant recovered is often reduced. Loss of supernatant reduces the ultimate RNA yield.

5. If your RNA pellet appears small, you might wish to rehydrate it in half of the recommended volume of rehydration solution in order to maximize the concentration of RNA that goes into the reverse-transcription step. Because the volume of RNA in the reverse-transcription step is fixed, it is advantageous to maximize the RNA concentration being reverse-transcribed, in order to detect the BCR/*abl* transcript should it be rare in your specimen.
6. Awareness of the ways in which a PCR reaction can become contaminated, as evidenced by a PCR product seen in the water-only control reaction, is always required when amplifying DNA. However, when a PCR reaction is nested, such as in this protocol, contamination can occur much more easily and must be more vigorously anticipated and guarded against. Because an aliquot of the water-only control reaction is reamplified in round 2, any slight otherwise undetectable contamination occurring in the round 1 step could be detected when an aliquot is reamplified in round 2.
7. Ways to avoid contamination include the following:
   a. Assembling the PCR mixes in a laboratory area dedicated to that purpose, using dedicated pipetmen and aerosol-resistant pipet tips
   b. Capping each tube after aliquoting the PCR master mix, keeping each tube capped except when adding each respective cDNA or PCR aliquot, and then recapping each tube prior to uncapping the next
   c. Adding cDNA or PCR product only in a laboratory area dedicated to that purpose, using dedicated pipetmen and aerosol-resistant pipet tips
8. Should contamination be detected in the blank lane, it is imperative that all solutions or reagents, including ddH_2O, dNTPs, primer dilutions, and *Taq* be discarded and new dilutions prepared.

References

1. Melo, J. V. (1996) The molecular biology of chronic myeloid leukemia. *Leukemia* **10,** 751–756.
2. McClure, J. S. and Litz, C. E. (1994) Chronic myelogenous leukemia: molecular diagnostic considerations. *Hum. Pathol.* **25,** 594–597.
3. Campana, D. and Pui, C.-H. (1995) Detection of minimal residual disease in acute leukemia: methodological advances and clinical significance. *Blood* **85,** 1416–1434.
4. Genset. (1991) *Oligonucleotide Handbook*, Genset, Vol. II, p. 171.
5. Oyama, T., Kanai, Y., Ochiai, A., et al. (1994) A truncated β-catenin disrupts the interaction between E-cadherin and α-catenin: a cause of loss of intercellular adhesiveness in human cancer cell lines. *Cancer Res.* **54,** 6282–6287.

14

TP53 Mutation Detection by SSCP and Sequencing

Jenni Hakkarainen, Judith A. Welsh, and Kirsi H. Vähäkangas

1. Introduction

1.1. TP53 Mutations and Their Significance

The TP53 tumor suppressor gene on chromosome 17p13.1 contains 11 exons and encodes a nuclear phosphoprotein of 53 kDa, a transcription factor involved in the regulation of the cell cycle ***(1)***. Normal p53 protein functions as a cell cycle checkpoint and is involved in DNA repair and/or apoptosis ***(2)***. The p53 protein acts as a powerful transcription factor that binds to as many as 300 different promoter elements in the genome, broadly altering patterns of specific gene expression ***(3)***. Loss of normal p53 function can lead to uncontrolled cell proliferation and neoplastic transformation. A *TP53* mutation, most commonly a missense mutation, may cause either a loss of tumor suppressor function or, in certain cases, a gain of oncogenic function ***(4–6)***. This functional duality may be one explanation for the high frequency of *TP53* mutations in human cancer ***(7–10)***, which makes the *TP53* gene especially suitable for mutational analysis. The modest size of the highly conserved *TP53* gene (p53 protein contains 393 amino acids in human) is an advantage in mutation analysis. Mutations in *TP53* are usually clustered within the most conserved regions in the area of exons 5–8, corresponding to the sequence-specific DNA-binding domain of the p53 protein ***(11,12)***.

At the clinical level, analysis of *TP53* mutations may serve as a marker of clonality of cancer lesions or to follow-up recurrences after treatment ***(6)***. In many cancers, such as breast cancer ***(13,14)*** and non-small-cell lung cancer ***(15)***, the presence of a specific *TP53* mutation predicts a poor prognosis. If *TP53* mutation analysis appears clinically significant (e.g., for the prognosis), it becomes important for an individual patient and attending physician to get an accurate result. The large variety of approaches and their practical applica-

From: *Methods in Molecular Medicine, vol. 97: Molecular Diagnosis of Cancer*
Edited by: J. E. Roulston and J. M. S. Bartlett © Humana Press Inc., Totowa, NJ

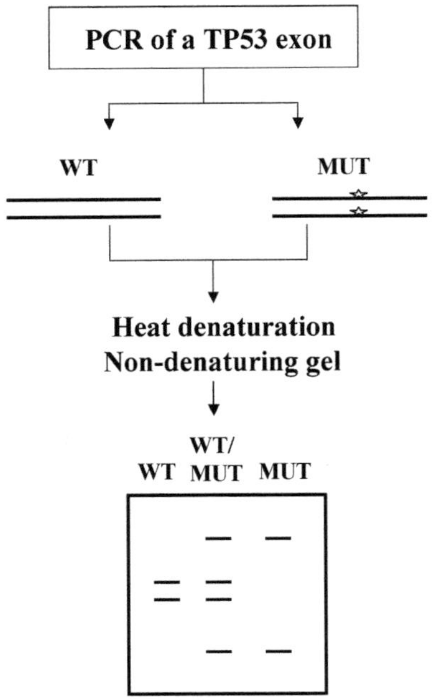

Fig. 1. Principle of SSCP. When the amplified DNA is heat denatured, both 3' and 5' strands of wild-type (WT) and the mutated (MUT) exon adopt different sequence-specific conformations, which show in electrophoresis on a nondenaturing gel.

tions, as well as the difficulty of getting fully characterized large sample sets, especially of rare tumors, have restricted the development of *TP53* mutation databases. From the mutation analysis methods for *TP53*, sequencing and PCR-SSCP (single-strand conformation polymorphism) have taken their place among those most frequently used for this purpose and serve as important reference methods in the validation of new and emerging high-throughput mutation analysis methodologies.

1.2. PCR-SSCP for TP53 Mutations

In SSCP, denaturated single-stranded DNA fragments are run on nondenaturating polyacrylamide gels ***(16,17)***. Under nondenaturating conditions, single-stranded DNA adopts a secondary structure that is dependent on its sequence. Point mutations modify the conformation and alter the electrophoretic mobility compared to wild-type DNA (*see* **Fig. 1**). Mutations that are detected using SSCP include base substitutions, small insertions, deletions, and rearrangements.

Optimization of the SSCP conditions is essential for specificity and efficiency ***(18–21)***. The critical factors include running conditions (e.g., the temperature), specificity of the primers for PCR, coverage by the used primers of full exons with splice sites, and positive and negative controls for all strands amplified. Theoretically, the simplest band pattern includes five bands if both mutated and wild-type sequences are present: one band per each single-stranded DNA sequence and one band for the double-stranded DNA, which, in some systems, may appear between single-stranded bands (*see* **ref. *21***). However, some mutations are detectable only in a very narrow window of temperatures and band patterns may be indiscernible at a certain temperature demanding confirmation in another. Because the conformation changes according to the temperature, more than one conformation may occur close to the critical transformation temperature and, therefore, several additional single-stranded bands may be seen ***(16,22)***. Despite these facts, most articles published with SSCP analysis use only one temperature to detect p53 mutations, one reason being the difficulty to maintain an exact temperature in larger gels (e.g., **refs. *23–25***).

The semiautomated electrophoretic system (PhastSystem®) and silver staining (**ref. *21*** and references within) are easier to handle, safer, and less expensive than radioactive SSCP originally developed by Orita and co-workers ***(16)***. Because the gel temperature is the most important parameter affecting the conformation and thus electrophoretic mobility of the single strand, one of the most important advantages of the SSCP technique using the PhastSystem is that the running temperature is precisely controlled, ensuring reproducible SSCP results. Furthermore, a relatively short time is required for analysis. One drawback in this technique is that only six samples can be analyzed on the same gel. We have developed complete conditions, using the Pharmacia PhastSystem® for temperature-controlled nonradioactive SSCP on amplified *TP53* exons 4–8, where mutations frequently occur in human tumors ***(21,26)***. Each *TP53* exon is amplified separately (primers in **Table 1**), and two temperatures are used for each. The original reagents for PhastSystem, developed by the company for the analysis of proteins, are still used and they work well on the short strands of p53 exons. New reagents for DNA also exist, but they are meant for longer strands.

Any mutation analysis method has a large variation in the quality of the results depending on how it is used ***(21,27)***. Thus, it is not enough to talk about PCR-SSCP, because this states only the principle that has been used, but also to specify how it was used (e.g., which detection method and how many temperatures were used).

1.3. PCR Sequencing for TP53 Mutations

Current manual and automated applications for sequencing the *TP53* gene are based on the dideoxy-chain-termination principle. The traditional detection of bands in manual sequencing is by radioactive labeling of nucleotides used in

Table 1
Primers Used for PCR in Orientation 5′ to 3′

Exon	Location	Primers with the orientation 5' to 3'
Outer primers		
X4:	Left	ACG TGA ATT CTG AGG ACC TGG TCC TCT GAC
	Right	ACG TGG ATC CAG AGG AAT CCC AAA GTT CCA
X5:	Left	ACG TGA ATT CGT TTC TTT GCT GCC GTG TTC
	Right	ACG TGG ATC CAG GCC TGG GGA CCC TGG GCA
X6:	Left	ACG TGA ATT CTG GTT GCC CAG GGT CCC CAG
	Right	ACG TGG ATC CTG GAG GGC CAC TGA CAA CCA
X7:	Left	ACG TGA ATT CAC CAT CCT GGC TAA CGG TGA
	Right	ACG TGG ATC CAG GGG TCA GCG GCA AGC AGA
X8:	Left	ACG TGA ATT CTT GGG AGT AGA TGG AGC CT
	Right	AGG CAT AAC TGC ACC CTT GG
Inner primers		
X4:	Left	TGC TCT TTT CAC CCA TCT AC
	Left for positive control	TGC TCT TTT CAC CC**<u>G</u>** TCT AC
	Right	ATA CGG CCA GGC ATT GAA GT
X5:	Left	TTC AAC TCT GTC TCC TTC CT
	Left for positive control	TT**<u>G</u>** AAC T**<u>G</u>**T GTC TC**<u>G</u>** TTC CT
	Right	CAG CCC TGT CGT CTC TCC AG
X6:	Left	GCC TCT GAT TCC TCA CTG AT
	Left for positive control	GCC TCT GAT TCC TC**<u>G</u>** CTG AT
	Right	TTA ACC CCT CCT CCC AGA GA
X7:	Left	CTT GCC ACA GGT CTC CCC AA
	Left for positive control	CTT GCC ACA G**<u>C</u>**T CTC CCC AA
	Right	TGT GCA GGG TGG CAA GTG GC
X8:	Left	TTC CTT ACT GCC TCT TGC TT
	Left for positive control	TTC CTT A**<u>G</u>**T GCC TC**<u>G</u>** TGC TT
	Right	CGC TTC TTG TCC TGC TTG CT

Note: Polymerase chain reaction is done in two sequences: first using the outer primers and the second reaction using the inner primers and sample from the first PCR as the template. Positive controls are amplified using the mutated primers in the place of the left primer. The changed nucleotide is bolded and underlined.

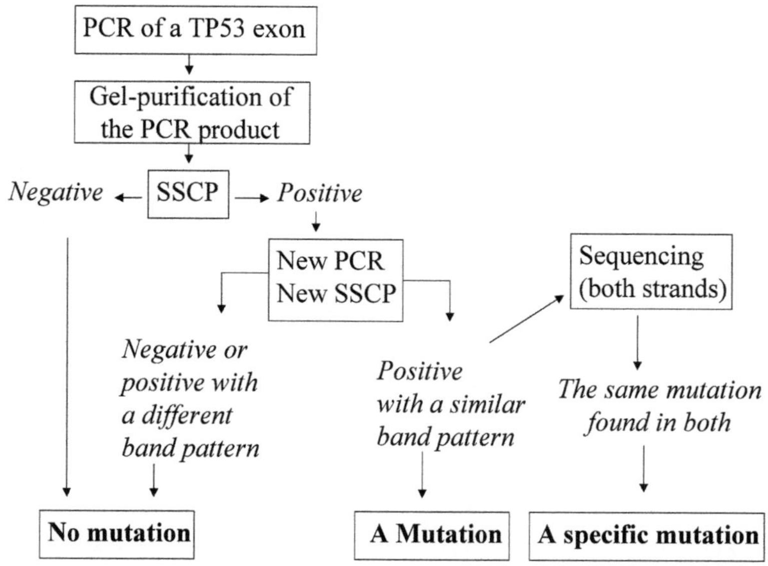

Fig. 2. Strategy of tumor sample analysis for TP53 mutations. (From **ref.** ***10.***)

the sequencing reaction (e.g., **refs.** ***10*** and ***28***). High-speed automatic sequencing and fluorescent probes are replacing manual radioactive sequencing ***(29)*** also in the analysis of *TP53* mutations ***(30,31)***. Although old-fashioned manual dideoxy sequencing is not sufficient for the future purposes of mutation detection, it is still useful as a reference point in the development and validation of newer methods. Also, small laboratories may have insufficient resources for new, more expensive methods and may have to rely on the traditional approaches for the near future.

2. Materials

2.1. Materials for PCR of p53 Exons and Purification of PCR Products

2.1.1. PCR Amplification

1. Enzyme: DyNAzyme II (Finnzymes, cat. no. F-501L).
2. 10X Buffer for DyNAzyme (Finnzymes, cat. no. F-511, comes with the enzyme).
3. Ultrapure dNTP set (Amersham Pharmacia, cat. no. 27-2035-02). For storage, add 250 µL of each dNTP to 12.3 mL of sterile H_2O and divide into 1 mL portions. Store at –20°C.
4. Sterile water.
5. Outer primers for the first PCR and inner primers for the nested, second PCR.
6. PCR machine (e.g., iCycler, Bio-Rad).
7. Heat block, 100°C.

8. Thin-wall PCR tubes, 0.6 mL (Robbins Scientific, cat. no. 1045-01-0).
9. Sterile Eppendorf tubes.

2.1.2. Minigel and Purification Gel

1. DNA markers 50–1000 bp (BMA, cat. no. 50461).
2. NuSieve 3:1 agarose (FMC, cat. no. 50090).
3. Stop solution (to be mixed with the sample for the gel runs), comes with the Sequenase kit or can be bought separately (USB, cat. no. 70724).
4. 10X TBE: 216 g Tris-HCl (ICN, cat. no. 819620), 110 g boric acid (Sigma, cat. no. B-7901), 160 mL of 0.25*M* EDTA, pH 8.0 Titriplex III, molecular weight (MW) 372.24 (Merck, cat. no. 1.08418), aqua distilled (2000 mL H_2O).
5. 0.5*M* Ammonium acetate (NH_4OAc), pH > 6.0, MW 77.08 (Sigma, cat. no. A-1542).
6. Ethanol, 100%.
7. Ethanol, 70% (400 mL of 99.5% ethanol + 168 mL H_2O).
8. Tris–EDTA buffer (10 m*M* Tris-HCl, 1 m*M* EDTA).
9. Minigel: Pharmacia Gel Electrophoresis Apparatus GNA-100 (Pharmacia Biotech).
10. Purification gel: Hoefer HE 99X Max (Amersham-Pharmacia Biotech).
11. Power supply: Biometra Power Pack P25.

2.2. Materials for SSCP

1. Absolute ethanol (100%).
2. Acetic acid (99.8%).
3. A Pharmacia PhastSystem electrophoresis and staining unit (Amersham-Pharmacia Biotech).
4. PhastGel Native Buffer Strips (Amersham-Pharmacia, cat. no. 17-0517-01).
5. PhastGel homogeneous gels (Amersham-Pharmacia, cat. no. 17-0624-01).
6. PhastGel Silver Staining Kit and solutions for staining (Amersham-Pharmacia, cat. no. 17-0617-01).
7. Solution 2 (numbers refer to the numbering of the places for tubes in the PhastSystem): In a 200-mL Erlenmeyer flask, mix 10 mL of acetic acid (99.8%), 50 mL of absolute ethanol, and 40 mL of distilled water.
8. Solution 3: In a 1000-mL Erlenmeyer flask, mix 25 mL of acetic acid (99.8%), 50 mL of absolute ethanol, and deionized water to a final volume of 500 mL.
9. Solution 4: 5% Glutaraldehyde solution (ready-made in the kit; half is used for one run; store at 4°C).
10. Solution 6: 0.4% Silver nitrate solution (ready-made in the kit; half is used for one run; store at 4°C).
11. Solution 7: 2.5% Sodium carbonate (ready-made) to which add 1 mL of formaldehyde (comes with the kit).
12. Solution 8: In a 200-mL Erlenmeyer flask, mix 100 mL of deionized water, 200 μL of 1*M* Tris-HCl, pH 8.0 (has to be prepared, adjusted by HCl), 1.6 g sodium

thiosulfate (comes with the kit). After the sodium thiosulfate has dissolved, the pH is lowered to 5.0–6.0 by a drop of acetic acid; check the final pH.

13. Tubings 5 and 9 from the PhastSystem development unit are inserted into bottles with deionized water. Tubing 0 is reserved for waste and 1 is not in use in this method.
14. Sample buffer for electrophoresis (95% formamide, 20 m*M* EDTA, 0.05% bromophenol blue, 0.05% xylene cyanol FF).
15. Heat block, 100°C.
16. Two metal weights, such as plumber's washers (e.g., round, 4 cm × 0.5 cm) to keep electrodes against the gels during the run; found in any hardware stores.
17. Gel-drying film and the frames (Promega, cat. no. V 7131).

2.3. Materials for Manual Sequencing

1. Sequencing reaction: Sequenase Kit, deaza (USB, cat. no. 70990).
2. Pyrophosphatase (USB, cat. no. 70950).
3. DS gel-purified PCR product (25–50 ng/μL).
4. 5' Primer, 1 pmol/μL.
5. 3' Primer, 1 pmol/μL.
6. Hot label at first base after sequencing primer (dNTP-^{33}P) (Perkin-Elmer/NEN).
7. Four colored 1.5-mL microcentrifuge tubes/sample (red, blue, green, yellow) for reactions.
8. 1.5-mL Microcentrifuge tubes.
9. Two heat blocks, 100°C and 42°C.
10. Ice.
11. Sequencing gel apparatus, includes two glass plates and spacers (LabRepCo, cat. no. S2), 64-well sharkstooth comb (VWR, cat. no. IB-80310).
12. SigmaCote (Sigma, cat. no. SL-2).
13. MOTS (methacryloxypropyltrimethoxy-silane) (Sigma, cat. no. M-6514).
14. SequaGel-8 (National Diagnostics, cat. no. EC-838).
15. Temed (Bio-Rad, cat. no. 161-0800).
16. Ammonium persulfate, 10% solution in H_2O (Bio-Rad, cat. no. 161-0700).
17. dH_2O (deionized water).
18. 95% Ethanol.
19. 100% Ethanol.
20. Lint-free paper towels.
21. Nine large bull-dog clips.
22. Power supply, capable of 3000 V.
23. 2000-mL fixative: 10% acetic acid, 10% methanol.
24. Oven set at 250°C.
25. BioMax MR1 film, 14 × 17 in. (Eastman Kodak, cat. no. 871-5187).
26. Film cassette, 35 × 43 cm (Kodak, cat. no. 177-1203).

3. Methods

3.1. PCR of p53 Exons

3.1.1. Amplification

1. For the first set of cycles, add all reagents into the PCR tubes, except the enzyme. Reagents for one 100-μL reaction are as follows:
   a. 10 μL of 10X enzyme buffer
   b. 16 μL of dNTPs
   c. 20 pmol of each primer
   d. 3 μL (200–500 ng) of template DNA
   e. 1 μL of enzyme
   f. Bring volume up to 100 μL using sterile water
2. Heat the tubes at 100°C for 10 min (hot start).
3. Add 1 μL of enzyme while samples are still in the heat block.
4. Start PCR: 97°C for 5 min, then 35 cycles of 94°C for 1 min, 60°C for 1 min, and 78°C for 30 s.
5. Keep at 4°C until collected from the thermocycler.
6. Repeat PCR as above (except the hot start) using 5 μL of the first reaction as the template.
7. Run 5 μL of the amplified sample on a 3% agarose minigel to check the result of amplification. Sizes of the bands are as follows: exon 5, 247 bp; exon 6, 180 bp; exon 7, 195 bp; exon 8, 200 bp.
8. Run the whole reaction volume on a 3% agarose thick preparative gel.

3.1.2. Extraction of the DNA From the Gel

1. Cut out the correct DNA band under long-wave ultraviolet (UV) light (short-wave UV light will destroy DNA).
2. Cut the gel piece into smaller pieces into an Eppendorf tube.
3. Add 450 μL of 0.5*M* ammonium acetate, pH >6.0.
4. Close the Eppendorf carefully and seal with Parafilm.
5. Incubate in a mixer at 37°C overnight.
6. Pipet the buffer into new tubes, add 950 μL of ice cold 100% ethanol, and let the DNA precipitate at –20°C at least overnight.
7. Pellet DNA by centrifuging 30 min at 11,000*g*.
8. Wash pellet three times with ice-cold 70% ethanol and let the pellet dry with the tube upside down on a paper towel at room temperature for at least 1 h. Be careful not to lose the pellet.
9. Dissolve the DNA pellet in 10–30 μL (depending on the strength of the band on the minigel) of Tris-EDTA buffer and store at –20°C.

3.2. SSCP Method

1. Mix 1 μL of the DNA sample and 1 μL of stop solution on ice.

2. Switch on the heat block (100°C).
3. Turn on the PhastSystem to appropriate temperature.
4. Mark the gels (e.g., by cutting an edge so that you can differentiate the left from the right gel, and in the case, that two machines are run at the same time, all gels can be identified).
5. Apply about 150 µL of water on each gel bed. Lay gel on top, making sure that there are no air bubbles under it, and press lightly with a paper towel to absorb extra water. Remove cellophane dustcover from the gels and set aside for later photography after staining.
6. Insert buffer strips in gel holder and lay on top of gels. Lower electrode assembly.
7. Start the prerun (400 V, 10 mA, 1 W) for 100 average volt hours (aVh).
8. Denature the samples in the heat block at 100°C for 3 min.
9. Apply 1 µL of the mixture to the grooves of the comb.
10. Pause the PhastSystem at 100 aVh and insert comb in the sample applicator. Be careful not to shake comb, thereby dropping samples prematurely.
11. Continue the run and wait until the aVh is 102 and the sample applicators rise from the gels.
12. Remove combs and lay metal weights on sample applicators to ensure electrodes are in contact with the gels at all times.
13. Start preparing the staining solution about 30 min before the end of running time.
14. Insert appropriately numbered tubing into correspondingly numbered solution bottles and cover openings with Parafilm.
15. Stop electrophoresis at the appropriate time and place gels in the wire holders in the developing chamber with gels facing each other. Be careful that gels do not touch each other. Close chamber carefully and start the staining program. Staining lasts 1 h and stops by itself.
16. Clean electrophoresis unit, including all separate parts (e.g., electrodes) with deionized water.
17. When staining is complete, remove gels and cover with the cellophane dustcovers and photograph.
18. To preserve the gels, wet the uncovered gels and the gel-drying films in deionized water. Place the film on an even surface and blot away extra water. Sandwich a gel between two sheets of Promega gel-drying film in drying frames, removing air bubbles as best you can. Air bubbles can crack the drying gels, making it impossible to read the bands correctly. Set aside overnight or until dry. Can be kept in a notebook for archiving.
19. For the washing program to clean the staining chamber, take the tubes out of the bottles and insert into bottles with deionized water. Place an unused gel in the chamber to cover the level sensor. After the run, wipe the chamber manually, first with deionized water and paper towel and then with absolute ethanol using a cotton swab.

3.3. Manual Sequencing Method

3.3.1. Setup of Reactions

1. Set up five denaturation tubes containing 8.0 µL template DNA (3 µL DNA + 5 µL H_2O), 3.0 µL sequencing primer.
2. Prepare cocktail (for five reactions): Add 7.6 µL enzyme dilution buffer, 2.5 µL Sequenase (13 U/µL), 9.6 µL of 5X reaction buffer, 5.5 µL dithiothreitol (DTT), 1.0 µL hot label, 0.8 µL pyrophosphatase.
3. Reaction tubes: Mark four reaction tubes per sample (one of each color).
4. Denature five denaturation tubes at 100°C for 3 min.
5. Move to a 42°C heat block for 2 min to cool.
6. Distribute 3.5 µL of labeled sample to each of the four colored reaction tubes.
7. Return to 42°C heat block for 5 min.
8. Add 2.5 µL stop solution from Sequenase kit to each reaction tube.
9. Store at –20°C.

3.3.2. Running Sequencing Gel

1. Clean both plates with dH_2O. Never use detergent on the glass.
2. Carefully apply 5 mL SigmaCote to one side of the large plate; spread to all edges using lint-free paper towel. Set aside for 10 min.
3. Prepare working MOTS solution: Mix 200 µL MOTS solution with 40 mL of 100% ethanol. Store at 4°C.
4. Add 90 µL of 10% acetic acid to 3 mL MOTS working solution and carefully apply to small plate; spread to all edges using lint-free paper towel. Set aside for 10 min.
5. Rinse large siliconized plate with 5 mL dH_2O and polish with lint-free paper towel until dry.
6. Rinse small MOTS plate with 5 mL of 95% ethyl alcohol and polish with lint-free paper towel until dry.
7. Sandwich the plates with treated sides facing each other and spacers inserted along sides. Keep sandwiched plates horizontal and level.
8. Prepare Sequagel-8% at room temperature according to manufacturer's directions.
9. Cast gel, slowly, allowing capillary action to fill plates, tapping out air bubbles should any arise.
10. Slide sharkstooth comb, even side down, along top of gel, creating a level edge.
11. Clamp three bull-dog clips on each spacer, not on gel, and three along the top, on comb. Do not clamp on bottom edge. Allow to set for 1 h at room temperature.
12. Put gel on S2 sequencing rig, with small plate against gel rig. Tighten screws, top and bottom.
13. Add 500 mL of 1X TBS in top compartment and 500 mL in bottom compartment of gel rig. Remove sharkstooth comb and clean with water.
14. Preheat gel rig at 2000 V for 15 min. Replace comb, tooth side down and 2–3 mm deep into gel. This creates wells.

15. Denature reaction tubes at 100°C for 3 min. Keep on ice and load 3 μL of each sample on gel, in the order A, C, G, T.
16. Turn on gel rig fan. Run gel at 2500 V until dark blue band reaches bottom of plates.
17. Turn off power, drain upper compartment of gel rig into bottom compartment, and remove plates to a staining box containing 2 L of fixative (10% acetic acid + 10% methanol).
18. Remove spacers and comb. Using a small spatula, pry plates apart, allowing small plate to lie, gel side up, in fixative for 20 min. Swish (gently mix) solution every 5–10 min or so.
19. Carefully drain fixative, add 1 L dH_2O, and set aside for 5 min.
20. Drain gel. Put into 250°C oven, gel side up, for about 25 min or until gel is dry.
21. Remove from oven and set aside until cool enough to handle.
22. In dark room, lay glass plate with gel side against Kodak film in Kodak cassette.
23. Develop film for one night and, if necessary, put down another film against gel for longer exposure. Mark film, if necessary, to distinguish between left and right, for reading purposes.
24. Read film from bottom to top.

4. Interpretation of the Results

A sample is judged to be positive for a *TP53* mutation only if two independent amplified products contain similar shifted band patterns (*see* **Figs. 2** and **3**). We achieve a 98% efficiency when using two temperatures in combination with other optimized conditions ***(21,26,32)***. Only 1 of the studied 33 samples with known *TP53* mutations remained undetected, and all of the artificially mutated positive controls were also detectable at least at one temperature ***(32)***. If only one temperature had been used, 16% (7 of 43) of the mutations would have been missed at higher temperatures (15°C for exon 4 and 20°C for other exons) and 28% (12 of 43) at 4°C.

The PCR-SSCP method allows the detection of 5% mutated alleles in the presence of the wild-type allele ***(25,32–33)***. We have found tumors with similar consistency, positive band patterns in SSCP analysis but negative by sequencing ***(10,32)***. These may represent real p53 mutations, because SSCP analysis has been reported to be more sensitive in detecting mutations than sequencing ***(33–35)***. The sensitivity of sequencing to detect mutated fragments against the wild-type background is such that more than 20% has to be mutated DNA ***(30,34)***. Thus, it may be that the lesions are reproducibly positive by SSCP, but negative in sequencing, representing cases where the relative concentration of mutated DNA in the amplification products was below the sensitivity of sequencing ***(33)***.

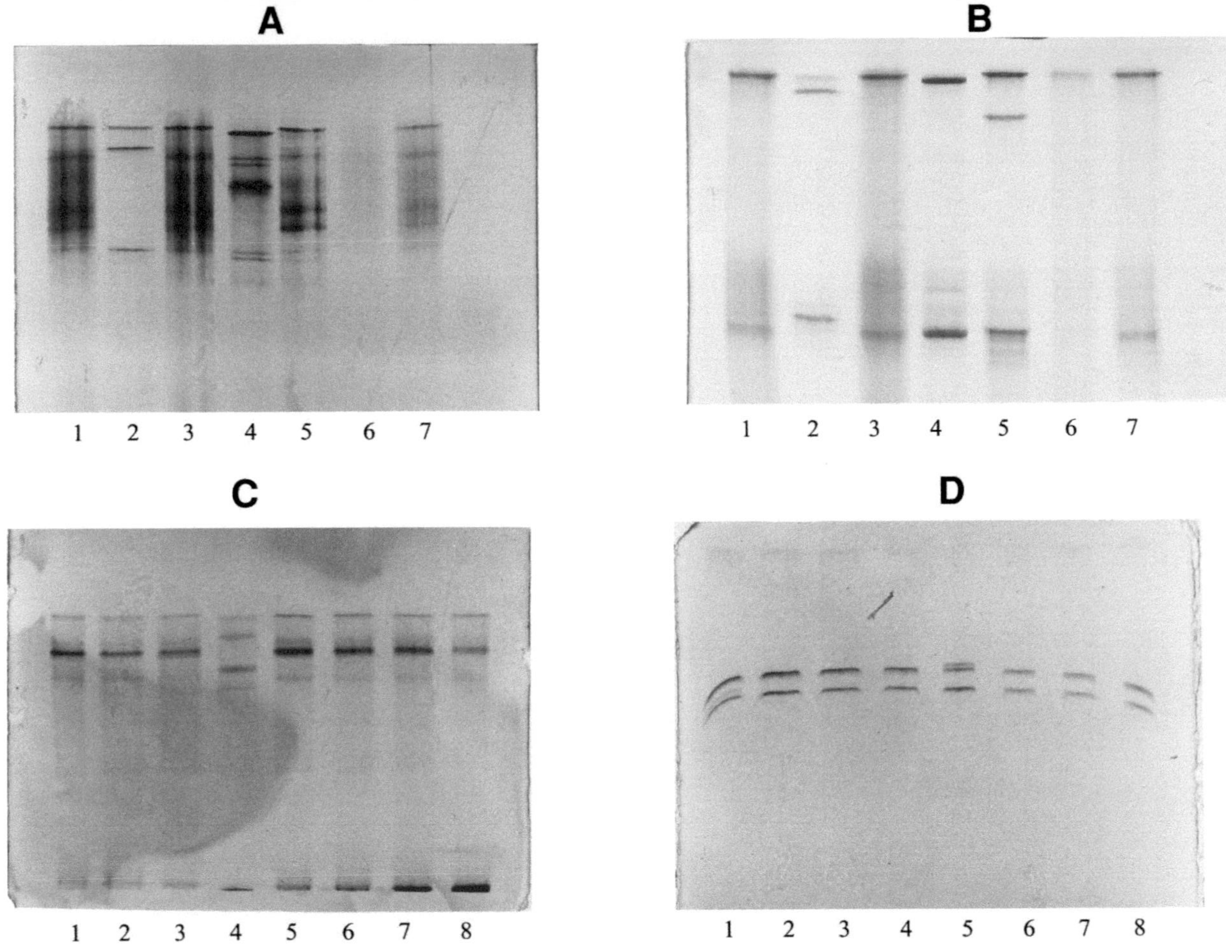

Fig. 3. SSCP of formalin-fixed, paraffin-embedded cancer samples for *TP53* exons 5 and 6: **(A)** exon 5, 4°C; **(B)** exon 5, 20°C; **(C)** exon 6, 4°C; **(D)** exon 6, 20°C. (A) and (B) contain the same samples in similar order, as do also (C) and (D). *Lane 3*: wild-type DNA negative control; *lane 4:* positive control amplified from wild-type DNA using a primer with a changed sequence. Changed band patterns indicating a mutation in the amplified product, either the result of a mutation in the tumor sample or an artifact as a result of a polymerase error, can be seen in *lane 2* in (A), *lanes 2 and 5* in (B), and *lane 8* in (D). The last mentioned mutation does not show in *lane 8* in (C) using the other temperature.

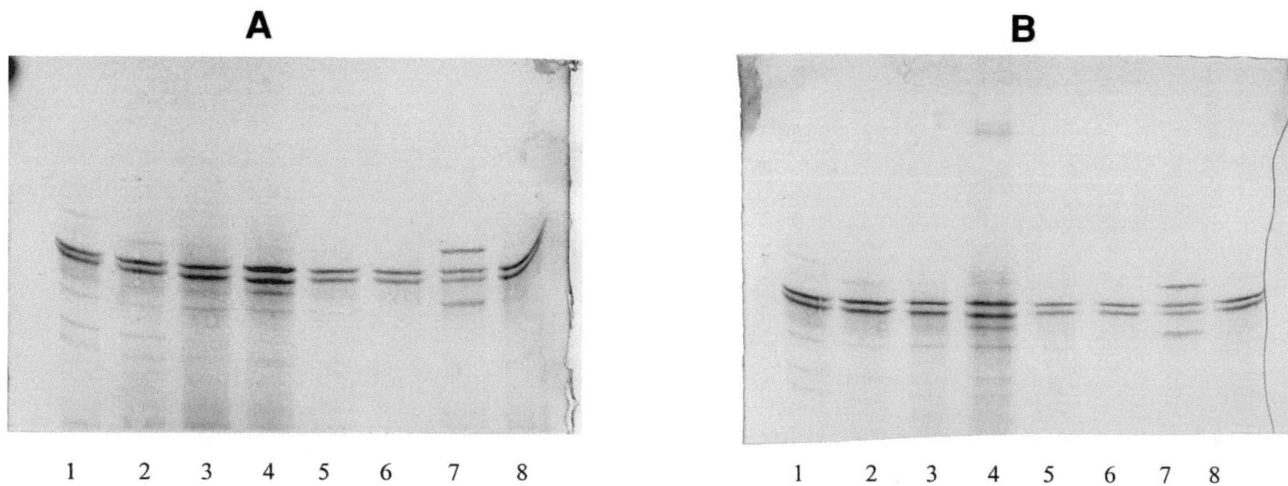

Fig. 4. SSCP for *TP53* exon 8 at +20°C. *Lane 3:* Wild-type DNA negative control; *lane 4:* positive control amplified from wild-type DNA using a primer with a changed sequence. *Lanes 7* in **(A)** and **(B)** show two independently amplified products from the same sample showing similarly changed band pattern and indicating a mutation in the original sample. Other lanes show negative samples.

We have adopted a strategy, when studying formalin-fixed, paraffin-embedded human tumor samples, where the existence of a *TP53* mutation is first confirmed with SSCP and the type of mutation is then separately analyzed in each studied exon by manual dideoxy sequencing (*see* **Fig. 4**) ***(10)***. In addition to sequencing both strands, it has been necessary in many cases to sequence at least two independent PCR products, as discovered by other authors ***(36)***, and to use deaza nucleotides to help with GC-rich areas ***(37)*** in the sequencing reactions. We have found clear mutations in SSCP (a similar band pattern in two or more independent amplified products that differ from the wild type) that have been, however, negative in sequencing ***(10,32)***. Because less mutated DNA in the wild-type DNA is required in our SSCP ***(21)*** than in manual sequencing, it is possible that they represent real mutations.

5. Notes

1. The most important point in PCR is the sterility. It applies to all reagents, supplies, and working habits. When repeating amplifying human p53 exons, the contamination is a major problem. It is absolutely necessary to run controls without the template at the beginning (to control for reagents) and at the end (to control pipetting) in every PCR series. If a right size band is seen in the minigel in controls, the whole series has to be considered contaminated and has to be thrown away. We set up the reactions in a laminar-flow hood where UV lamp is on at least for half an hour before starting the work (contaminating DNA is not destroyed by heat). If the laminar-flow hood (including the airways) is not cleaned on regular basis, it can serve as a source of contamination as well (has been experienced!).
2. For amplification of several samples for the same p53 exon, it is easiest to prepare a mixture of all the reagents (except the enzyme in the mixture for the first PCR, and the templates, of course) and divide it in the PCR tubes after that.
3. To save time, you can prepare the tubes with reagents (including the enzyme) for the second nested PCR reaction at the same time as you prepare the first PCR reaction mixture, and store refrigerated for the 2–3 h that the first amplification runs.
4. Program "4°C indefinitely" in the PCR machine as the last cycle so that you do not have to wait at the machine for the program to end.
5. It is important to realize that the developed SSCP method requires exactly the same primers for PCR that were used for the development. If primer sequences are changed, the conditions and controls have to be amended as well.
6. For a good background and readable result in the SSCP, it is extremely important to run a cleaning run in the development unit after each experiment. Furthermore, manual cleaning with a cotton wipe of the staining chamber and especially the level sensor after the cleaning run is also needed.
7. Another important factor is the purity of the starting material. The PCR product has to be carefully gel-purified before SSCP.

8. Program the PhastGel machine beforehand. Use a separate number for each of the running conditions (prerun and each of the temperatures).
9. Always write down the lot numbers of the reagents. If a problem is the result of a bad reagent, it is impossible to locate it otherwise.
10. Negative and positive controls ensure the quality of the run. As negative controls, gel-purified, amplified normal DNA is used. We amplify 6–10 tubes at the same time and use those that look the same as the former negative controls. The PCR products should not be pooled because some of them may contain a PCR error that have to be excluded from the set. As positive controls, DNA is amplified using mutated primers, and only runs where the positive controls are clearly visible are accepted.
11. If the DNA sample is very dilute, the mixing ratio can be increase up to 4:1 of DNA to stop solution.
12. Silver-stained gels should be dried between sheets of the Promega gel-drying film immediately after the SSCP because they are very sensitive to light and will fade quickly if not stored properly. On the other hand, the bands in the gels stored properly get more visible within about 1 wk after the run. The interpretation of the gels is thus best done after such a storage period.
13. Although the gels can be stored for long periods (up to 4 yr according to our experience), it is advisable to photograph or scan the successful experiments for storage.
14. The DNA sample has to be gel-purified after PCR amplification for a good sequencing results as well.
15. It is necessary to clean the sequencing apparatus carefully after each run to keep the temperature even during the runs.
16. Both strands should be sequenced to be sure of the existence of a mutation in a gel (*see* **Fig. 2**).
17. The rest of the sequencing reaction can be stored overnight at –20°C for another run next day.
18. Sequenase should not be left outside the freezer for more than is necessary. While working with it, keep on ice.
19. Reading of the sequencing result is done from the bottom of the film to the top using a chart with the wild-type sequence. It is easier to record the result on an available chart of the wild-type sequence. In this way, the result can be documented on the same page.

References

1. Lane, D. P. and Lain, S. (2002) Therapeutic exploitation of the p53 pathway. *Trends Mol. Med.* **8(4),** 38–42.
2. Vousden, K. H. (2002) Activation of the p53 tumor suppressor protein. *Biochim. Biophys. Acta* **1602,** 47–59.
3. Zhao, R., Gish, K., Murphy, M., et al. (2000) Analysis of p53 regulated gene expression patterns using oligonucleotide arrays. *Genes Dev.* **14,** 981–993.

4. Sigal, A. and Rotter, V. (2000) Oncogenic mutations of the p53 tumor suppressor: the demons of the guardian of the genome. *Cancer Res.* **60,** 6788–6793.
5. van Oijen, M. G. C. T. and Slootweg, P. J. (2000) Gain-of-function mutations in the tumor suppressor gene p53. *Clin. Cancer Res.* **6,** 2138–2145.
6. Guimaraes, D. P. and Hainaut, P. (2002) TP53: a key gene in human cancer. *Biochimie* **84,** 83–93.
7. Hollstein, M., Sidransky, B., Vogelstein, C., et al. (1991) P53 mutations in human cancers. *Science* **253,** 49–53.
8. Greenblatt, M. S., Bennett, W. P., Hollstein, M., et al. (1994) Mutations in the p53 tumor suppressor gene: clues to cancer etiology and molecular pathogenesis. *Cancer Res.* **54,** 4855–4878.
9. Hainaut, P., Soussi, T., Shomer, B., et al. (1997) Database of p53 gene somatic mutations in human tumors and cell lines: updated compilation and future prospects. *Nucleic Acid Res.* **25,** 151–157.
10. Vähäkängas, K. H., Bennett, W. P., Castren, K., et al. (2001) P53 gene and K-ras mutations in lung cancers from former and never-smoking women. *Cancer Res.* **61,** 4350–4356.
11. Levine, A. J. (1997) P53, the cellular gatekeeper for growth and division. *Cell* **88,** 323–331.
12. Hainaut, P. and Vähäkangas, K. (1997) P53 as a sensor of carcinogenic exposures: mechanisms of p53 protein induction and lessons from p53 gene mutations. *Pathol.–Biolog.* **45,** 833–844.
13. Borresen, A.-L., Anderson, T. I., Eyfjörd, J. E., et al. (1995) TP53 mutations and breast cancer prognosis: particularly poor survival rates for cases with mutations in the zinc-binding domains. *Genes Chromosomes Cancer* **14,** 71–75.
14. Valgardsdottir, R., Tryggvadottir, L., Steinarsdottir, M., et al. (1997) Genomic instability and poor prognosis associated with abnormal TP53 in breast carcinomas. Molecular and immunohistochemical analysis. *APMIS* **105,** 121–130.
15. Huang, C., Taki, T., Adachi, M., et al. (1998) Mutations in exon 7 and 8 of p53 as poor prognostic factors in patients with non-small cell lung cancer. *Oncogene* **16,** 2469–2477.
16. Orita, M., Iwahana, H., Kanazawa, H., et al. (1989) Detection of polymorphisms of human DNA by gel electrophoresis as single strand conformation polymorphisms. *Proc. Natl. Acad. Sci. USA* **86,** 2766–2770.
17. Hayashi, K. (1992) PCR-SSCP: a method for detection of mutations. *GATA* **9,** 73–92.
18. Hayashi, K. and Yandell, D. W. (1993) How sensitive is PCR-SSCP? *Hum. Mutat.* **2,** 338–346.
19. Glavac, D. and Dean, M. (1993) Optimization of the single-strand conformation polymorphism (SSCP) technique for detection of point mutations. *Hum. Mutat.* **2,** 404–414.
20. Moyret, C., Theillet, C., Puig, P. L., et al. (1994) Relative efficiency of denaturing

gradient gel electrophoresis and single-strand conformation polymorphism in the detection of mutations in exon 5 to 8 of the p53 gene. *Oncogene* **9,** 1739–1743.

21. Welsh, J. A., Castren, K., and Vahakangas, K. (1997) Single-strand conformation polymorphism analysis to detect p53 mutations: characterization and development of controls. *Clin. Chem.* **43,** 2251–2255.
22. Sheffield, V. C., Cox, D. R., Lerman, L. S., et al. (1989) Attachment of a 40-base-pair G + C-rich sequence (GC-lamp) to genomic DNA fragments by the polymerase chain reaction results in improved detection of single-base changes. *Proc. Natl. Acad. Sci. USA* **86,** 232–236.
23. Meinhold-Heerlein, I., Ninci, E., Ikenberg, H., et al. (2001) Evaluation of methods to detect p53 mutations in ovarian cancer. *Oncology* **60,** 176–188.
24. Ryu, J.-W., Lee, M.-C., and Jang, W.-C. (2000) Detecting p53 gene mutation of breast cancer and defining differences between silver staining PCR-SSCP and immunohistochemical staining. *J. Korean Med. Sci.* **15,** 73–77.
25. Pinheiro, N. A., Moura, R. P., Monteiro, E., et al. (1999) Detection of point mutations by non-isotopic single strand conformation polymorphism. *Brazil J. Med. Biol. Res.* **32,** 55–58.
26. Vähäkangas, K. H., Castren, K., and Welsh, J. A. (2000) Single-strand conformation polymorphism analysis of mutations in exons 4–8 of the TP53 gene, in *Methods in Molecular Medicine, Volume 49: Molecular Pathology Protocols* (Killeen, A. A., ed.), Humana, Totowa, NJ, pp. 15–27.
27. Wikman, F. P., Lu, M.-L., Thykjaer, T., et al. (2000) Evaluation of the performance of a p53 sequencing microarray chip using 140 previously sequenced bladder tumor samples. *Clin. Chem.* **46,** 1555–1561.
28. Vähäkangas, K. H., Samet, J. M., Metcalf, R. A., et al. (1992) Mutations of the p53 and ras genes in radon-associated lung cancer from uranium miners. *Lancet* **339,** 576–580.
29. Shi, M. M. (2001) Enabling large-scale pharmacogenetic studies by high-throughput mutation detection and genotyping technologies. *Clin. Chem.* **47,** 164–172.
30. Worsham, M. J., Pals, G., Raju, U., et al. (2002) Establishing a molecular continuum in breast cancer: DNA microarrays and benign breast disease. *Cytometry* **47,** 56–59.
31. Schaefer K. L., Wai, D., Poremba, C., et al. (2002) Analysis of TP53 mutations in pediatric tumor patients using microarray-based sequencing technology. *Med. Pediatr. Oncol.* **38(4),** 247–253.
32. Castren, K., Ranki, A., Welsh, J., et al. (1998a) Infrequent p53 mutations in arsenic-related skin lesions. *Oncol. Res.* **10,** 475–482.
33. Chaubert, P., Beautista, D., and Benhattar J. (1993) An improved method for rapid screening of DNA mutations by nonradioactive single-strand conformational polymorphism procedure. *Biotechniques* **15,** 586.
34. Cheng, J. and Haas, M. (1992) Sensitivity of detection of heterozygous point mutations in p53 cDNAs by direct PCR sequencing. *PCR Methods Appl.* **1,** 199–201.

35. Wu, J. K., Ye, Z., and Darras, B. T. (1993) Sensitivity of single-strand conformation polymorphism (SSCP) analysis in detecting p53 point mutations in tumours with mixed cell populations. *Am. J. Hum. Genet.* **52,** 1273–1275.
36. Conway, K., Edmiston, S. N., Cui, L., et al. (2002) Prevalence and spectrum of p53 mutations associated with smoking in breast cancer. *Cancer Res.* **62,** 1987–1995.
37. Mizusawa, S., Nishimura, S., and Seela, F. (1986) Improvement of the dideoxy chain termination method of DNA sequencing by use of deoxy-7-deazaguanosine triphosphate in place of dGTP. *Nucleic Acids Res.* **14,** 1319–1324.

15

PCR Diagnosis of T-Cell Lymphoma in Paraffin-Embedded Bone Marrow Biopsies

Jean Benhattar and Sandra Gebhard

1. Introduction

Management of T-cell lymphoma patients requires bone marrow examination for the assessment of stage and prognosis *(1,2)*. Bone marrow biopsy (BMB) is mandatory when bone marrow aspirate is not successful (e.g., in cases of patchy lymphomatous infiltration or induction of fibrosis ["dry aspirate"]) *(3)*. Moreover, BMB has some advantages over aspirate, such as examination of a greater volume of tissue with preserved architecture, assessment of cellularity, and application of immunohistochemistry.

The distinction between reactive T-cell infiltrate and T-cell lymphoma on BMB can be very difficult, even with the use of extensive immunohistochemistry, mainly because monoclonality of T-cells cannot be reliably established by immunohistochemistry *(4)*. Loss of T-cell-antigen expression or aberrant expression of B-cell antigen creates additional pitfalls. Moreover, intense nonspecific reactive changes, sometimes with necrosis, are common features in T-cell lymphomas. They are probably induced by a variety of cytokines produced by neoplastic T-cells. As a consequence, tumor cells may constitute only a minor part of an infiltrate, including lymphocytes, plasma cells, histiocytes, granulomas, macrophages, and eosinophils.

Molecular genetic analysis of T-cell receptor (TCR) gene rearrangement is considered a reliable tool in the determination of T-cell clonality *(5)*. Rearrangement of TCR-γ gene is frequently investigated because it occurs at an early stage of T-cell development *(6)* and is present in almost all of normal and neoplastic T-cells. Detection of monoclonal rearrangement of TCR-γ gene by polymerase chain reaction (PCR) has been shown to be a simple and rapid

From: *Methods in Molecular Medicine, vol. 97: Molecular Diagnosis of Cancer*
Edited by: J. E. Roulston and J. M. S. Bartlett © Humana Press Inc., Totowa, NJ

method for analysis of clonality in frozen and in paraffin-embedded tissues *(7–13)*.

Compared to lymph node biopsy, BMB usually requires special fixation and decalcification, which creates additional problems for PCR analysis. BMB is preferentially fixed in mercuric chloride-containing fixatives, such as formaldehyde sublimate or B5 (mercuric chloride and formaldehyde) to improve morphological details. An alternative fixative is alcoholic Bouin (Dubosq-Brasil). Conflicting results have been reported concerning the effects of these fixatives on DNA preservation ***(13–16)***. However, it has recently been shown in a series of 46 paraffin-embedded, shortly decalcified, formaldehyde-sublimate or alcoholic Bouin-fixed BMBs that DNA could be amplified in 98% of the cases, confirming the overall good tissue preservation ***(13)***. This study has shown that TCR-γ PCR is a complementary tool for the assessment of T-cell lymphoma in BMB, particularly useful when histological and immunohistochemistry examination of BMB did not firmly establish a diagnosis of T-cell lymphoma.

2. Materials and Reagents

2.1. Specimen

Paraffin-embedded BMSs lightly decalcified during 1 h in an acidic decalcifier, such as the Surgipath Decalcifier II (Surgipath Medical Industries, Richmond, IL).

2.2. DNA Extraction and PCR

1. Sterile scalpels.
2. Water bath (65°C).
3. Xylene.
4. Ethanol.
5. DNeasy tissue kit (Qiagen, Hilden, Germany).
6. Proteinase K (stock of 15–20 mg/mL, in 10 m*M* Tris-HCl, pH 7.5).
7. Incubators (55°C and 70°C).
8. Thermocycler.
9. 10X PCR buffer (100 m*M* Tris-HCl [pH 8.3]), 500 m*M* KCl).
10. 50 m*M* $MgCl_2$.
11. 5 m*M* deoxynucleoside triphosphate mix (dNTP).
12. 50 ng/μL Each primer.
13. 5 U/μL *Taq* DNA polymerase (Invitrogen).
14. Primer sequences *(17)*:
    TVγ 5'- AGG GTT GTG TTG GAA TCA GG -3'
    TJγ 5'- CGT CGA CAA CAA GTG TTG TTC CAC -3'

2.3. Electrophoresis

1. Horizontal gel electrophoresis apparatus (e.g., Danaphor type 100 from Danaphor, Grandvaux, Switzerland).
2. Standard agarose (Eurobio, Les Ulis, France).
3. 10X TBE buffer: 900 m*M* Tris-HCl, 900 m*M* boric acid, 20 m*M* disodium EDTA (pH 8.0).
4. Ethidium bromide (10 mg/mL, in distillated water).
5. 2X Ficoll loading dye: 100 mg of Ficoll 400 (Pharmacia Bioteck), 60 μL of 1% xylene cyanol FF, add water up to 1 mL. Store at 4°C.
6. 30-cm vertical gel electrophoresis apparatus (e.g., SE600 series from Hoefer [Hoefer Scientific, San Francisco, CA]).
7. 6% Nondenaturing polyacrylamide gel (acrylamide/bisacrylamide, 29:1): 22.8 g of acrylamide, 1.2 g of bis-acrylamide, 40 mL of 1X TBE, add H_2O to make the volume up to 400 mL. After dissolution, filtrate and store at 4°C. (*Note*: acrylamide is a neurotoxin; if required, use commercially prepared solutions.)
8. 6X Blue/orange loading dye (Promega): 10% Ficoll 400, 0.25% xylene cyanol FF, 0.25% bromophenol blue, 0.4% orange G, 10 m*M* Tris-HCl (pH 7.5), 50 m*M* EDTA.
9. SYBR Gold gel stain (Molecular Probes, Eugene, OR).
10. Gel documentation system with a charge-coupled device (CCD) camera (e.g., the AlphaImager from Alpha Innotech Corporation, San Leandro, CA).

3. Methods

3.1. DNA Extraction

Extraction of DNA from paraffin-embedded tissues with the DNeasy tissue kit is performed using a modified version of the manufacturer's protocol (*see* **Note 1**).

1. Carefully scrape each paraffin block with a sterile scalpel to remove a small part of the tissue of interest (5–20 mg). Place the thin slices of tissue obtained in a microcentrifuge tube (*see* **Note 2**).
2. Add 1 mL xylene and heat at 65°C in a water bath for 5 min to remove the paraffin. Vortex vigorously. Centrifuge at full speed (12,000*g*–15,000*g*) for 5 min in a microfuge. Remove and discard the supernatant.
3. Repeat **step 2** once.
4. Add 1 mL of 100% ethanol to the pellet to remove residual xylene, and mix gently. Centrifuge for 3 min at full speed in a microfuge, remove, and discard supernatant.
5. Rehydrate the pellet by addition of 1 mL of 70% ethanol. Vortex and centrifuge for 3 min. Remove and discard the supernatant. Air-dry the pellet for 10–15 min until the residual ethanol has evaporated.
6. Resuspend the tissue pellet in 180 μL of ATL lysis buffer contained in the DNeasy tissue kit and add 10 μL of proteinase K (15–20 mg/ μL). Mix well and incubate overnight (14–18 h) at 55°C.

7. Add a further 10 μL proteinase K and incubate for 1 h at 55°C.
8. Add 10 μL of RNaseA (10 mg/μL) and incubate 5 min at room temperature.
9. Add 200 μL of buffer AL (contained in the DNeasy tissue kit), vortex, and incubate 10 min at 70°C to yield a homogeneous solution.
10. Add 220 μL ethanol, mix well, load into a DNeasy minicolumn sitting in a microcentrifuge tube, and spin for 1 min at 7000*g*. Discard flowthrough and collection tube.
11. Place the DNeasy minicolumn in a clean microcentrifuge tube, add 600 μL of buffer AW1 (contained in the DNeasy tissue kit), and spin for 1 min at 12,000*g*–15,000*g*. Discard flowthrough and collection tube.
12. Add 600 μL of buffer AW2 and spin for 1 min at 12,000*g*–15,000*g*. Discard flowthrough. Rotate the tube and spin again to dry the column.
13. Place the DNeasy minicolumn in a clean microcentrifuge tube, add directly on the column 80 μL of buffer AE (contained in the DNeasy tissue kit), incubate 15 min at 70°C, and then centrifuge for 2 min at 12,000*g*–15,000*g* to elute.
14. Keep the DNA solution at –20°C.

3.2. PCR Reaction

1. Prepare the PCR master mix in a separate area. The volume prepared is based on the number of reaction tubes desired. For 18 reaction tubes (20 μL for each PCR reaction), add to a microcentrifuge tube the following: 214 μL of water, 40 μL of 10X PCR buffer, 26 μL of primer TVγ, 26 μL of primer TJγ, 15 μL of 50 m*M* $MgCl_2$, 20 μL of 5 m*M* dNTP, and 2 μL of *Taq* DNA polymerase (*see* **Note 3**).
2. Place 3 μL of each DNA solution in 0.5-mL microcentrifuge tubes on ice and aliquot 17 μL of the master mix into each tube. Each sample is prepared in duplicate. Include a negative control containing 3 μL of H_2O instead of DNA and a positive control containing 3 μL of DNA obtained from a tumor with a clonal TCR-γ gene rearrangement.
3. Prepare the program for amplification. Use an initial denaturation step of 95°C for 5 min, followed by a three-step profile: denaturation at 94°C for 30 s, annealing at 55°C for 45 s, and extension at 72°C for 75 s, for a total of 40 cycles (*see* **Note 4**). Store tubes at 15°C at the end of the last cycle.
4. Start the thermocycler and place tubes in the block when the temperature reaches 95°C.
5. Perform amplification.
6. Remove the tubes from the block and store at 4°C until the reactions are run on gels.

3.3. Detection of Amplification Products

3.3.1. Control of PCR Amplification

1. Prepare a 2% agarose gel in 1X TBE buffer containing 1 μg of ethidium bromide per milliliter. Use electrophoresis to separate the amplification products. Add 10 μL to each well (5 μL of PCR product and 5 μL of 2X Ficoll loading dye) and

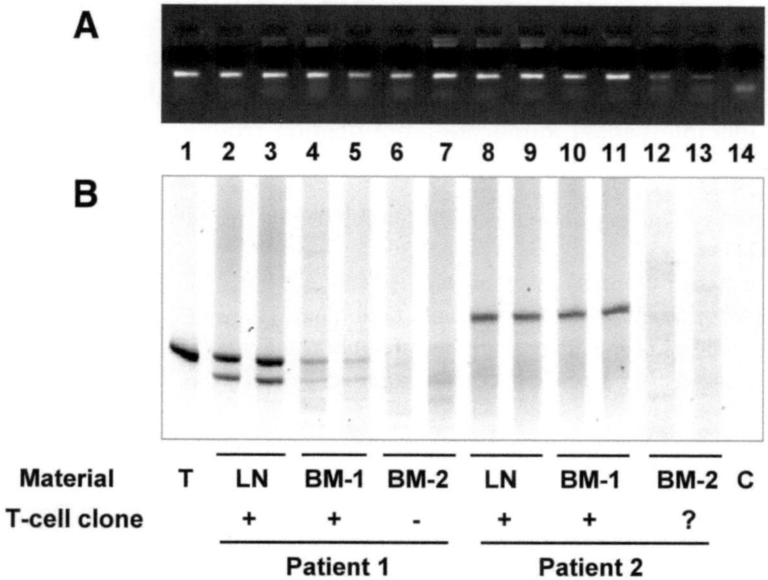

Fig. 1. Analysis of rearranged TCR-γ products on agarose and polyacrylamide gels. After PCR amplification, DNA extracted from extramedullar (LN: lymph node) and consecutive paraffin-embedded bone marrow (BM) biopsies are analyzed on 2% agarose (**A**) and 6% polyacrylamide (**B**) gels. Except for the last sample (*lanes 12* and *13*), brief electrophoresis on agarose gel confirms the correct amplification of the analyzed samples (A). For patient 1, the clonal bands are present only in the first BMB (BM-1). For patient 2, an identical clonal rearrangement is detected in the LN and in the BM-1. For the BM-2, the interpretation is complicated as a consequence of poor PCR amplification. Positive and negative controls: T, well-characterized T-cell lymphoma; C, water in place of DNA in the PCR reaction.

electrophorese at 80 mA for a short time (migration of 0.5–1 cm of the xylene cyanol indicator).

2. Place the gel on the ultraviolet (UV) transilluminator to visualize the PCR products (*see* **Fig. 1A**) (*see* **Notes 5–7**).

3.3.2. Detection on Acrylamide Gel

1. Prepare a 6% nondenaturing polyacrylamide gel in TBE buffer. Add 6 μL to each well (2 μL of PCR product, 3 μL of H_2O, and 1 μL of 6X blue/orange loading dye) and electrophorese at 600 V in a 30-cm-long gel until the xylene cyanol indicator is approx 4 cm from the bottom of the gel (about 2.5 h).
2. Carefully release the gel from the glass plates and stain for 20 min in the dark with a SYBR Gold gel stain diluted 1:10,000 in 1X TBE buffer (*see* **Note 8**).
3. Visualize by UV transillumination using a CCD camera. Photograph the gel and save the image (*see* **Fig. 1B**).

3.4. Interpretation of Data

To provide confidence in the results, duplicate amplifications should be performed. Furthermore, with a nonconvincing result (weak amplification or nonreproducible bands), duplicate amplification from a new extracted DNA must be performed.

1. A clonal T-cell population is identified by one or two discrete bands (*see* **Notes 9–11**).
2. Bone marrow biopsy is considered negative when PCR products show either smears or nonreproducible multiple faint bands (*see* **Fig. 1B**, *lanes 6* and *7*).
3. The analysis is considered noninterpretable when no or only weak amplification is observed after electrophoresis on agarose gel (**Fig. 1B**, *lanes 12* and *13*).

4. Notes

1. Alternative DNA extraction procedures can be used. Our experience indicates that recovery of DNA with the DNeasy tissue kit is comparable to that provided by the standard phenol/chloroform extraction or by other similar approaches. However, it offers the benefit of superior elimination of inhibitory molecules, such as heavy metals (as those contained in some fixatives; e.g., mercury), and the recovery of larger DNA molecules from fixed tissues.
2. To avoid cross-contamination of DNA, the use of serial tissue sections is not recommended. Indeed, when cutting sections from paraffin-embedded blocks, the microtome's blade and tweezers should be extensively cleaned between samples, which is time-consuming and not always feasible.
3. In creating the master mix, it is useful to overestimate the volume required by one or two reactions to allow for pipetting inaccuracies and other losses of volume. Make up the master mix on ice just before dispensing it into the individual tubes and add the *Taq* DNA polymerase last.
4. When genomic DNA extracted from frozen tissue has to be amplified, it is sufficient to perform 35 cycles with an extension time of 45 s in place of 75 s.
5. This rapid electrophoresis on agarose gel is an easy method to confirm the correct amplification of the extracted DNA. Under these conditions, all of the amplified rearranged TCR-γ gene products migrate together (*see* **Fig. 1A**). The primers used in this approach generate PCR products of about 160–200 bp. This procedure clearly reduces the number of false-negative results that are generally caused by either a high DNA degradation level or a bad amplification reaction (*see* **Fig. 1A**, *lanes 12* and *13*).
6. For samples with too weak or even no amplification, it is advised to repeat the analysis, but from an additional DNA extraction. Indeed, the fixative and the decalcifier act more strongly at the surface of the tissue block. Thus, by sampling the tissue more deeply within the block, it is possible to obtain a less pronounced DNA degradation.
7. Our laboratory has applied this DNA extraction and PCR approaches to more

than 250 clinical fixed BMB specimens. Under these conditions, PCR amplification was successful in 94% of samples.

8. Numerous methods can be used to detect the amplified products, such as ethidium bromide staining or ^{32}P-labeling of PCR products. However, SYBR Gold staining is rapid, simple to perform, and provides good sensitivity and high resolution, and its solution can be reused several times.
9. Detection of a clonal rearrangement of TCR-γ does not automatically imply malignancy. Indeed, clonal T-cell populations have been described in a very few number of benign situations, as in old-age patients or in association with viral infections ***(17,18)***. Therefore, to avoid false-positive results and misdiagnoses, it is of the highest importance to integrate all available results from morphology, immunohistochemistry, molecular biology, and clinical data to make a diagnosis of T-cell lymphoma in BMB. On the other hand, when the monoclonal rearrangement obtained from BMB and those observed in other diagnostic materials (i.e., lymph node or even other BMB) are identical, the presence of the same lymphoproliferative disease can be certified in bone marrow.
10. Monoclonal TCR-γ gene rearrangement is not detected in some of the BMBs, morphologically and immunohistochemically positive for T-cell lymphoma ***(13)***. The uneven distribution of malignant T-cells in BMB resulting in sample variation, PCR artifacts, or TCR-γ gene rearrangement undetectable by our set of primers may account for at least some of the negative results ***(19)***. However, the occurrence of false-negative results may also result from the absence of clonal TCR gene rearrangement (γ- and β-chains) as observed in some anaplastic large-cell lymphomas (40–60%), as well as in a few peripheral T-cell lymphomas not otherwise characterized.
11. The TCR-γ PCR technique allows identification of a clonal population of cells as low as 1–3% of the cells examined, presumably below the morphological threshold ***(6)***.

Acknowledgments

The authors thank C. Bricod for excellent technical assistance and help in the improvement of this approach. The authors also thank Dr. F. Delacrétaz for helpful discussion and continuous support.

References

1. Ansell, S. M., Habermann, T. M., Kurtin, P. J., et al. (1997) Predictive capacity of the international prognostic factor index in patients with peripheral T-cell lymphoma. *J. Clin. Oncol.* **15,** 2296–2301.
2. Caulet, S., Delmer, A., Audouin, J., et al. (1990) Histopathological study of bone marrow biopsies in 30 cases of T-cell lymphoma with clinical, biological and survival correlations. *Hematol. Oncol.* **8,** 155–168.
3. Bain, B. J., Clark, D. M., and Lampert, I. A. (1996) In: *Bone Marrow Pathology*, 2nd ed., (Bain, B. J., ed.), Blackwell Science, London, pp. 1–50.

4. Jaffe, E. S. (1990) The role of immunophenotypic markers in the classification on non-Hodgkin's lymphomas. *Semin. Oncol.* **17,** 11–19.
5. Griesser, H. (1995) Gene rearrangements and chromosomal translocations in T cell lymphoma—diagnostic applications and their limits. *Virchows Arch.* **426,** 323–338.
6. Abbas, A. K., Lichtman, A. H., and Pober, J. S. (1994) In: *Cellular and Molecular Immunology*, 2nd ed., (Abbas, A. K., ed.), Saunders, Philadelphia, pp. 166–186.
7. Benhattar, J., Delacrétaz, F., Martin, P., et al. (1995) Improved polymerase chain reaction detection of clonal T-cell lymphoid neoplasms. *Diagn. Mol. Pathol.* **4,** 108–112.
8. Diss, T. C., Watts, M., Pan, L. X., et al. (1995) The polymerase chain reaction in the demonstration of monoclonality in T cell lymphomas. *J. Clin. Pathol.* **48,** 1045–1050.
9. Weirich, G., Funk, A., Hoepner, I., et al. (1995) PCR-based assays for detection of monoclonality in non-Hogkin's lymphoma: application to formalin-fixed, paraffin-embedded tissue and decalcified bone marrow samples. *J. Clin. Med.* **73,** 235–241.
10. Lorenz, J., Jux, G., Zhao-Hohn, M., et al. (1994) Detection of T-cell clonality in paraffin-embedded tissues. *Diagn. Mol. Pathol.* **3,** 93–99.
11. Chhanabhai, M., Adomat, S., Gascoyne, R., et al. (1997) Clinical utility of heteroduplex analysis of TCR gamma gene rearrangements in the diagnosis of T-cell lymphoproliferative disorders. *Am. J. Clin. Pathol.* **108,** 295–301.
12. Signoretti, S., Murphy, M., Cangi, M., et al. (1999) Detection of clonal T-cell receptor γ gene rearrangements in paraffin-embedded tissue by polymerase chain reaction and non-radioactive single-strand conformation polymorphism analysis. *Am. J. Pathol.* **154,** 67–75.
13. Gebhard, S., Benhattar, J., Bricod, C., et al. (2001) Polymerase chain reaction in the diagnosis of T-cell lymphoma in paraffin-embedded bone marrow biopsies: a comparative study. *Histopathology* **38,** 37–44.
14. Mies, C. (1992) Molecular pathology of paraffin-embedded tissue. *Diagn. Mol. Pathol.* **1,** 206–211.
15. Coad, J. E., Olson, D. J., Christensen, D. R., et al. (1997) Correlation of PCR-detected clonal gene rearrangements with bone marrow morphology in patients with B-lineage lymphomas. *Am. J. Pathol.* **21,** 1047–1056.
16. Scholte, G., van Doorn, L., Quint, W., et al. (1997) Polymerase chain reaction for the detection of *Helicobacter pylori* in formaldehyde-sublimate fixed, parrafin-embedded gastric biopsies. *Diagn. Mol. Pathol.* **6,** 238–243.
17. Malik, U. R., Oleksowicz, L., Dutcher, J. R., et al. (1996) Atypical clonal T-cell proliferation in infectious mononucleosis. *Med. Oncol.* **13,** 207–213.
18. Posnett, D., Sinha, R., Kabak, S., et al. (1994) Clonal populations of T cells in normal elderly humans: the T cell equivalent to "benign monoclonal gammapathy." *J. Exp. Med.* **179,** 609–618.
19. Krafft, A. E., Taubenberger, J. K., Sheng, Z. M., et al. (1999) Enhanced sensitivity with a novel TCR gamma PCR assay for clonality studies 569 formalin-fixed, paraffin-embedded (FFPE) cases. *Mol. Diagn.* **4,** 119–133.

16

Circulating DNA Analysis

Protocols and Clinical Applications Using Taqman Assays

Kwan-Chee Allen Chan and Yuk-Ming Dennis Lo

1. Introduction

In recent years, the application of circulating nucleic acids as a clinical diagnostic tool has aroused the interest of many clinicians and biomedical scientists. Circulating nucleic acids refer to the DNA and RNA species that are present in the plasma or serum portion of a blood sample. Although the existence of circulating nucleic acids was described more than half a century ago, the potential clinical implication of circulating nucleic acid analysis has only been realized by the global scientific community in the past 5 yr. In this chapter, current developments of circulating DNA analysis will be discussed. The clinical applications of circulating Epstein–Barr virus (EBV) DNA in cancer detection and monitoring will be discussed in detail to illustrate the important technical issues of performing circulating DNA analysis.

1.1. Discovery of Circulating DNA

The presence of circulating cell-free nucleic acids was first described by Mandel and Metais in 1948 *(1)*. They demonstrated that DNA and RNA could be recovered from the noncellular compartment of the blood of healthy and sick individuals. This report was published 4 yr after the demonstration that DNA was the material of inheritance and even preceded the classic article of Watson and Crick on the double helical structure of DNA *(2)*. However, this interesting phenomenon did not arouse much attention at that time. Further development of the field had to await some 30 yr when Leon and Shapiro demonstrated in 1977 that the concentrations of circulating DNA were much higher in patients suffering from cancers than in patients with nonmalignant diseases

From: *Methods in Molecular Medicine, vol. 97: Molecular Diagnosis of Cancer*
Edited by: J. E. Roulston and J. M. S. Bartlett © Humana Press Inc., Totowa, NJ

(3). In some patients, the level of circulating DNA decreased after successful anticancer therapy *(3)*. Although this work had already suggested that tumor-derived nucleic acids may be present in the plasma or serum of cancer patients, the precise cellular origin of the extracellular DNA in cancer patients could not be determined because of the technological limitations at that time.

In 1989, Stroun et al. showed that DNA found in the plasma of cancer patients carried certain neoplastic characteristics of tumor DNA, such as decreased strand stability *(4)*. In 1994, the presence of tumor-derived DNA in the circulation was confirmed by Sorenson et al. and Vasioukhin et al., who detected specific oncogene mutations in the plasma/serum and the tumor tissues of patients suffering from pancreatic cancer *(5)* and myelodysplastic syndrome and acute myelogenous leukemia *(6)*. Significant progress was made 2 yr later when two groups simultaneously reported that microsatellite alterations, such as loss of heterozygosity (LOH), could be detected from the plasma/serum of some cancer patients when corresponding changes were detectable in the primary tumors *(7,8)*. Since then, several groups have reported the detection of cancer-derived DNA and RNA in the circulation of cancer patients through different approaches *(9–12)*.

The application of circulating DNA went beyond cancer detection when Lo et al. demonstrated that fetal DNA could be detected in the plasma of pregnant women in 1997 *(13)*. Recently, circulating DNA analysis has also been shown to be valuable in prenatal diagnosis *(14,15)*, the monitoring of organ-transplantation recipients *(16)*, and trauma patients *(17)*.

1.2. Clinical Applications: Cancer Detection

1.2.1. Oncogene and Tumor Suppressor Gene Mutations in Plasma and Serum

The first piece of concrete evidence of the presence of tumor-derived DNA in the circulation came from the study of oncogene mutations. In 1994, Sorenson et al. demonstrated that the mutated, *KRAS* gene could be detected in the plasma of pancreatic cancer patients *(5)*, whereas Vasioukhin et al. reported the presence of point mutations of the *NRAS* gene in the plasma of patients with myelodysplastic syndrome or acute myelogenous leukemia *(6)*. Since then, different groups have reported that matched oncogene mutations could be detected in the primary tumors and the plasma/serum of patients suffering from a wide variety of malignant diseases *(12,18–20)*.

The detection rates of oncogene or tumor suppression gene mutations in the plasma/serum of cancer patients are highly variable and dependent on several factors, including the genes being studied, the detection methods, the stages of the disease, the sample types, and the preparation protocols. In general, patients with more advanced diseases and having distant metastases are more likely to have mutated oncogene sequences detected in their plasma/serum ***(18,21–24)***.

1.2.2. Microsatellite Analysis

Following the demonstration of oncogene mutations in plasma/serum, scientists began to look for other tumor-associated genetic changes in plasma. As microsatellite instability and loss of heterozygosity (LOH) are frequently demonstrated in tumor tissues, the possibility of detecting similar changes in plasma was investigated. Two groups simultaneously described the presence of LOH in the plasma of cancer patients in 1996 ***(7,8)***. Chen et al. showed that LOH could be demonstrated in the plasma of patients suffering from small-cell lung carcinoma ***(7)*** and Nawroz et al. reported LOH changes in the plasma of head and neck cancer patients ***(8)***. Their findings confirmed the presence of tumor-derived DNA in plasma of cancer patients and also suggested that tumor DNA could constitute a major proportion of the circulating nucleic acids.

As in the study of microsatellite alterations in tumor tissues, multiple microsatellite markers are used in the analysis of circulating DNA. This approach can increase the detection rate of LOH or microsatellite instability in the plasma. Because different groups of investigators have used different numbers and locations of microsatellite markers, their results are very heterogeneous ***(12,25–27)***. In general, patients having invasive tumors, regional spreads, or distant metastases are more likely to give positive results ***(12,28–30)***. On the other hand, LOH can sometimes be seen in the plasma of patients having small tumors or *in situ* carcinomas ***(25,26)***. This observation indicates that a substantial amount of DNA may be liberated by small and noninvasive tumors. The mechanism underlying tumoral DNA release remains unclear.

1.2.3. Mitochondrial DNA Mutations

Mitochondrial DNA (mtDNA) mutations have been documented in a number of cancers ***(31)***. The presence of circulating mtDNA mutations was first reported in the plasma of patients suffering from type 2 diabetes mellitus in 2000 ***(32)***. In 2001, Jeronimo et al. showed that identical mtDNA mutations could be detected in the plasma and tumor tissues of three prostate cancer patients ***(33)***. One major concern in the study of mtDNA by polymerase chain reaction (PCR) is the potential amplification of nuclear-encoded pseudogenes. This can be overcome by choosing primer sets with longer amplicons when tumor tissues are studied. However, this strategy may not be applicable to the analysis of circulating mtDNA because reports have suggested that circulating DNA molecules mainly exist as short fragments with lengths of around 200–400 bp ***(34,35)***. Recently, Nomoto et al., by using a more sensitive method (viz., oligonucleotide mismatch ligation assay), were able to detect tumor-associated mtDNA mutations in the plasma of 8 out of 10 patients suffering from hepatocellular carcinoma ***(36)***.

1.2.4. Aberrantly Methylated DNA in Plasma

DNA methylation is an epigenetic characteristic associated with gene expression silencing. Alterations of DNA methylation patterns, including global genome hypomethylation and regional hypermethylation of tumor suppressor genes, DNA repairing genes, and metastasis inhibitor genes or their promoters, are increasingly found in different types of tumor. Methylation-specific PCR (MSP) has been developed for the study of aberrant DNA methylation patterns ***(37)***. The principle of MSP relies on the chemical modification of DNA by bisulfite treatment. After bisulfite treatment, the unmethylated cytosine residues in the DNA sequence are deaminated and converted to uracil while the methylated cytosine residues remain unaltered. Thus, the sequence of the treated DNA with different methylation patterns can be amplified by PCR using sequence-specific primers. Because MSP allows the detection of small amounts of aberrantly methylated DNA sequences in a background of wild-type sequences, it is the method of choice for the detection of tumor-associated aberrant methylation in plasma.

Currently, detection of cancer-associated epigenetic changes in the plasma/serum of patients suffering from carcinoma of the lung ***(38)***, esophagus ***(39,40)***, liver ***(41)***, breast ***(42)***, and leukemia ***(43)*** have been reported. The presence of hypermethylated *APC* sequences in the plasma have also been shown to be associated with poor prognosis in patients suffering from carcinoma of the esophagus ***(40)***. Real-time quantitative MSP has also been developed and was shown to be able to detect down to 10 genome equivalents of methylated and unmethylated *p16* sequences ***(11)***. Simultaneous quantification of methylated sequences, unmethylated sequences, and any residual sequences that are not converted by bisulfite conversion is particularly important in the methylation study, as the efficiency of bisulfite conversion is variable and a substantial amount of DNA molecules could be destroyed during the process ***(44)***.

1.3. Analysis of Plasma EBV DNA

1.3.1. Association Between EBV Infection and Malignant Diseases

Epstein–Barr (EBV) infection has been implicated in the pathogenesis of several malignant diseases, including nasopharyngeal carcinoma (NPC) and certain lymphomas ***(45)***. In particular, EBV is an important etiological factor for NPC, and the EBV genome is detectable in almost all NPC tissues obtained in Hong Kong ***(45)***. Thus, serological tests for antibodies against EBV antigens are frequently used for the screening of NPC ***(46)***.

1.3.2. Plasma EBV DNA in NPC Patients

Following the demonstration of the presence of tumor-derived DNA in the plasma of cancer patients, Mutirangura et al. have shown that EBV DNA could be detected in the serum of NPC patients ***(47)***. In 1998, they studied 42 NPC patients and found that EBV could be detected in the serum of one-third of them and in none of the plasma of 82 control subjects ***(47)***. Their finding of the absence of EBV DNA in healthy subjects is particularly striking because over 95% of adults in Southeast Asia have previously been infected with EBV, and some of the circulating B-lymphocytes of these individuals carry the EBV genome ***(45)***. This suggests that the composition of serum DNA is quite different from that of the cellular components and the circulating EBV DNA in NPC patients is more likely to be tumor derived.

1.3.3. Quantitative Analysis of EBV DNA

In 1999, Lo et al. developed a real-time quantitative assay for the detection of EBV DNA in the plasma of NPC patients ***(10)*** and this has markedly improved the sensitivity of circulating EBV DNA analysis. By this approach, they were able to detect EBV DNA in the plasma of 96% of NPC patients but in only 7% of normal individuals ***(10)***. The latter healthy individuals had much lower EBV DNA concentrations than the NPC patients. Plasma concentrations of EBV DNA in the two groups are shown in **Figure 1**. Moreover, EBV DNA concentrations were shown to be positively correlated with the clinical stages of the NPC patients ***(10)***. In patients with more advanced disease (stages III and IV), the median plasma EBV concentrations were approximately eight times higher than that of early-stage patients (stages I and II) (*see* **Fig. 2**) ***(10)***.

1.3.4. Disease Monitoring for NPC Patients

Following the demonstration of the presence of EBV DNA in the plasma of NPC patients, Lo et al. investigated the circulating EBV DNA levels of these patients after they had received radiotherapy and demonstrated that the levels of plasma EBV DNA in patients with NPC recurrence were much higher than the levels of those who remained in continuous clinical remission ***(48)***.

They also monitored the serial changes of plasma EBV DNA concentrations in another group of patients after they had received radiotherapy ***(48)***. All but one of these patients showed a significant drop in EBV DNA concentrations after the completion of radiotherapy ***(48)***. In patients who remained in remission, their serum EBV DNA levels were continuously low or undetectable ***(48)***. On the other hand, elevation of EBV DNA levels could be detected after the initial drop in those patients who subsequently developed local recurrence or

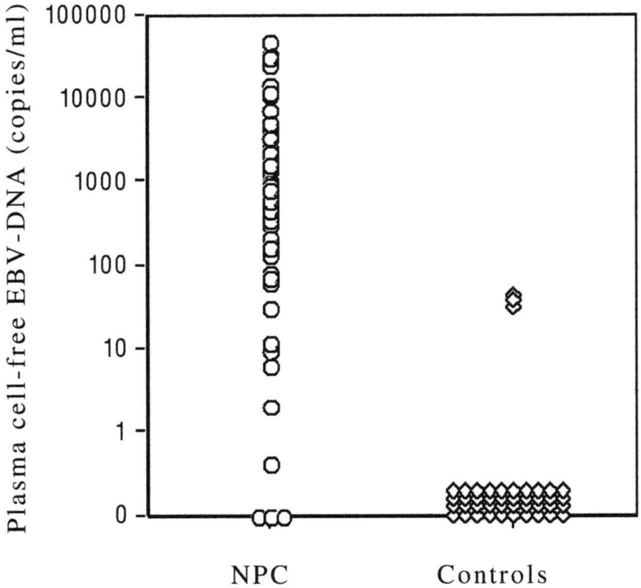

Fig. 1. Comparison of plasma cell-free EBV DNA in NPC patients and control subjects. The categories (NPC patients and control subjects) are plotted on the *x*-axis. Results from NPC patients and control subjects are indicated by ○ and ◇, respectively. The *y*-axis denotes the concentration of cell-free EBV DNA (copies of EBV DNA/mL of plasma) detected by the *Bam*HI-W region PCR system). (Adapted from **ref. *10*.**)

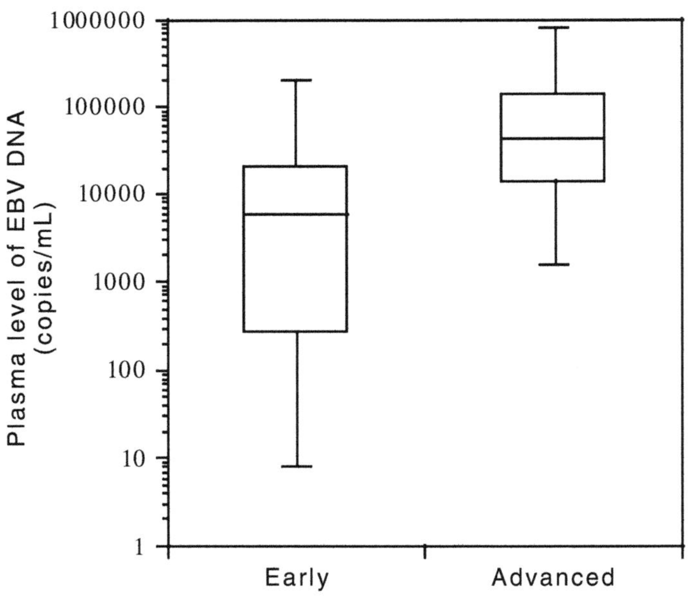

Fig. 2. Comparison between the plasma EBV DNA level between patients suffering from early-stage (stages I and II) and advanced-stage (stages III and IV) NPC (Mann-Whitney rank sum test, $p < 0.001$).

distant metastasis. In some of these patients, the rise in EBV DNA level could precede the clinical relapse by up to 6 mo ***(48)***.

1.3.5. Kinetics of EBV DNA Following Radiotherapy

The demonstration of the disappearance of circulating EBV DNA in NPC patients after they have received radiotherapy is good evidence that the concentrations of EBV DNA could directly reflect the tumor burden in such patients. As mentioned earlier, the circulating EBV DNA concentrations in NPC patients would decrease after receiving radiotherapy. In 2000, Lo et al. demonstrated that a surge of EBV DNA concentration preceded the reduction in NPC patients after radiotherapy ***(49)***. However, the timing of the surge was variable in different patients. In 80% of the patients, the surges occurred within 3 d after radiotherapy, whereas in the remaining 20%, the surges appeared in the second week after radiotherapy ***(49)***. However, the factors determining the timing of the surge and the clinical significance of the timing remains unclear. Following the initial surge, the EBV DNA concentrations decrease following first-order kinetics and their median half-life was determined to be 3.8 d ***(49)***.

1.3.6. Prognostication of NPC Patients

It has been shown that pretreatment EBV DNA is a powerful prognosticator for early disease recurrence, independent of stage, within 1 yr of treatment ***(50)***. The relative risk of every 10-fold increase in plasma EBV DNA level is 3.8 ***(50)***. **Figure 3** shows a Kaplan–Meier survival curve on patients having different pretreatment levels of circulating EBV DNA. In patients having stage III and stage IV disease, those who have lower pretreatment circulating EBV DNA levels did better in terms of disease-free survival than those who have higher levels ***(50)***.

1.3.7. Advantages of Real-Time Quantitative Assay for EBV DNA Analysis

Real-time quantification using fluorescence detection appears to be more sensitive than gel electrophoresis in the detection of circulating EBV DNA. We are able to detect down to five copies of the EBV genome with the real-time TaqMan assay targeting the *Bam*H1-W region. This quantitative EBV DNA assay also has the advantage of greater flexibility. As there is a several-fold difference between the concentrations of circulating EBV DNA in NPC patients and in a small proportion of plasma EBV DNA-positive healthy subjects ***(10)***, we can choose a suitable threshold of EBV DNA level so as to optimize the sensitivity and specificity required for a particular diagnostic or monitoring purpose. Moreover, the closed system design can reduce the chance

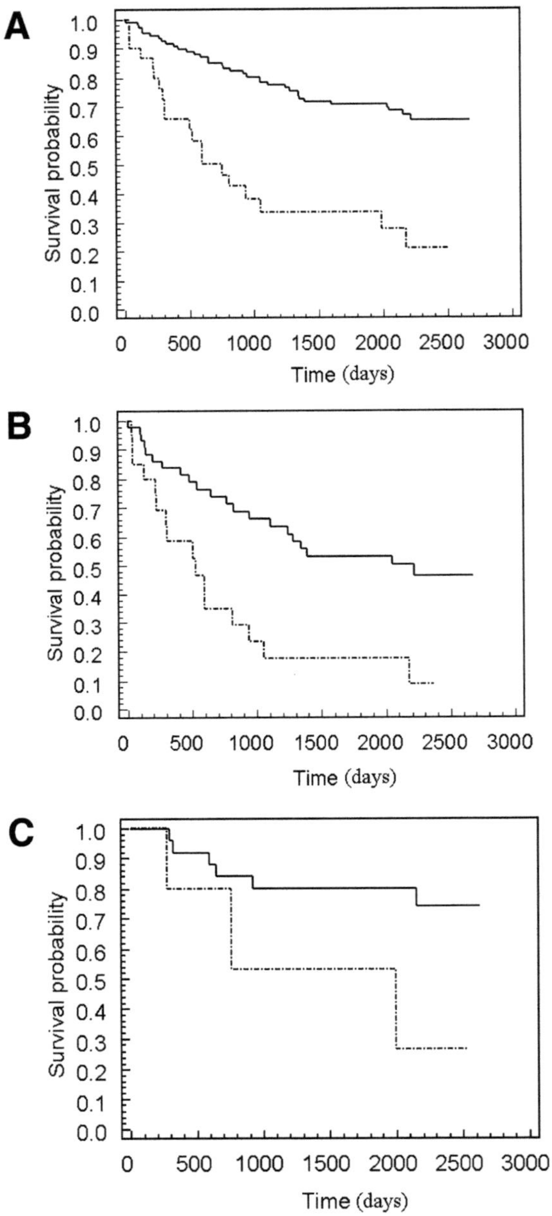

Fig. 3. Kaplan–Meier survival analysis for NPC patients: **(A)** all AJCC/UICC stages; **(B)** stage IV only; (C) stage III only. The solid and dotted lines indicate results from patients with serum EBV DNA <40,568 and >40,568 copies/mL, respectively. (Adapted from **ref. *50***.)

of contamination when large numbers of specimens are handled. Therefore, the robustness of this assay is ideal for high-throughput clinical services.

2. Materials and Equipment

2.1. Equipment for Plasma Preparation (see *Note 1*)

1. Disposable plastic syringe.
2. 21-Gage needle.
3. Blood collection bottle with EDTA.
4. Disposable transfer pipets.
5. Polypropylene tubes.
6. Eppendorf centrifuge (e.g., model 5804).
7. Eppendorf centrifuge (e.g., model 5415D).

2.2. Reagents and Consumables for DNA Extraction

The introduction of DNA extraction kits that consist of a DNA-binding matrix has improved the robustness of DNA extraction and has obviated the tedious procedure of phenol–chloroform extraction. We have been using the QIAamp DNA Mini Kit (Qiagen, Hilden, Germany) for DNA extraction from plasma.

1. Protease.
2. Buffer AL.
3. Wash buffer AW1.
4. Wash buffer AW2.
5. QIAamp spin column.
6. Qiagen 2-mL collection tube for spin column.
7. 100% Ethanol.
8. Molecular-grade H_2O.

Note: **Items 1–5** are supplied in the QIAamp DNA Mini Kit.

2.3. Establishing the Standards With Known Amounts of EBV DNA

The preparation of plasma DNA has been discussed previously. For the quantification of circulating EBV DNA, we need to establish a calibration curve. DNA solutions with known quantities of EBV DNA can be prepared from the Namalwa cell line [American Type Culture Collection no. CRL-1432, ***(51)***]. The Namalwa cell line is a diploid cell line containing two integrated EBV genomes/cell and it is incapable of producing free EBV. A conversion factor of 6.6 pg of DNA per diploid cell is used for copy number conversion.

2.3.1. Preparation of EBV DNA Standards

1. Harvest Namalwa cells following tissue culture.
2. Extract the DNA from these cells using the QIAamp Mini Kit (Qiagen, Hilden, Germany) following the blood protocol.

3. Measure the concentration of total DNA (D µg/mL) by spectrophotometry.
4. Translate the concentration of total DNA into EBV genome equivalents in each microliter of solutions (N genomes/5 µL) by using the formula $N = (D \times 1000 \times 2 \times 5)/6.6$.
5. Dilute the DNA solution to obtain a standard concentration of 10,000 genomes/µL. Then, dilute the standard (10,000 genomes/µL) serially to obtain DNA solutions with concentrations of 1000, 500, 100, 50, 25, 12.5, 6.25, 3.13, 1.57, and 0.78 EBV genomes/µL.

2.4. Real-Time PCR Assay

2.4.1. Reagents for the Real-Time PCR Assay

1. AmpliTaq Gold polymerase (5 U/µL).
2. $MgCl_2$ (25 m*M*).
3. dCTP, dATP, dGTP (200 µM each).
4. dUTP (400 µ*M*).
5. Uracil-*N*-glycosylase (1 U/µL).
6. 10X TaqMan buffer A.
7. Forward primer for the *Bam*H1-W region W-44F (5'-CCCAACACTCCA CCACACC-3') (10 pmol/µL).
8. Reverse primer for the *Bam*H1-W region W-119R (5'-TCTTAGGAGCTGT CCGAGGG-3') (10 pmol/µL).
9. Dual-labeled fluorescent probe W-67T [5'-(FAM)CACACACTACACACAC CCCACCCGTCTC(TAMRA)-3'] (0.625 µ*M*).
10. Molecular-grade H_2O.

Items 1–6 are supplied in the TaqMan PCR Reagent Kit (Perkin-Elmer Corp.). Fluorogenic probes are custom synthesized by Perkin-Elmer Applied Biosystems (*see* **Note 2**).

2.4.2. Equipment for the Real-Time Assay

1. Perkin-Elmer ABI PRISM 7700 sequence detector.
2. Perkin-Elmer Applied Biosystems MicroAmp Optical 96-well reaction plates.
3. Perkin-Elmer Applied Biosystems optical caps (eight caps/strip).

3. Methods

3.1. Protocol for Plasma Preparation

1. Collect peripheral blood from the antecubital vein of a subject with a 21-gage needle and a plastic syringe.
2. Put the blood into a bottle containing EDTA as the anticoagulant.
3. Centrifuge the bottle at 1600*g* at 4°C to separate the plasma from the cellular components.

4. Carefully transfer the supernatant into a 1.5-mL polypropylene tube without disturbing the cellular components.
5. Centrifuge the 1.5-mL microcentrifuge tube at 16,000*g* to ensure the removal of all cells.
6. Transfer the supernatant (cell-free plasma) into a clean polypropylene tube for subsequent DNA extraction.

3.2. Protocol for DNA Extraction (Modified From the Manufacturer's Protocol of the QIAamp DNA Mini Kit)

1. Pipet 800 µL of plasma and 80 µL of protease (provided in the Qiagen kit) into a clean polypropylene tube (*see* **Note 3**). Mix the contents by pulse-vortexing.
2. Add 800 µL of buffer AL (provided) into the mixture and vortex.
3. Incubate the mixture at 56°C in a heating block for 10 min for the digestion of plasma proteins by protease.
4. Briefly centrifuge the polypropylene tube so as to remove the condensed solution on the cover of the tube.
5. Add 800 µL of absolute ethanol to the tube and mix again by pulse-vortexing. After mixing, briefly centrifuge the tube.
6. Apply 600 µL of the mixture in **step 5** into the QIAamp spin column. Close the cap and centrifuge at 6000*g* for 1 min. Then, place the spin column in a clean 2-mL tube and discard the tube containing the filtrate.
7. Repeat **step 6** until all of the mixture in **step 5** has been passed through the spin column.
8. Carefully open the QIAamp spin column and add 500 µL of the first washing buffer, buffer AW1, to the spin column. Close the cap and centrifuge at 6000*g* for 1 min. Then, place the spin column in a clean 2-mL tube and discard the tube containing the filtrate.
9. Carefully open the QIAamp spin column and add 500 µL of the second washing buffer, buffer AW2, to the spin column. Close the cap and centrifuge the spin column at maximum speed for 3 min so as to remove all of the residual washing buffer.
10. Carefully transfer the QIAamp spin column into a new 1.5-mL collection tube and discard the tube containing the filtrate.
11. Add 50 µL autoclaved double-distilled water to the spin column.
12. Stand the column at room temperature for 5 min to allow redissolving of DNA into the water.
13. Centrifuge the spin column at 6000*g* and collect the DNA solution from the 1.5-mL collection tube.

3.3. Detection and Quantification of Targeted Sequences in Plasma

As the DNA concentration is very low in plasma, the detection methods used for plasma DNA analysis must be very sensitive. PCR has provided a convenient way for amplifying the sequence of interest and thus is a good method for the analysis of circulating DNA. Conventionally, gel electrophoresis is used for the post-PCR analysis. However, one of the major concerns with gel electrophoresis is carryover contamination because target sequence is amplified thousands to millions of times after PCR. Therefore, any carryover of PCR products can have disastrous effects on subsequent plasma DNA analysis. Moreover, this method is only qualitative and it cannot provide accurate information concerning the concentration of the target sequences. Although the amount of the initial template can be estimated by coamplifying known amounts of target DNA sequences and comparing their band intensities, this quantification method is imprecise. The development of real-time quantitative PCR ***(52,53)*** has improved the sensitivity and the precision of the quantification of plasma DNA ***(54)***. Furthermore, because the detection and PCR amplification take place at the same time in a closed system, real-time quantitative PCR obviates any post-PCR handling and decreases the chance of carryover contamination.

3.3.1. Principles of Real-Time Quantitative PCR

Real-time quantitative PCR was first described by Higuchi et al. in 1993 ***(53)***. In their experiment, ethidium bromide was used to bind the double-stranded PCR products and the fluorescence signal emitted by this complex is continuously monitored by a video camera. Quantification of the initial target copy number can then be achieved by plotting the increase in fluorescence versus the cycle number.

In 1996, this system was improved by Heid et al., who introduced a fluorescent TaqMan assay and a sequence detector capable of measuring fluorescence in real time ***(52)***. The TaqMan assay consists of a dual-labeled fluorogenic hybridization probe. This hybridization probe is an oligonucleotide with a 5'-reporter dye such as FAM (6-carboxyfluorescein) and a 3'-quencher dye such as TAMRA (6-carboxytetramethylrhodamine). The principle underlying this method is the fluorescence resonance energy transfer (FRET) system ***(55)***. During FRET, a donor fluorophore is excited by an external light source and emits light that is absorbed by a second acceptor fluorophore. Therefore, as long as the hybridization probe is intact and the reporter dye and quencher dye are in close proximity, the fluorescence signal emitted by the reporter dye cannot be detected. **Figure 4** illustrates the principle of the TaqMan assay. During the annealing phase of each PCR cycle, the fluorogenic probe anneals to a sequence in between the forward and the reverse primers, and during the extension phase, the *Taq* polymerase cleaves the fluorogenic probe and frees the reporter dye from the quencher dye because of its 5' to 3' nuclease activity ***(56)***. The separation of the reporter dye from the quencher dye results in an

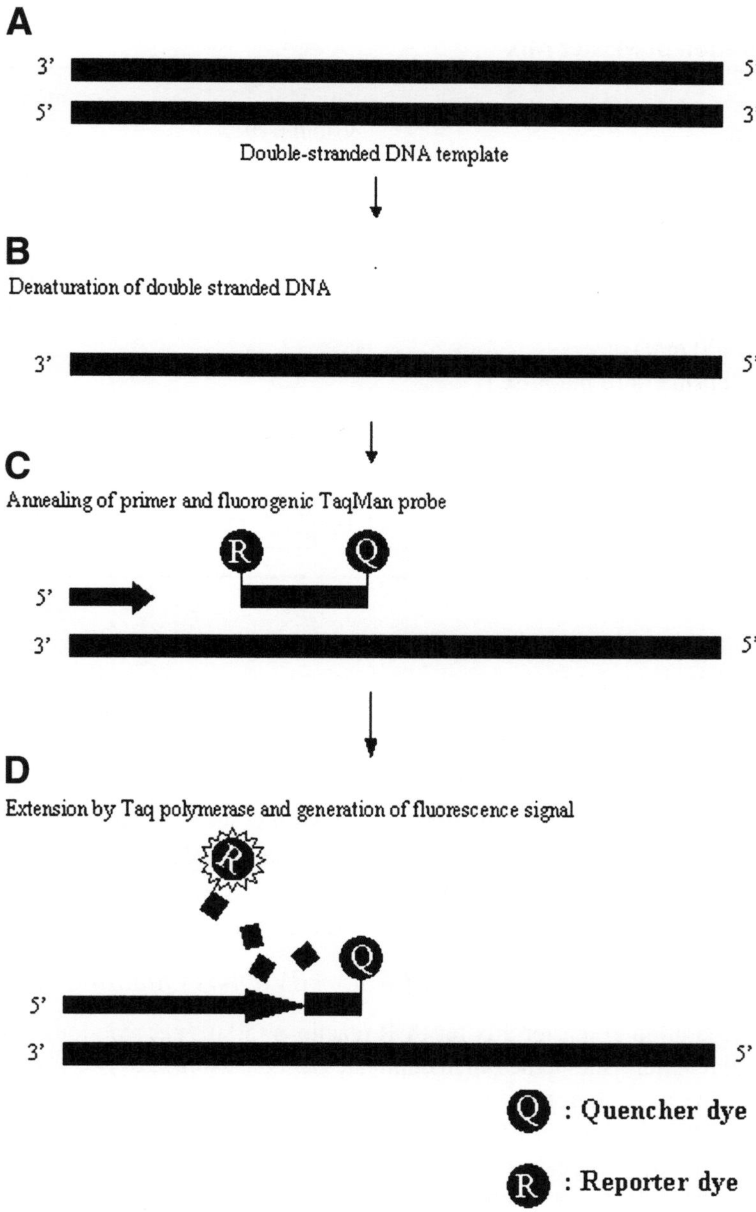

Fig. 4. Principle of TagMan assay: **(A)** double-stranded lDNA template; **(B)** denaturation of double-stranded DNA; **(C)** annealing of fluorogenic probe to the target DNA sequence 3' to annealing site of the forward primer; **(D)** cleaving of fluorogenic probe by *Taq* polymerase and the generation of fluorescence signal during DNA replication.

Table 1
Preparation of Master Mix

Reagent	Volume (μL)	Volume enough for *N* reactions (μL)
10X TaqMan buffer A	5	5*N*
$MgCl_2$ (25 m*M*)	4	4*N*
dATP (200 m*M*)	2	2*N*
dCTP (200 m*M*)	2	2*N*
dGTP (200 m*M*)	2	2*N*
dUTP (400 m*M*)	2	2*N*
Forward primer (10 pmol/μL)	1.5	1.5*N*
Reverse primer (10 pmol/μL)	1.5	1.5*N*
TaqMan probe (0.625 μmol/μL)	2	2*N*
Uracil-*N*-glycosylase (1 U/μL)	0.5	0.5*N*
AmpliTaq Gold (5 U/μL)	0.25	0.25*N*
H_2O (molecular grade)	22.25	22.25*N*

increase in fluorescence signal. The reporter fluorescent signal generated at every cycle is captured by a charged-coupled device (CCD) camera. The data are then stored by a computer and analyzed with proprietary software. The threshold cycle, which is defined as the number of PCR cycles required to generate a fixed-intensity fluorescence signal, is then determined for each sample. The threshold cycle (C_T) values of the samples with known quantities are used to construct a standard curve and the quantities of test samples can be estimated by matching their C_T values to the standard curve.

3.3.2. Protocol for Real-Time PCR for EBV DNA Quantification

1. Preparation of master mix for PCR reactions (50 μL per reaction) (*see* **Table 1**). All reactions should be run in duplicates and the average of two C_T values is used for the analysis for each sample of unknown quantity and for each calibration sample. Multiple water blanks are also required as negative controls, and extra volume for compensation for pipetting errors (200 μL) is required when preparing the master mix. Therefore, the number of reactions *N* is equal to 2 × (number of unknown samples + 14).
2. Pipet 45 μL of master mix into each well of a MicroAmp Optical 96-well reaction plate.
3. Pipet 5 μL of each sample in duplicate (including the calibration standard and plasma DNA samples of unknown concentrations) into each well in which the master mix has been added.
4. Seal the 96-well reaction plate with optical caps.

5. Put the 96-well reaction plate in the reaction chamber of the ABI 7700 sequence detector.
6. Input the sample names and types to the sequence detector program and start the program.

   Thermal cycling profile.
   a. 50°C for 2 min (*see* **Note 4**)
   b. 95°C for 10 min
   c. 95°C for 15 s } 40 cycles
   d. 56°C for 1 min }

3.3.3. Conversion of EBV DNA Concentration From Raw Data

$$C = Q\frac{V_{\text{DNA}}}{V_{\text{PCR}}}\frac{1}{V_{\text{ext}}}$$

where C represents concentration of EBV DNA in plasma (genome-equivalents/mL plasma), Q represents the target quantity (copies/5 µL) determined by a sequence detector in a PCR, V_{DNA} represents the total volume of DNA obtained after extraction (50 µL in our case), V_{PCR} represents the volume of DNA solution used for PCR (5 µL in our case), and V_{ext} represents the volume of plasma/serum extracted (0.8 mL in our case).

4. Notes

1. Specimen types and preparation protocols used for circulating DNA analysis have not yet been standardized. Both serum and plasma have been used for the analysis of circulating DNA by different groups ***(10,47)***. This has made the comparison between studies difficult because the DNA concentrations in serum samples are more than 10 times higher than those of plasma samples ***(57,58)***. Therefore, results from similar studies may be very different when different sample types and preparation protocols are employed. For instance, the detection rates of EBV DNA in NPC patients vary from 31% to 96% with different sample types, preparation protocols, and detection methods ***(10,47,59,60)***. In general, we use plasma as the material for DNA analysis and adopt a more vigorous centrifugation protocol because Chiu et al. have shown that centrifugation at a low speed is inadequate to separate all cellular components from the plasma ***(61)***. Furthermore, Lui et al. have shown that the excess DNA in serum mainly comes from hematopoietic cells and this suggests that DNA may be released from blood cells during the clotting process ***(57)***. Concerning the choice of anticoagulants, we usually use ethylenediamine tetra-acetic acid (EDTA) because the use of heparin may potentially inhibit the PCR process during downstream analysis.
2. In the initial study that utilized real-time quantitative PCR for EBV DNA analysis, two regions of the EBV genome were studied, one of which is the *Bam*HI-W region and the other the *EBNA-1* region. These two regions were chosen because they are relatively conserved in different serotypes of EBV. There are several

copies of the *Bam*HI-W region in the EBV genome, whereas *EBNA-1* is a single copy gene. In that study, the results using the *Bam*HI-W region and the *EBNA-1* region for EBV DNA analysis were concordant. However, the threshold cycle (C_T) number was lower when the *Bam*H1-W region was analyzed and, therefore, the *Bam*HI-W region was adopted in subsequent studies by our group.
3. The recommended volume of whole blood and buffy coat used for each DNA binding column is 200 μL for the QIAamp DNA Mini Kit. As the DNA concentration in plasma is much lower than that of whole blood, a comparatively larger amount (e.g., 800 μL) of plasma is loaded to each DNA-binding column for DNA extraction and the volume of eluting solvent is reduced to 50 μL. The time allowed for the redissolving of DNA has also been increased from 1 min to 5 min to increase the yield of extraction. These adjustments can increase the concentration of the DNA solution.
4. The addition of Uracil-*N*-glycosylase (UNG) into the reaction mixture and the use of dUTP instead of dTTP is an anticontamination strategy ***(62)***. Because dUTP is used in all PCR reactions carried out in our laboratory, all carryover PCR products would be destroyed by enzymatic digestion by the UNG during the 2-min incubation at 50°C (**step 1**). In **step 2**, the UNG is degraded and the AmpliTaq Gold polymerase is activated.

References

1. Mandel, P. and Metais, P. (1948) Les acides nucleiques du plasma sanguin chez l'homme. *C.R. Acad. Sci. Paris* **142,** 241–243.
2. Watson, J. and Crick, F. (1953) A structure for deoxyribose nucleic acid. *Nature* **171,** 737.
3. Leon, S. A., Shapiro, B., Sklaroff, D. M., et al. (1977) Free DNA in the serum of cancer patients and the effect of therapy. *Cancer Res.* **37,** 646–650.
4. Stroun, M., Anker, P., Maurice, P., et al. (1989) Neoplastic characteristics of the DNA found in the plasma of cancer patients. *Oncology* **46,** 318–322.
5. Sorenson, G. D., Pribish, D. M., Valone, F. H., et al. (1994) Soluble normal and mutated DNA sequences from single-copy genes in human blood. *Cancer Epidemiol. Biomarkers Prev.* **3,** 67–71.
6. Vasioukhin, V., Anker, P., Maurice, P., et al. (1994) Point mutations of the N-ras gene in the blood plasma DNA of patients with myelodysplastic syndrome or acute myelogenous leukaemia. *Br. J. Haematol.* **86,** 774–779.
7. Chen, X. Q., Stroun, M., Magnenat, J. L., et al. (1996) Microsatellite alterations in plasma DNA of small cell lung cancer patients. *Nature Med.* **2,** 1033–1035.
8. Nawroz, H., Koch, W., Anker, P., et al. (1996) Microsatellite alterations in serum DNA of head and neck cancer patients. *Nature Med.* **2,** 1035–1037.
9. Jackson, P. E., Qian, G. S., Friesen, M. D., et al. (2001) Specific p53 mutations detected in plasma and tumors of hepatocellular carcinoma patients by electrospray ionization mass spectrometry. *Cancer Res.* **61,** 33–35.
10. Lo, Y. M., Chan, L. Y., Lo, K. W., et al. (1999) Quantitative analysis of cell-free Epstein–Barr virus DNA in plasma of patients with nasopharyngeal carcinoma. *Cancer Res.* **59,** 1188–1191.

11. Lo, Y. M., Wong, I. H., Zhang, J., et al. (1999) Quantitative analysis of aberrant p16 methylation using real-time quantitative methylation-specific polymerase chain reaction. *Cancer Res.* **59,** 3899–3903.
12. Gonzalez, R., Silva, J. M., Sanchez, A., et al. (2000) Microsatellite alterations and TP53 mutations in plasma DNA of small-cell lung cancer patients: follow-up study and prognostic significance. *Ann. Oncol.* **11,** 1097–1104.
13. Lo, Y. M., Corbetta, N., Chamberlain, P. F., et al. (1997) Presence of fetal DNA in maternal plasma and serum. *Lancet* **350,** 485–487.
14. Lo, Y. M. D., Hjelm, N. M., Fidler, C., et al. (1998) Prenatal diagnosis of fetal RhD status by molecular analysis of maternal plasma. *N. Engl. J. Med.* **339,** 1734–1738.
15. Lo, Y. M. D., Lau, T. K., Zhang, J., et al. (1999) Increased fetal DNA concentrations in the plasma of pregnant women carrying fetuses with trisomy 21. *Clin. Chem.* **45,** 1747–1751.
16. Lo, Y. M., Tein, M. S., Pang, C. C., et al. (1998) Presence of donor-specific DNA in plasma of kidney and liver-transplant recipients. *Lancet* **351,** 1329–1330.
17. Lo, Y. M., Rainer, T. H., Chan, L. Y., et al. (2000) Plasma DNA as a prognostic marker in trauma patients. *Clin. Chem.* **46,** 319–323.
18. Sorenson, G. D. (2000) A review of studies on the detection of mutated KRAS2 sequences as tumor markers in plasma/serum of patients with gastrointestinal cancer. *Ann. NY Acad. Sci.* **906,** 13–16.
19. Gocke, C. D., Benko, F. A., Kopreski, M. S., et al. (2000) p53 and APC mutations are detectable in the plasma and serum of patients with colorectal cancer (CRC) or adenomas. *Ann. NY Acad. Sci.* **906,** 44–50.
20. Mayall, F., Jacobson, G., Wilkins, R., et al. (1998) Mutations of p53 gene can be detected in the plasma of patients with large bowel carcinoma. *J. Clin. Pathol.* **51,** 611–613.
21. Yamada, T., Nakamori, S., Ohzato, H., et al. (1998) Detection of K-ras gene mutations in plasma DNA of patients with pancreatic adenocarcinoma: correlation with clinicopathological features. *Clin. Cancer Res.* **4,** 1527–1532.
22. Silva, J. M., Dominguez, G., Silva, J., et al. (2001) Detection of epithelial messenger RNA in the plasma of breast cancer patients is associated with poor prognosis tumor characteristics. *Clin. Cancer Res.* **7,** 2821–2825.
23. Kopreski, M. S., Benko, F. A., Kwee, C., et al. (1997) Detection of mutant K-ras DNA in plasma or serum of patients with colorectal cancer. *Br. J. Cancer.* **76,** 1293–1299.
24. Castells, A., Puig, P., Mora, J., et al. (1999) K-ras mutations in DNA extracted from the plasma of patients with pancreatic carcinoma: diagnostic utility and prognostic significance. *J. Clin. Oncol.* **17,** 578–584.
25. Nunes, D. N., Kowalski, L. P., and Simpson, A. J. (2001) Circulating tumor-derived DNA may permit the early diagnosis of head and neck squamous cell carcinomas. *Int. J. Cancer.* **92,** 214–219.
26. Chen, X., Bonnefoi, H., Diebold-Berger, S., et al. (1999) Detecting tumor-related alterations in plasma or serum DNA of patients diagnosed with breast cancer. *Clin. Cancer Res.* **5,** 2297–2303.

27. Coulet, F., Blons, H., Cabelguenne, A., et al. (2000) Detection of plasma tumor DNA in head and neck squamous cell carcinoma by microsatellite typing and p53 mutation analysis. *Cancer Res.* **60,** 707–711.
28. Fujiwara, Y., Chi, D. D., Wang, H., et al. (1999) Plasma DNA microsatellites as tumor-specific markers and indicators of tumor progression in melanoma patients. *Cancer Res.* **59,** 1567–1571.
29. Taback, B., Fujiwara, Y., Wang, H. J., et al. (2001) Prognostic significance of circulating microsatellite markers in the plasma of melanoma patients. *Cancer Res.* **61,** 5723–5726.
30. Silva, J. M., Dominguez, G., Garcia, J. M., et al. (1999) Presence of tumor DNA in plasma of breast cancer patients: clinicopathological correlations. *Cancer Res.* **59,** 3251–3256.
31. Penta, J. S., Johnson, F. M., Wachsman, J. T., et al. (2001) Mitochondrial DNA in human malignancy. *Mutat. Res.* **488,** 119–133.
32. Zhong, S., Ng, M. C., Lo, Y. M., et al. (2000) Presence of mitochondrial tRNA(Leu(UUR)) A to G 3243 mutation in DNA extracted from serum and plasma of patients with type 2 diabetes mellitus. *J. Clin. Pathol.* **53,** 466–469.
33. Jeronimo, C., Nomoto, S., Caballero, O. L., et al. (2001) Mitochondrial mutations in early stage prostate cancer and bodily fluids. *Oncogene* **20,** 5195–5198.
34. Jahr, S., Hentze, H., Englisch, S., et al. (2001) DNA fragments in the blood plasma of cancer patients: quantitations and evidence for their origin from apoptotic and necrotic cells. *Cancer Res.* **61,** 1659–1665.
35. Giacona, M. B., Ruben, G. C., Iczkowski, K. A., et al. (1998) Cell-free DNA in human blood plasma: length measurements in patients with pancreatic cancer and healthy controls. *Pancreas* **17,** 89–97.
36. Nomoto, S., Yamashita, K., Koshikawa, K., et al. (2002) Mitochondrial D-loop mutations as clonal markers in multicentric hepatocellular carcinoma and plasma. *Clin. Cancer Res.* **8,** 481–487.
37. Herman, J. G., Graff, J. R., Myohanen, S., et al. (1996) Methylation-specific PCR: a novel PCR assay for methylation status of CpG islands. *Proc. Natl. Acad. Sci. USA* **93,** 9821–9826.
38. Esteller, M., Sanchez-Cespedes, M., Rosell, R., et al. (1999) Detection of aberrant promoter hypermethylation of tumor suppressor genes in serum DNA from non-small cell lung cancer patients. *Cancer Res.* **59,** 67–70.
39. Hibi, K., Taguchi, M., Nakayama, H., et al. (2001) Molecular detection of p16 promoter methylation in the serum of patients with esophageal squamous cell carcinoma. *Clin. Cancer Res.* **7,** 3135–3138.
40. Kawakami, K., Brabender, J., Lord, R. V., et al. (2000) Hypermethylated APC DNA in plasma and prognosis of patients with esophageal adenocarcinoma. *J. Natl. Cancer Inst.* **92,** 1805–1811.
41. Wong, I. H., Lo, Y. M., Zhang, J., et al. (1999) Detection of aberrant p16 methylation in the plasma and serum of liver cancer patients. *Cancer Res.* **59,** 71–73.
42. Silva, J. M., Dominguez, G., Villanueva, M. J., et al. (1999) Aberrant DNA methylation of the p16INK4a gene in plasma DNA of breast cancer patients. *Br. J. Cancer* **80,** 1262–1264.

43. Wong, I. H., Ng, M. H., Huang, D. P., et al. (2000) Aberrant p15 promoter methylation in adult and childhood acute leukemias of nearly all morphologic subtypes: potential prognostic implications. *Blood* **95,** 1942–1949.
44. Grunau, C., Clark, S. J., and Rosenthal, A. (2001) Bisulfite genomic sequencing: systematic investigation of critical experimental parameters. *Nucleic Acids Res.* **29,** E65–E65.
45. Rickinson, A. B. and Kieff, E. (1996) Epstein–Barr virus, in *Fields Virology* (Fields, B. N., Knipe, D. M., and Howley, P. M., eds.), Lippincott–Raven, Philadelphia, pp. 2397–2446.
46. Tam, J. S. and Murray, H. G. (1990) Nasopharyngeal carcinoma and Epstein–Barr virus—associated serologic markers. *Ear Nose Throat J.* **69,** 261–267.
47. Mutirangura, A., Pornthanakasem, W., Theamboonlers, A., et al. (1998) Epstein–Barr viral DNA in serum of patients with nasopharyngeal carcinoma. *Clin. Cancer Res.* **4,** 665–669.
48. Lo, Y. M., Chan, L. Y., Chan, A. T., et al. (1999) Quantitative and temporal correlation between circulating cell-free Epstein–Barr virus DNA and tumor recurrence in nasopharyngeal carcinoma. *Cancer Res.* **59,** 5452–5455.
49. Lo, Y. M., Leung, S. F., Chan, L. Y., et al. (2000) Kinetics of plasma Epstein–Barr virus DNA during radiation therapy for nasopharyngeal carcinoma. *Cancer Res.* **60,** 2351–2355.
50. Lo, Y. M., Chan, A. T., Chan, L. Y., et al. (2000) Molecular prognostication of nasopharyngeal carcinoma by quantitative analysis of circulating Epstein–Barr virus DNA. *Cancer Res.* **60,** 6878–6881.
51. Klein, G., Dombos, L., and Gothoskar, B. (1972) Sensitivity of Epstein–Barr virus (EBV) producer and non-producer human lymphoblastoid cell lines to superinfection with EB-virus. *Int. J. Cancer* **10,** 44–57.
52. Heid, C. A., Stevens, J., Livak, K. J., et al. (1996) Real time quantitative PCR. *Genome Res.* **6,** 986–994.
53. Higuchi, R., Fockler, C., Dollinger, G., et al. (1993) Kinetic PCR analysis: real-time monitoring of DNA amplification reactions. *Biotechnology (NY)* **11,** 1026–1030.
54. Lo, Y. M. D., Tein, M. S., Lau, T. K., et al. (1998) Quantitative analysis of fetal DNA in maternal plasma and serum: implications for noninvasive prenatal diagnosis. *Am. J. Hum. Genet.* **62,** 768–775.
55. Stryer, L. (1978) Fluorescence energy transfer as a spectroscopic ruler. *Annu. Rev. Biochem.* **47,** 819–846.
56. Holland, P. M., Abramson, R. D., Watson, R., et al. (1991) Detection of specific polymerase chain reaction product by utilizing the 5'–3' exonuclease activity of *Thermus aquaticus* DNA polymerase. *Proc. Natl. Acad. Sci. USA* **88,** 7276–7280.
57. Lui, Y. Y., Chik, K. W., Chiu, R. W., et al. (2002) Predominant hematopoietic origin of cell-free DNA in plasma and serum after sex-mismatched bone marrow transplantation. *Clin. Chem.* **48,** 421–427.
58. Lee, T. H., Montalvo, L., Chrebtow, V., et al. (2001) Quantitation of genomic DNA in plasma and serum samples: higher concentrations of genomic DNA found in serum than in plasma. *Transfusion* **41,** 276–282.

59. Hsiao, J. R., Jin, Y. T., and Tsai, S. T. (2002) Detection of cell free Epstein–Barr virus DNA in sera from patients with nasopharyngeal carcinoma. *Cancer* **94,** 723–729.
60. Shotelersuk, K., Khorprasert, C., Sakdikul, S., et al. (2000) Epstein–Barr virus DNA in serum/plasma as a tumor marker for nasopharyngeal cancer. *Clin. Cancer Res.* **6,** 1046–1051.
61. Chiu, R. W. K., Poon, L. L. M., Lau, T. K., et al. (2001) Effects of blood-processing protocols on fetal and total DNA quantification in maternal plasma. *Clin. Chem.* **47,** 1607–1613.
62. Pang, J., Modlin, J., and Yolken, R. (1992) Use of modified nucleotides and uracil-DNA glycosylase (UNG) for the control of contamination in the PCR-based amplification of RNA. *Mol. Cell Probes* **6,** 251–256.

17

Microsatellite Instability

Theory and Methods

Gillian Gifford and Robert Brown

1. Introduction

Microsatellites are short sequences of 1–5 bp repeated in tandem throughout the genome, and because of their polymorphic nature, they have been widely used as genetic markers *(1)*. The basis of microsatellite analysis is the PCR amplification across the microsatellite locus of interest with specific primers based on unique DNA sequences flanking the microsatellite repeat. This is followed by electrophoresis of the polymerase chain reaction (PCR) product to determine the size and, therefore, the numbers of repetitions of the basic motif in the alleles present *(2)*.

Mutations can occur within the sequence of these microsatellites as a result of the slippage of DNA polymerase during DNA synthesis, resulting in small expansions or deletions within the repeat sequence manifesting as loss or gain of simple repetitive units *(3)*. This is a common phenomenon, and in healthy cells, this is repaired by the cell DNA mismatch repair (MMR) system. In cells defective in MMR (e.g., as a result of mutation or hypermethylation of one or more of the MMR genes) *(4–6)*, these expansions/deletions are not repaired. Microsatellite analysis of DNA from such MMR-deficient cells may show the appearance of a new microsatellite PCR product on an electrophoretic gel, either higher or lower than the normal alleles, and the concomitant loss of intensity of one of the normal alleles. This is defined as allelic shift, and if this occurs at a substantial proportion of microsatellite loci, it is representative of microsatellite instability (MSI), often taken as diagnostic of loss of DNA MMR (*see* **Fig. 1**).

From: *Methods in Molecular Medicine, vol. 97: Molecular Diagnosis of Cancer*
Edited by: J. E. Roulston and J. M. S. Bartlett © Humana Press Inc., Totowa, NJ

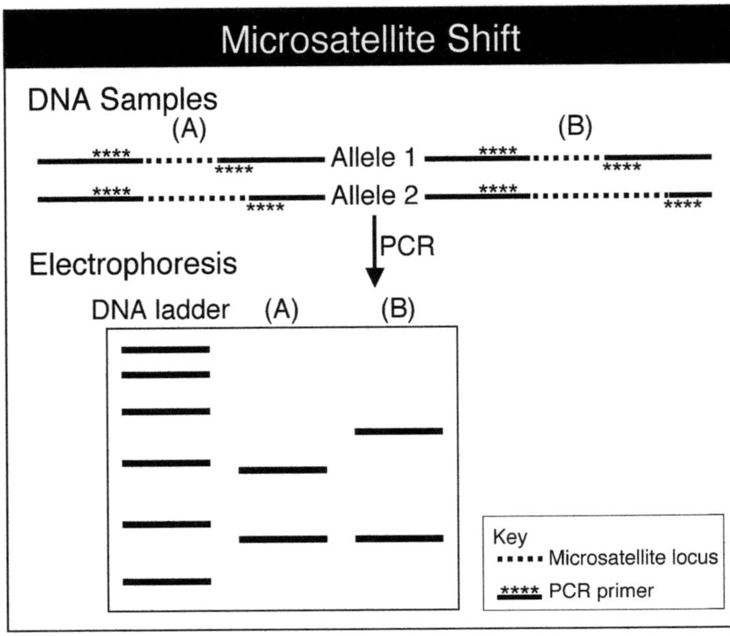

Fig. 1. Schematic of detection of allelic shifts. Unique sequences surrounding the microsatellite can be used to PCR amplify the DNA. In many normal samples, microsatellite show two alleles of differing size as a result of the polymorphic nature of microsatellites. Allelic shift is defined as an alteration in size of one of the alleles (as shown in sample B) compared to the normal (sample A).

In 1993, the MSI phenotype was shown to occur in colorectal tumors of patients with the cancer susceptibility syndrome, hereditary nonpolyposis colorectal cancer (HNPCC) *(7)*. HNPCC is a familial form of colon cancer that also predisposes to endometrial, urinary, gastric, renal, and ovarian malignancies *(8)*. HNPCC was later characterized by mutations in genes of the MMR system and, therefore, this MSI was regarded as an important phenotype in cells deficient in MMR activity and, consequently, as a marker of high risk of cancer *(9)*. The MSI phenotype is found in up to 90% of tumors of the HNPCC syndrome *(10)* because of germline mutations within the specific human MMR proteins MLH1 *(11,12)* and MSH2 *(13,14)*. Carriers of a mutation in MLH1 or MSH2 have up to 70% lifetime risk of developing colorectal and other forms of cancer *(15)*. Microsatellite analysis of colorectal tumors from early-onset cases or those with a family history is a strong predictor of germline mutations in MMR genes such as MLH1 and MSH2 *(16,17)*. This early detection can predict HNPCC, allowing for preventative or early treatment for all family members. MSI cannot, however, be used to definitively diagnose HNPCC among unselected colorectal carcinoma cases because around 20% of sporadic cases are microsatellite unstable ***(18–20)***.

Another clinically important observation is the link between MSI and survival in colorectal cancer. In 1993, Thibodeau et al. reported that in cancer of the proximal colon, the presence of MSI predicted for enhanced patient survival ***(7)***, which has subsequently been confirmed by large population studies ***(21)***. The mechanistic basis of this enhanced survival remains unclear, although the influence of mutations induced by loss of MMR ***(22)***, effects of loss of MMR on apoptosis or cell cycle arrest ***(23)***, and the activation of cytotoxic lymphocytes in MMR-deficient tumors ***(24)*** have all been speculated to have a role.

Microsatellite instability has now been reported to a varying degree in a range of tumor types, including lung ***(25)***, bladder ***(26)***, ovarian ***(27,28)***, and breast ***(29)*** and is the hallmark of MMR deficiency. MSI in sporadic colorectal tumors is mainly the result of loss of MMR because of methylation of the hMLH1 gene ***(30,31)***. Methylation of hMLH1 has been reported in a wide variety of types of tumors ***(32)*** and appears to be selected for during chemotherapy in some tumor types ***(33)***.

Several different techniques have been used to detect MMR defects. These include identification of mutation or epigenetic inactivation of MMR genes, in vitro assays of MMR activity in cell extracts, mRNA levels of MMR genes by reverse transcription (RT)–PCR, expression of MMR proteins by Western or immunohistochemistry, and MSI analysis. These various techniques have their advantages and disadvantages, which are summarized in **Table 1**. Of these various techniques, MSI and immunohistochemistry are the most frequently used for analyzing clinical tissue samples. MSI has the major advantage of measuring MMR function, but it cannot account for tissue heterogeneity and only detects complete loss of MMR activity. Immunohistochemistry allows tissue heterogeneity of expression of specific MMR proteins to be assessed and is semiquantitative, but it is not a measure of MMR function and scoring can be less objective than other methods.

One of the most exciting potential diagnostic uses of microsatellite analysis in cancer lies not in testing the tumors directly, but through an indirect, less invasive procedure to demonstrate the presence of mutant tumor cells or DNA in bodily fluids. Tumor cells are continuously sloughed off and are detectable in body fluids that drain from the organ affected by the tumor ***(34)***, including sputum ***(35)*** and urine ***(36,37)***. Furthermore, many studies now show that free circulating tumor DNA can be isolated from the serum/plasma of cancer patients by taking a simple blood sample and that these samples can contain microsatellite alterations compared to normal DNA. First investigations of microsatellite alterations in serum/plasma were shown in two separate studies

Table 1
Methods of Assaying MMR in Tissue Samples

Method	Advantage	Disadvantage
Mutation detection of MMR genes	Robust methodology, applicable to tumors	Labor intensive No account of tissue heterogeneity Does not measure MMR function Majority of sporadic tumors have gene inactivation as a result of methylation rather than mutation
DNA methylation of MMR genes	Rapid and easy Robust methodology, applicable to tumors	No account of tissue heterogeneity Does not measure MMR function Semiquantitative Not all tumors have lost MMR as a result of methylation
In vitro assay of MMR activity	Does measure MMR function Quantitative	Labor intensive No account of tissue heterogeneity Challenging methodology, not readily applicable to tumors
RT-PCR of MMR mRNA	Rapid and easy Sensitive (too sensitive?) and robust methodology, applicable to tumors, if good quality RNA can be isolated Quantitative	No account of tissue heterogeneity Does not measure MMR function
Western of MMR proteins	Rapid and easy Robust methodology, applicable to tumors	No account of tissue heterogeneity Does not measure MMR function Semiquantitative
Immunohistochemistry of MMR proteins	Rapid and easy Allows for tissue heterogeneity Robust methodology, applicable to tumors	Does not measure MMR function Semiquantitative
MSI	Does measure MMR function Robust methodology, applicable to tumors	No account of tissue heterogeneity Not quantitative (i.e., only measures complete loss of MMR activity) Needs to be clonal event in order to detect

in patients with head and neck and lung cancer. In head and neck squamous cell carcinoma, 6/21 patients showed identical allelic shift in paired tumor and serum DNA ***(38)***. Similarly, in patients with small-cell lung cancer, 16/21 patients displayed allelic shift in at least one locus examined. The same shifts were present in the plasma DNA of 93% of these cases ***(39)***. Since then, MSI in serum of cancer patients has been reported in renal ***(40)***, breast ***(41–43)***, and ovarian cancers ***(44)***. One drawback of this approach is the dilution by normal DNA, which can mean that changes detectable in the tumor are not always seen in the corresponding serum. It remains unclear from which cells this tumor DNA is derived, although it has been suggested to originate from cells undergoing apoptosis. This approach remains controversial. For instance, in one study in colorectal cancer in which 80% of DNA from primary tumors showed allelic shifts, no alterations were seen in the paired serum DNA ***(45)***. Microsatellite analysis also relies on the availability of a corresponding "normal" for comparison, although it has been suggested that analysis of the Bat 26 locus does not necessitate this ***(46,47)***.

Detecting MSI in cells or tumor DNA isolated from body fluids may provide a powerful means of early detection and diagnosis of cancer. The association of MSI with differences in prognosis or response to chemotherapy has the potential to provide a clinically useful means of further defining the molecular pathology of a variety of tumor types.

2. Materials

2.1. Polymerase Chain Reaction

1. *Taq* DNA polymerase (e.g., AmpliTaq Gold), 5 U/μL supplied with Geneamp 10X PCR buffer II: 150 m*M* Tris-HCl, 500 m*M* KCl, pH 8.0 (Applied Biosystems).
2. $MgCl_2$ solution supplied at 25 m*M* (Applied Biosystems).
3. dNTP mixture containing dATP, dCTP, dGTP, and dTTP, 10m*M* each (Applied Biosystems).
4. Microsatellite primers, fluorescently labeled with, for example, 5'-FAM, HEX (Oswel DNA Service, Southampton, UK; *see* **Table 2**).
5. Template DNA samples.
6. Sterile water.

2.2. Sample Preparation Prior to Polyacrylamide Gel Electrophoresis

1. 100% Ethanol.
2. Glycogen, molecular biology grade (Roche).

2.3. Semiautomated Polyacrylamide Gel Electrophoresis Using the 373XL DNA Sequencer (Genescanning)

1. Sequagel 6 monomer solution supplied with Sequagel Complete Buffer solution (Flowgen).

Table 2
A Suggested List of Primers for Microsatellite Analysis

Primer	Primer sequence 5' → 3'	T_m (°C)	Product size (bp)	Chromosome location
Mfd15	GGAAGAATCAAATAGACAAT GCTGGCCATATATATATTTAAACC	52	150	17Q11.2-q12
D2S123	AAACAGGATGCCTGCCTTTA GGACTTTCCACCTATGGGAC	60	197–227	2p16
MYCL1	TGGCGAGACTCCATCAAAG CTTTTTAAGCTGCAACAATTTC	53	140–209	1p32
P53	GAATCCGGGAGGAGGTTG AACAGCTCCTTTAATGGCAGCGG GAGGAGGTTG	55	104–175	17p13.1
APC	ACTCACTCTAGTGATAAATCG AGCAGATAAGACAGTATTACTAGTT	55	96–122	5q21/22
D18S69	CTCTTTCTCTGACTCTGACC GACTTTCTAAGTTCTTGCCAG	60	110	18q21
D18S58	GCTCCCGGCTGGTTTT GCAGGAAATCGCAGGAACTT	53	144–160	18q22.3
Bat 26	TGACTACTTTTGACTTCAGCC AACCATTCAACATTTTTAACCC	58	80–10	2p

2. 10% Ammonium persulfate made fresh with distilled water as required (Fisher).
3. Deionized formamide sample loading buffer: 1 mL deionized formamide, 200 µL dextran blue: (50 m*M* EDTA, pH 8.0, 30 mg/mL blue dextran).
4. Genescan DNA internal lane size standard (e.g., GS500XL ROX) (Applied Biosystems).
5. 10X TBE: 216 g Tris-HCl, 110 g boric acid, 16.9 g EDTA in 1 L distilled water. Dilute to 1X for use.
6. Glass plates for Applied Biosystems 373 DNA Sequencer, appropriate spacers (0.3 mm) and bull-dog clips.

3. Methods

3.1. PCR (see Note 1)

A suggested list of microsatellite primers are displayed in **Table 2**.

1. Determine the quantity of DNA master mix required for the (Number of samples) + (No template negative control) + 1, using the following recipes, which are dependent on the primer being used (*see* **Note 2**). *P53*: 25 µL reaction volume containing 1X PCR buffer, 1.5 m*M* $MgCl_2$, 0.2 m*M* dNTPs, 0.5 U AmpliTaq Gold, 12.5 pmol each forward and reverse primer. *Others*: 50 µL reaction vol-

ume containing 1X PCR buffer, 1.5 m*M* $MgCl_2$, 0.2 m*M* dNTPs, 1.25 U AmpliTaq Gold, 150 ng each forward and reverse primer. It is appropriate to PCR the tumor and normal samples from the same patient at the same time.

2. Thaw DNA samples and reagents at room temperature and transfer to wet ice. Make up master mix according to the calculations in **step 1**. Vortex and briefly pulse in a benchtop centrifuge. Store on wet ice until use. Add 2 µL of each DNA sample to the base of a well in a 96-well plate. Add the appropriate amount of master mix and cover with an adhesive plate sealer. Centrifuge briefly to move any liquid clinging to the walls to the base of the well.
3. Perform PCR reaction using the following protocol, adjusting the annealing temperature dependent on the locus being amplified: 95°C, 10 min, 1 cycle; 95°C, 45 s, T_m (*see* **Table 2** for individual primers), 45 s, 72°C, 45 s, for a total of 30 cycles; 72°C, 5 min, 1 cycle; 4°C hold (*see* **Note 3**).
4. Store product at –20°C until required.

3.2. PCR Product Preparation Prior to Electrophoresis

1. Transfer 1 µL of each PCR sample to another 96-well plate. Add 0.5 µL glycogen and 3 µL of 100% ethanol. Cover with adhesive film and centrifuge briefly. Store at –20°C, preferably overnight (*see* **Note 4**).
2. Prior to electrophoresis, centrifuge at 400*g* for 10 min. Remove cover and air-dry for several hours or until all ethanol has evaporated. This can be speeded up by placing in a 37°C incubator, for example.
3. Once dry and just before loading the gel, add 1 µL of deionized formamide and 0.5 µL of Genescan size standard to each sample (*see* **Note 5**). This can be made up as a master mix for the number of samples + 1, adding 1.5 µL to each well to resuspend the DNA. Denature at 95°C for 5 min and place on ice while loading.

3.3. Electrophoresis Using the 373XL DNA Sequencer With Genescan 3.1 Software

3.3.1. Gel Casting

1. Wash glass plates, one plain and one notched, in hot water and rinse in distilled water. Stand upright and allow to air-dry. To assemble, place the plain plate, etched side facing downward, on top of a raised platform (e.g., two tip boxes). Place the spacers along the two long edges using a few drops of distilled water under each to anchor securely. Place the notched plate on top, etched side facing upward and ensure all edges are flush with the bottom plate (*see* **Note 6**). Clamp with three bull-dog clips along each long edge, positioning these to grip in the center of the spacer.
2. To make the gel, combine 40 mL of Sequagel 6 monomer solution, 10 mL of Sequagel complete buffer, and 400 µL of fresh 10% ammonium persulfate solution. Swirl gently to mix.
3. To cast the gel, take up the gel mix in a 50-mL syringe and inject slowly but steadily between the glass plates. Tap gently on the glass in front of the flow of

gel to ease progression and prevent the formation of air bubbles.
4. Insert a well-forming comb and secure by clamping with two bull-dog clips.
5. Leave to polymerize for a minimum of 2 h.

3.3.2. Polyacrylamide Gel Electrophoresis

1. Assemble the polymerized gel in the sequencer and perform the plate check and prerun steps according to the manufacturer's instructions using 1X TBE buffer. Similarly, create a specific sample sheet detailing which sample is to be loaded in which lane. It is preferable to run tumor and normal samples from the same patient on the same gel. During the prerun stage, it is appropriate to carry out **step 3** of **Subheading 3.2.**
2. Load all 1.5 μL of the resuspended product into each well in the gel using duck-billed pipet tips. Electrophoresis is carried out for 12 h at 2500 V, after which, a "virtual gel" is produced for analysis showing bands representing both the size standard and products.

3.3.3. Gel Analysis

Analyze according to manufacturer's instructions. The software will determine the size of the product bands by comparing them to the known sizes of the bands in the internal lane size standard. This information is displayed in the form of electropherograms with bands represented as peaks, the height of each peak being the relative amount of each allele present. The paired tumor and normal sample electropherogram profiles for each patient should be presented on the same display for ease of comparison. A typical display is shown in **Figure 2**.

4. Defining Microsatellite Instability: Factors to Consider

1. Microsatellite sequences amplified by PCR, particularly those involving mononucleotide and dinucleotide repeats, tend to show a cluster of fragments of different lengths, seen as a series of peaks surrounding the major peak. This is attributed partly to the *Taq* polymerase used in the PCR reaction, which has terminal deoxynucleotidyl transferase (TDT) activity. TDT activity adds one extra base to the products in a sequence-dependent manner, leading to a variety of PCR products differing by one base ***(48,49)***. In addition, *Taq* polymerase is susceptible to slippage while replicating long stretches of similar sequence, resulting in the addition or subtraction of complete repeat units ***(52)***. For purposes of analysis in our laboratory, we have taken the major peak to be the main allele.
2. Allelic shift is identified when alleles of a different size are detected in the microsatellites of the tumor DNA that are not detected in the normal samples of the same patient. In practice, the normal allele is not completely lost, presumably the result of the presence of DNA from some contaminating normal cells in the extract that will still contain the normal allele lost in the tumor. With this in mind, we record a shift only when there is the appearance of a new allele peak

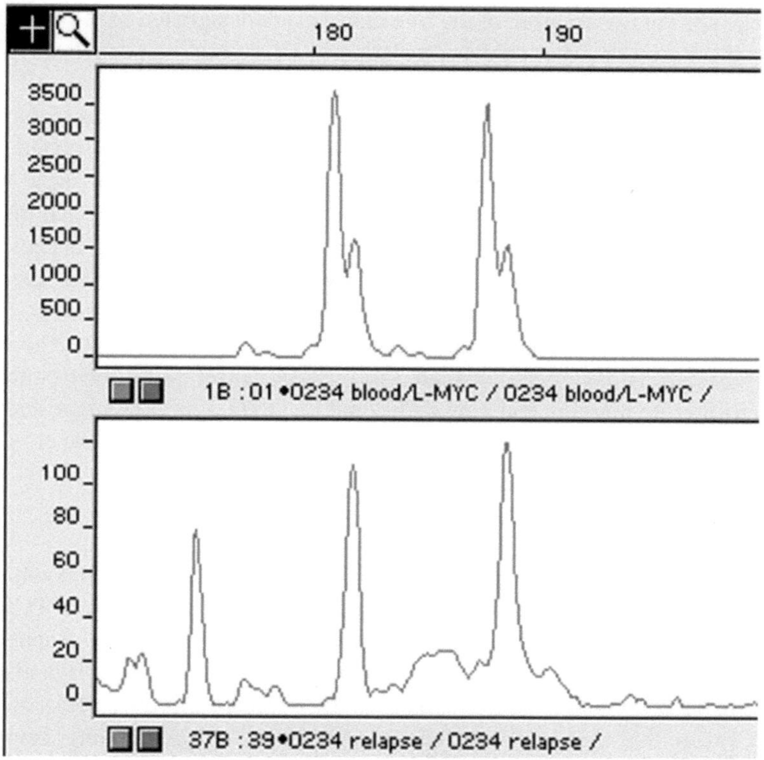

Fig. 2. Example of allelic shift. The panel displays two normal allele peaks at the MYCL1 locus of 181- and 188-bp size from DNA extracted from blood lymphocytes. The lower panel, tumor DNA, shows retention of the two normal peaks with appearance of a new allele peak of size 153 bp. The retention of the two normal alleles is the result of "contamination" of the tumor sample with normal cells.

and concomitant reduction in the size of the retained allele. Examples of allelic shift are shown in **Fig. 2**. Because of the complicated clustering of peaks (*see* **Note 1**), we recommend caution in scoring minor shifts of 1–2 bp.

3. For the majority of tumor types, there are no definitive guidelines for defining a microsatellite-unstable tumor, resulting in highly variable reports of MSI incidence. Several hundred markers have been used for analysis and it is unclear how many markers should be analyzed, which chromosomal locations these should occupy, which type of repeats should be included, and what percentage need to show a shift to define MSI. To standardize the markers used for colorectal cancer diagnosis, the National Cancer Institute (NCI) sponsored The International Workshop on Microsatellite Instability and RER Phenotypes in Cancer Detection and Familial Predisposition to review the field and define uniform criteria ***(50)***. Recommendations in colorectal cancer were for a panel of five microsatellite markers (Bat 25, Bat 26, D5S346 [APC], D2S123, and D17S250). Tumors displaying

allelic shift at two or more of the five markers are designated MSI-high and MSI-low if only one marker showed variation in microsatellite sequence. If no shift was identified at any of the loci, the tumor is characterized as microsatellite stable. To be confident that a tumor is MSI-low versus MSI-high, it was recommended that if only one of the five markers tested was positive, then a second panel of five markers be tested; however, specific recommendations for these were not made. If more than five markers are tested, it was recommended that the criteria be modified to assess the percentage of markers demonstrating instability. The MSI-high group would be defined as showing shift at ≥30–40% of the markers and the MSI-low group would exhibit shift at <30–40%.

4. The optimal panel of markers for other tumor types is not known. The NCI recommendations have been evaluated in ovarian cancer using their panel of five microsatellite markers and nine additional loci ***(51)***. Findings suggested that the addition of the NME1 locus may be required in addition to the panel of five for optimal detection of MSI.

5. Notes

1. In order to prevent cross-contamination when performing PCR, it is important to have separate pre-PCR and post-PCR areas. We suggest the use of PCR hoods, which provide a self-contained environment and ultraviolet (UV) capabilities to sterilize pipets and other equipment from contaminating DNA. It is also advisable to have a set of pipets exclusively for PCR. Keep your own stocks of reagents and ensure that they are vortexed and centrifuged before opening, bringing the reagent down from the sides of the tube and underneath the lid, to prevent aerosol formation.
2. We have described PCR reactions for the microsatellite loci specifically analyzed in our laboratory. These are tailored for high-throughput analysis and, therefore, the same PCR reaction is used for almost all primers. It may be necessary to optimize these reactions when transferring to another laboratory and other thermocyclers. There are a number of troubleshooting approaches and one of the most critical factors is magnesium concentration. This may vary from 0.5 to 5 m*M* and a panel should be tested for each primer. Other factors to consider are primer concentration, template DNA concentration, amount of *Taq* polymerase and cycling conditions.
3. The described PCR program is tailored for AmpliTaq Gold polymerase that requires activation at 95°C for a recommended 10 min. It may be necessary to adjust the program to give longer cycling steps or more cycles, but we do not recommend more than a total of 35 cycles because of the increased risk of false positives.
4. It is possible to use liquid PCR product for Genescanning, but because of the limited volume capacity of the wells (approx 2 μL if using the 64-well comb), it is preferable to precipitate DNA samples prior to loading. We have found that 1 μL of PCR product is sufficient in most cases, although this can be scaled up accordingly.

5. A range of size standards is available from Applied Biosystems and should be chosen according to the size of your product.
6. It is important that the glass plates be used in the same orientation for each Genescan run. Using a diamond pen, etch the corner of one side of both the bottom and top plates and ensure that these sides face the outside for every run. The rubber seal on the instrument can leave an invisible mark on the outside of the notched plate. If this then becomes the internal surface, it can impede the flow of gel when casting and cause the formation of large air bubbles or stop the flow entirely.

References

1. Hearne, C. M., Ghosh, S., and Todd, J. A. (1992) Microsatellites for linkage analysis of genetic traits. *Trends Genet.* **8,** 288–294.
2. Weber, J. L. and May, P. E. (1989) Abundant class of human DNA polymorphisms which can be typed using the polymerase chain reaction. *Am. J. Hum. Genet.* **44,** 388–396.
3. Strand, M., Prolla, T. A., Liskay, R. M., et al. (1993) Destabilization of tracts of simple repetitive DNA in yeast by mutations affecting DNA mismatch repair. *Nature* **365,** 274–276.
4. Thibodeau, S. N., French, A. J., Roche, P. C., et al. (1996) Altered expression of hMSH2 and hMLH1 in tumors with microsatellite instability and genetic alterations in mismatch repair genes. *Cancer Res.* **56,** 4836–4840.
5. Kane, M. F., Loda, M., Gaida, G. M., et al. (1997) Methylation of the hMLH1 promoter correlates with lack of expression of hMLH1 in sporadic colon tumors and mismatch repair-defective human tumor cell lines. *Cancer Res.* **57,** 808–811.
6. Herman, J. G., Umar, A., Polyak, K., et al. (1998) Incidence and functional consequences of hMLH1 promoter hypermethylation in colorectal carcinoma. Proc. Natl. Acad. Sci. USA **95,** 6870–6875.
7. Thibodeau, S. N., Bren, G., and Schaid, D. (1993) Microsatellite instability in cancer of the proximal colon. *Science* **260,** 816–819.
8. Lynch, H. T., Smyrk, T. C., Watson, P., et al. (1993) Genetics, natural history, tumor spectrum, and pathology of hereditary nonpolyposis colorectal cancer: an updated review. *Gastroenterology* **104,** 1535–1549.
9. Peltomaki, P., Lothe, R. A., Aaltonen, L. A., et al. (1993) Microsatellite instability is associated with tumors that characterize the hereditary non-polyposis colorectal carcinoma syndrome. *Cancer Res.* **53,** 5853–5855.
10. Aaltonen, L. A., Peltomaki, P., Leach, F. S., et al. (1993) Clues to the pathogenesis of familial colorectal cancer. *Science* **260,** 812–816.
11. Bronner, C. E., Baker, S. M., Morrison, P. T., et al. (1994) Mutation in the DNA mismatch repair gene homologue hMLH1 is associated with hereditary nonpolyposis colon cancer. *Nature* **368**, 258–261.
12. Papadopoulos, N., Nicolaides, N. C., Wei, Y. F., et al. (1994) Mutation of a mutL homolog in hereditary colon cancer. *Science* **263**, 1625–1629.
13. Fishel, R., Lescoe, M. K., Rao, M. R., et al. (1993) The human mutator gene

homolog MSH2 and its association with hereditary nonpolyposis colon cancer. *Cell* **75,** 1027–1038.

14. Leach, F. S., Nicolaides, N. C., Papadopoulos, N., et al. (1993) Mutations of a mutS homolog in hereditary nonpolyposis colorectal cancer. *Cell* **75,** 1215–1225.
15. Aarnio, M., Sankila, R., Pukkala, E., et al. (1999) Cancer risk in mutation carriers of DNA-mismatch-repair genes. *Int. J. Cancer* **81,** 214–218.
16. Farrington, S. M., Lin-Goerke, J., Ling, J., et al. (1998) Systematic analysis of hMSH2 and hMLH1 in young colon cancer patients and controls. *Am. J. Hum. Genet.* **63,** 749–759.
17. Liu, T., Wahlberg, S., Burek, E., et al. (2000) Microsatellite instability as a predictor of a mutation in a DNA mismatch repair gene in familial colorectal cancer. *Genes Chromosomes Cancer* **27,** 17–25.
18. Aaltonen, L. A., Salovaara, R., Kristo, P., et al. (1998) Incidence of hereditary nonpolyposis colorectal cancer and the feasibility of molecular screening for the disease. *N. Engl. J. Med.* **338,** 1481–1487.
19. Dietmaier, W., Wallinger, S., Bocker, T., et al. (1997) Diagnostic microsatellite instability: definition and correlation with mismatch repair protein expression. *Cancer Res.* **57,** 4749–4756.
20. Thibodeau, S. N., French, A. J., Cunningham, J. M., et al. (1998) Microsatellite instability in colorectal cancer: different mutator phenotypes and the principal involvement of hMLH1. *Cancer Res.* **58,** 1713–1718.
21. Samowitz, W. S., Curtin, K., Ma, K.-N., et al. (2001) Microsatellite instability in sporadic colon cancer is associated with an improved prognosis at the population level. *Cancer Epidemiol. Biomarkers Prev.* **10,** 917–923.
22. Parsons, R., Myeroff, L., Liu, B., et al. (1995) Microsatellite instability and mutations of the transforming growth factor beta type II receptor in colorectal cancer. *Cancer Res.* **55,** 5548–5550.
23. Jacob, S., Aguado, M., Fallik, D., et al. (2001) The role of the DNA mismatch repair system in the cytotoxicity of the topoisomerase inhibitors camptothecin and etoposide to human colorectal cancer cells. *Cancer Res.* **61,** 6555–6562.
24. Guidoboni, M., Gafa, R., Viel, A., et al. (2001) Microsatellite instability and high content of activated cytotoxic lymphocytes identify colon cancer patients with a favourable prognosis. *Am. J. Pathol.* **159,** 297–304.
25. Shridhar, V., Siegfried, J., Hunt, J., et al. (1994) Genetic instability of microsatellite sequences in many non-small cell lung carcinomas. *Cancer Res.* **54,** 2084–2087.
26. Gonzalez-Zulueta, M., Ruppert, J. M., Tokino, K., et al. (1993) Microsatellite instability in bladder cancer. *Cancer Res.* **53,** 5620–5623.
27. Sood, A. K. and Buller, R. E. (1996) Genomic instability in ovarian cancer: a reassessment using an arbitrarily primed polymerase chain reaction. *Oncogene* **13,** 2499–2504.
28. Cass, I., Kholodilov, N., Runowicz, C., et al. (1996) Microsatellite instability in ovarian carcinoma. *Proc. Am. Assoc. Cancer Res.* **37,** 544.
29. Patel, U., Grundfest-Broniatowski, S., Gupta, M., et al. (1994) Microsatellite

instabilities at five chromosomes in primary breast tumors. *Oncogene* **9,** 3695–3700.

30. Kane, M. F., Loda, M., Gaida, G. M., et al. Methylation of the hMLH1 promoter correlates with lack of expression of hMLH1 in sporadic colon tumors and mismatch repair-defective human tumor cell lines. *Cancer Res.* **57,** 808–811.
31. Kuismanen, S. A., Holmberg, M. T., Salovaara, R., et al. Genetic and epigenetic modification of MLH1 accounts for a major share of microsatellite-unstable colorectal cancers. *Am. J. Pathol.* **156,** 1773–1779.
32. Esteller, M. and Herman, J.G. (2002) Cancer as an epigenetic disease: DNA methylation and chromatin alterations in human tumors. *J. Pathol.* **196,** 1–7.
33. Strathdee, G., Mackean, M. J., Illand, M., et al. A role for methylation of the hMLH1 promoter in loss of hMLH1 expression and drug resistance in ovarian cancer. *Oncogene* **18,** 2335–2341.
34. Sidransky, D. (1997) Nucleic acid-based methods for the detection of cancer. *Science* **278,** 1054–1059.
35. Miozzo, M., Sozzi, G., Musso, K., et al. (1996) Microsatellite alterations in bronchial and sputum specimens of lung cancer patients. *Cancer Res.* **56,** 2285–2288.
36. Mao, L., Schoenberg, M. P., Scicchitano, M., et al. (1996) Molecular detection of primary bladder cancer by microsatellite analysis. *Science* **271,** 659–662.
37. Steiner, G., Schoenberg, M. P., Linn, J. F., et al. (1997) Detection of bladder cancer recurrence by microsatellite analysis of urine. *Nature Med.* **3,** 621–624.
38. Nawroz, H., Koch, W., Anker, P., et al. (1996) Microsatellite alterations in serum DNA of head and neck cancer patients. *Nature Med.* **2,** 1035–1037.
39. Chen, X. Q., Stroun, M., Magnenat, J. L., et al. (1996) Microsatellite alterations in plasma DNA of small cell lung cancer patients. *Nature Med.* **2,** 1033–1035.
40. Goessl, C., Heicappell, R., Munker, R., et al. (1998) Microsatellite analysis of plasma DNA from patients with clear cell renal carcinoma. *Cancer Res.* **58,** 4728–4732.
41. Chen, X., Bonnefoi, H., Diebold-Berger, S., et al. (1999) Detecting tumor-related alterations in plasma or serum DNA of patients diagnosed with breast cancer. *Clin. Cancer Res.* **5,** 2297–2303.
42. Shaw, J. A., Smith, B. M., Walsh, T., et al. (2000) Microsatellite alterations plasma DNA of primary breast cancer patients. *Clin. Cancer Res.* **6,** 1119–1124.
43. Mayall, F., Fairweather, S., Wilkins, R., et al. (1999) Microsatellite abnormalities in plasma of patients with breast carcinoma: concordance with the primary tumor. *J. Clin. Pathol.* **52,** 363–366.
44. Hickey, K. P., Boyle, K. P., Jepps, H. M., et al. (1999) Molecular detection of tumor DNA in serum and peritoneal fluid from ovarian cancer patients. *Br. J. Cancer* **80,** 1803–1808.
45. Hibi, K., Robinson, C. R., Booker, S., et al. (1998) Molecular detection of genetic alterations in the serum of colorectal cancer patients. *Cancer Res.* **58,** 1405–1407.
46. Hoang, J. M., Cottu, P. H., Thuille, B., et al. (1997) BAT-26, an indicator of the replication error phenotype in colorectal cancers and cell lines. *Cancer Res.* **57,** 300–303.

47. Zhou, X. P., Hoang, J. M., Li, Y. J., et al. (1998) Determination of the replication error phenotype in human tumors without the requirement for matching normal DNA by analysis of mononucleotide repeat microsatellites. *Genes Chromosomes Cancer* **21,** 101–107.
48. Hu, G. (1993) DNA polymerase-catalyzed addition of nontemplated extra nucleotides to the 3' end of a DNA fragment. *DNA Cell Biol.* **12,** 763–770.
49. Ginot, F., Bordelais, I., Nguyen, S., et al. (1996) Correction of some genotyping errors in automated fluorescent microsatellite analysis by enzymatic removal of one base overhangs. *Nucleic Acids Res.* **24,** 540–541.
50. Boland, C. R., Thibodeau, S. N., Hamilton, S. R., et al. (1998) A National Cancer Institute Workshop on Microsatellite Instability for cancer detection and familial predisposition: development of international criteria for the determination of microsatellite instability in colorectal cancer. *Cancer Res.* **58,** 5248–5257.
51. Sood, A. K., Holmes, R., Hendrix, M. J., et al. (2001) Application of the National Cancer Institute international criteria for determination of microsatellite instability in ovarian cancer. *Cancer Res.* **61,** 4371–4374.
52. Litt, M., Hauge, X., Sharma, V. (1993) Shadow bands seen when typing polymorphic dinucleotide repeats: some causes and cures. *Biotechniques* **15,** 280–284.

18

Diagnostic and Prognostic Significance of the Methylation Status of *Myf-3* in Lymphoproliferative Disorders

Jeremy M. E. Taylor, Peter H. Kay, and Dominic V. Spagnolo

1. Introduction

Methylation of DNA plays a major role in many biological processes throughout phylogeny. Generally, methylated DNA is associated with inactive gene transcription and compact chromatin structure. In mammalian DNA, typically cytosine residues within the 5'-CpG-3' dinucleotide have the potential to be methylated. By contrast, methylation of cytosine residues within the context of other nucleotide sequences such as 5'-CCTGG-3' is infrequent *(1)*.

DNA methylation is catalyzed by a series of 5-methyltransferases. A methyl group is transferred from the sole methyl donor *S*-adenosylmethionine to the 5-carbon position of cytosine to form 5-methylcytosine (5MC) *(2)*. Four 5-methyltransferases have been found thus far *(3)*. DNMT1 (maintenance methyltransferase) predominantly methylates hemimethylated double-stranded DNA and thus replicates the pattern of methylated cytosines on the nascent DNA strand during the S-phase. The function of DNMT2 is unknown, whereas DNMT3a and DNMT3b methylate new CpG sites (*de novo* methylation), and during embryogenesis, they might establish new patterns of methylation that are necessary for tissue differentiation. It is postulated that deregulated DNMT3 activity leads to *de novo* DNA methylation found in malignant cells and, furthermore, that DNMT1 maintainance methylation replicates the pattern of increased methylation in daughter cells.

In the last two decades, a role for DNA methylation has been identified in X-chromosome inactivation, parental genomic imprinting, and embryonic development. It is also thought that some elements of the DNA-methylating

From: *Methods in Molecular Medicine, vol. 97: Molecular Diagnosis of Cancer*
Edited by: J. E. Roulston and J. M. S. Bartlett © Humana Press Inc., Totowa, NJ

Table 1
Effect of Cytosine Methylation on Restriction-Site Cleavage by *Msp*I and *Hpa*II

Recognition sequence[a]	*Msp*I	*Hpa*II
5'- C C G G -3'	+	+
5'- C mC G G -3'	+	–
5'- mC C G G -3'	–	–

[a]In mammalian DNA, typically only the internal cytosine is methylated.

Note: mC: methylated cytosine; +: enzyme cleaves recognition sequence; –: enzyme does not cleave recognition sequence.

machinery may be involved in the inactivation of intragenomic parasitic DNA. It is not surprising, therefore, that in neoplasia, the DNA-methylating system is frequently deregulated and is characterized by regional hypermethylation, global hypomethylation, and increased activity of DNA-methylating enzymes ***(4)***. One hot spot of DNA hypermethylation is the short arm of chromosome 11 ***(5)***, a region known to include tumor suppressor genes ***(6)***.

There are several techniques for assessing the methylation status of specific DNA sequences and these have been reviewed by Oakeley ***(7)***. Although relatively cumbersome, the Southern-blot (SB)-based technique, as described below, has been used for many years and provides clear unequivocal information on the methylation status of DNA sequences under investigation. Other methods are polymerase chain reaction (PCR)-based and have the advantage of requiring small amounts of DNA for analysis; however, they have the disadvantage of analyzing relatively short DNA sequences. Furthermore, incomplete reactions prior to PCR may result in misinterpretation of the findings; for example, the Singer–Sam method depends on complete *Hpa*II digestion of the DNA target ***(8)***, and the methylation-sensitive PCR method depends on complete conversion of cytosine to thymine ***(9)***.

The myogenic gene *Myf-3* maps to 11p15, a hot spot of methylation. *Myf-3* is expressed in myoblasts and establishes myogenic differentiation during embryonic development. There is no evidence however, that *Myf-3* is expressed in lymphoid cells; thus, its biologic significance in lymphoproliferative disorders (LPDs) is uncertain. It has an extensive internal CpG island that is unmethylated in DNA from benign lymphoid tissue and other normal tissues, but it is methylated in DNA from a high proportion of lymphoid neoplasms ***(10)***. Increased *Myf-3* methylation is also found in colorectal, breast, ovarian, and bladder neoplasms, indicating that in some types of malignant disease, *Myf-3* methylation status is a sensitive and specific marker of malignancy ***(11–15)***.

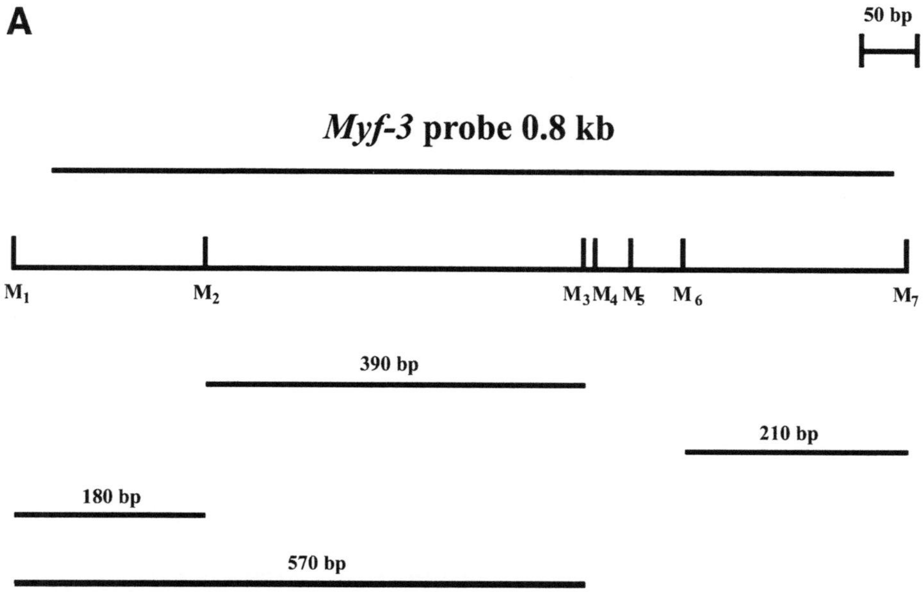

Fig. 1. **(A)** The expected sizes of *Myf-3*-digestion fragments showing how comparison of *Msp*I and *Hpa*II digested DNA is used to analyze cytosine methylation of 5'-CCGG-3' recognition sequences. Restriction sites M_1–M_7 are shown and the extent of sequences that hybridize to the *Myf-3* probe is indicated ***(16)***. *Msp*I-digested DNA from benign and malignant LPD samples has hybridizing fragments of approx 180 bp, 210 bp, and 390 bp. *Hpa*II-digested DNA from benign and malignant LPDs has larger hybridizing fragments e.g., an approx 0.6-kb *Hpa*II fragment is found in DNA from benign LPDs. This fragment might result from methylation at the M_2 restriction site, which is predicted to produce a 570-bp hybridizing fragment. In malignant LPDs, progressively larger hybridizing fragments are found that are predicted to result from methylation of additional flanking restriction sites (*see* **Fig. 2**). (Reprinted from **ref.** ***10*** by permission of Nature Publishing Group.)

The SB technique can be used to assess the methylation status of cytosine residues that occur within methylation-sensitive restriction enzyme-recognition sequences. The *Myf-3* methylation-status can be assessed by digesting DNA with the methylation-sensitive and methylation-insensitive isoschizomers *Hpa*II and *Msp*I, respectively (*see* **Table 1**) and then comparing the sizes of *Myf-3*-hybridizing fragments following Southern blotting of digested DNA fragments (*see* **Figs. 1** and **2**). In some genes, the level of DNA methylation may vary with age or tissue type ***(17)***, and findings show that in colonic tissue, the level of *Myf-3* methylation increases with age ***(12,18)***. However, in DNA from patients with benign LPDs, the level of *Myf-3* methylation remained con-

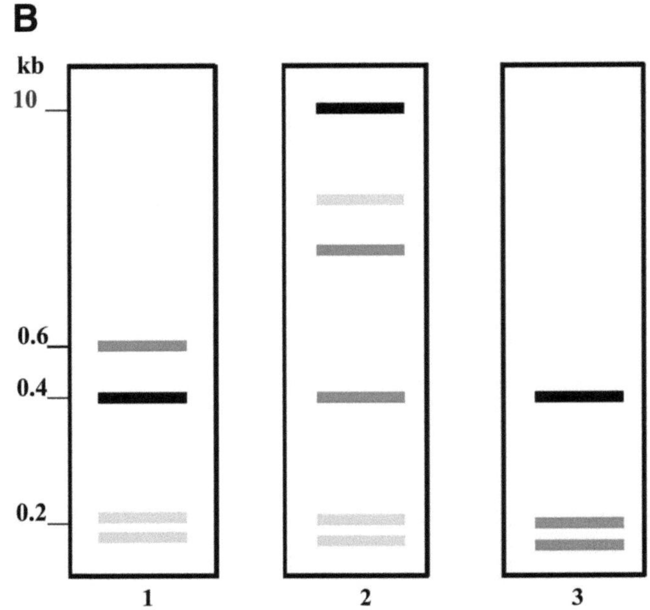

Fig. 1. *(continued)* **(B)** The predicted sizes, shown in **(A)**, of *Myf-3*-hybridizing fragments in a Southern blot. Lane 1 represents *Hpa*II digested DNA from a benign LPD. There are two faint hybridizing fragments of approx 0.2 kb, dense fragments of 0.4 kb, and less dense fragments of 0.6 kb. The 0.6-kb fragments are predicted to result from methylation, in a proportion of cells, at the *Msp*I restriction site M_2. Lane 2 shows three hypermethylated *Hpa*II-digested *Myf-3* fragments up to 10 kb that have varying densities. It is predicted that the hypermethylated fragments result from methylation of *Msp*I sites M_1–M_7 and flanking *Msp*I sites. Lane 3 shows *Msp*I-digested hybridizing fragments. There is a dense band of 0.4-kb fragments and two less dense bands of approx 0.2-kb fragments.

stant through a wide age range and in different types of lymphoid tissue (*see* **Figs. 3** and **4**).

2. Materials

2.1. DNA Extraction

1. Milli-Q purified water.
2. White cell lysis buffer (WCLB): Mix 10 mL of 1 *M* Tris-HCl, pH 7.6, 20 mL of 0.5 *M* EDTA, pH 8.0, 50 mL of 1 *M* NaCl, 10 mL of 20% sodium dodecyl sulfate (SDS), pH 7.2, and 910 mL of water.
3. 10 mg/mL Proteinase K.
4. 10 mg/mL RNase A: Dissolve 100 mg RNase A in 100 µL of 1 *M* Tris-HCl, pH

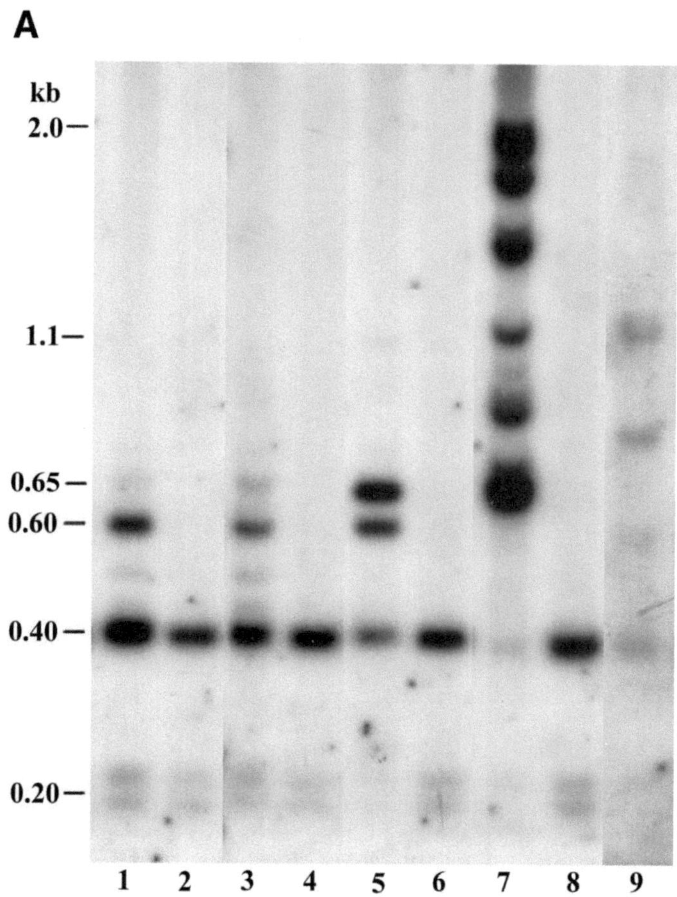

Fig. 2. **(A)** A Southern blot of *Hpa*II- (*lanes 1, 3, 5, 7,* and *9*) and *Msp*I- (*lanes 2, 4, 6,* and *8*) digested DNA hybridized with the *Myf-3* probe. All *Msp*I digests have hybridizing fragments of approx 0.4 kb and 0.2 kb. In addition, *Hpa*II digests of DNA from normal peripheral blood leukocytes (*lane 1*) and a benign lymph node (*lane 3*) have a 0.6-kb hybridizing fragment (*see* **Fig. 1**). *Hpa*II-digested DNA from a lymphoma has a dense 0.65-kb hybridizing fragment (*lane 5*) that is absent in nonmalignant samples and indicates a minor increase of *Myf-3* methylation. By contrast, hypermethylated *Myf-3* fragments are found in DNA from the lymphomas in *lanes 7* and *9* (*see* **Note 1**). Normal peripheral blood leukocytes: *lanes 1* and *2*; nonspecific reactive hyperplasia: *lanes 3* and *4*; low-grade follicular lymphoma: *lanes 5* and *6*; diffuse large B-cell lymphoma: *lanes 7* and *8*; extranodal natural killer (NK)-cell lymphoma of nasal type: *lane 9*.

7.5, and 150 µL of 1 *M* NaCl. Adjust volume to 10 mL with water and heat in a boiling water bath for 15 min. Cool, aliquot, and store at –20°C.

5. Phenol: Equilibrated with Tris-HCl, pH 8.0.

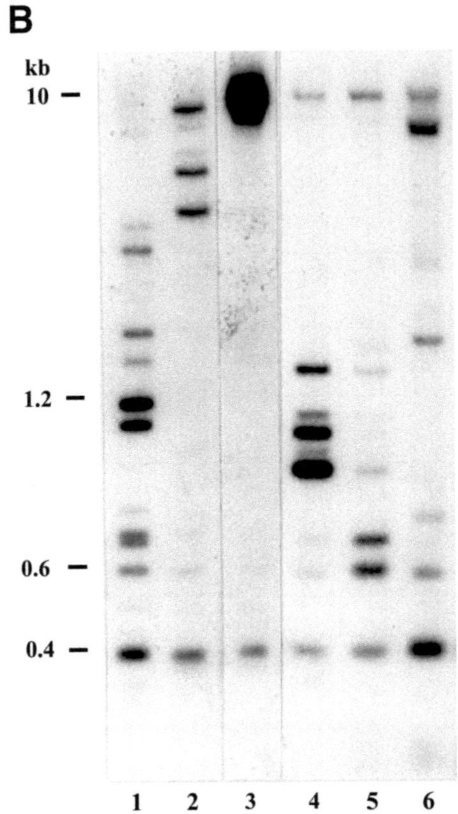

Fig. 2. *(continued)* (**B**) A Southern blot of *Hpa*II-digested DNA from NHL hybridized to the *Myf-3* probe; hypermethylated *Myf-3* fragments are seen in all lanes (*see* **Note 1**). DNA from lymphomas in *lanes 1, 2,* and *4–6* has multiple hypermethylated *Myf-3* fragments that have different densities. This indicates that although the lymphoma cells have monoclonal antigen–receptor gene rearrangements, not all of the clonal cells have identical sites of *Myf-3* methylation. By contrast, the single, dense 10-kb fragment in *lane 3* indicates that the lymphoma cells have monoclonal *Myf-3* methylation and that both gene copies are identically methylated. The *Myf-3* methylation profile varied in three biopsies taken at intervals of 1 and 3 yr from the same patient. The first two samples (*lanes 4* and *5*) have fragments of common size but different relative density, whereas the third sample (*lane 6*) has novel large fragments. These findings indicate there are different proportions of lymphoma cell subclones whereby each is identified by its level of *Myf-3* hypermethylation and might indicate increasing *Myf-3* methylation during the course of the disease. (Reprinted from **ref. *10*** by permission of Nature Publishing Group.)

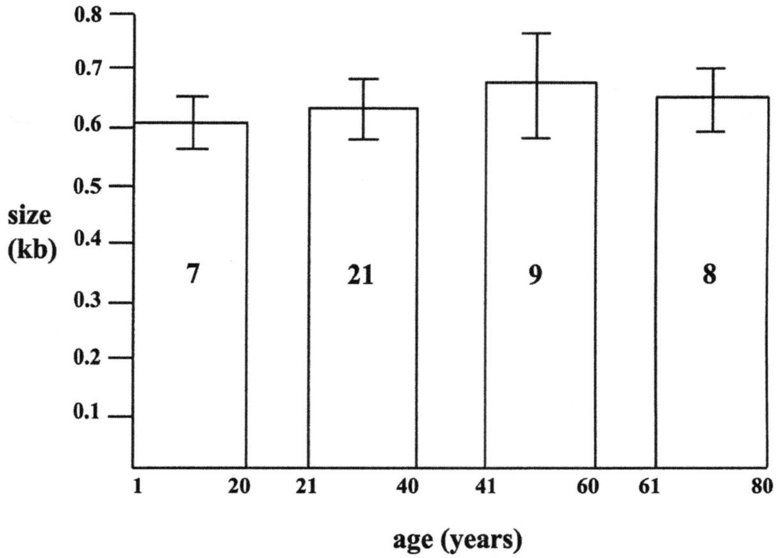

Fig. 3. The maximum level of *Myf-3* methylation in *Hpa*II-digested DNA from benign LPDs was compared between patients of different age. The maximum level of *Myf-3* methylation does not alter with age. Sample numbers are shown within each age group; the bar indicates the mean ± 1 standard deviation.

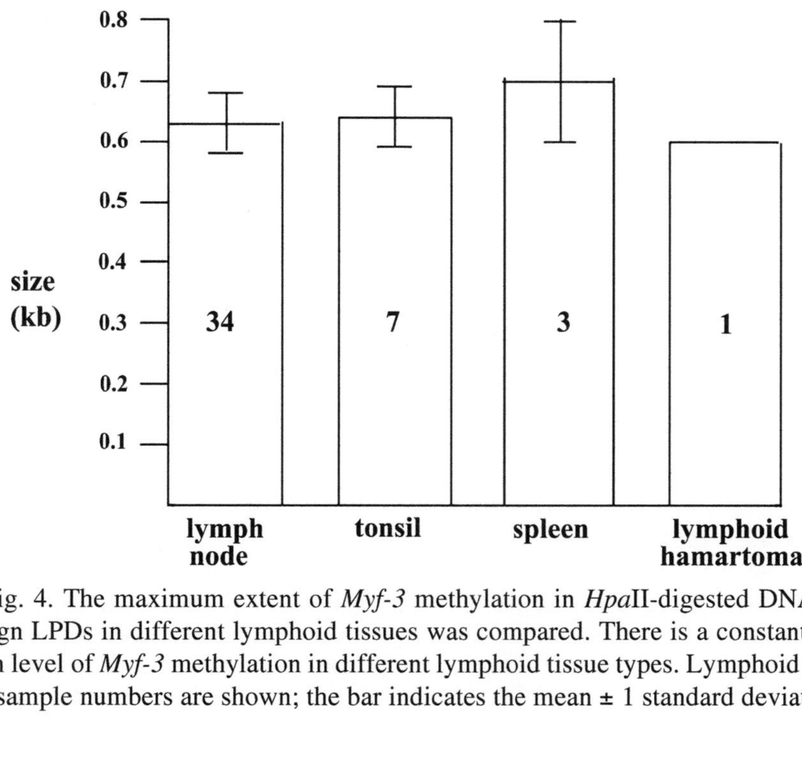

Fig. 4. The maximum extent of *Myf-3* methylation in *Hpa*II-digested DNA from benign LPDs in different lymphoid tissues was compared. There is a constant maximum level of *Myf-3* methylation in different lymphoid tissue types. Lymphoid tissues and sample numbers are shown; the bar indicates the mean ± 1 standard deviation.

6. Chloroform-isoamyl alcohol: A mixture of 24:1 (v/v) chloroform and isoamyl alcohol.
7. 1X TE buffer, pH 8.0: 10m*M* Tris-HCI, pH 8.0, and 1m*M* EDTA, pH 8.0, and 1m*M* EDTA, pH 8.0.

2.2. Southern Blot Analysis

1. *Hpa*II and *Msp*I restriction enzymes (Promega, Australia).
2. 10X Restriction enzyme buffer (Promega, Australia).
3. 10 mg/mL Bovine serum albumin (BSA) (Promega, Australia).
4. 1.8% Agarose dissolved in 1X TAE buffer with ethidium bromide. Concentrated stock 50X TAE buffer: 242 g Tris, 57.1 mL glacialacetic acid, and 100 mL of 0.5*M* EDTA, pH 8.0 dissolved in Milli-Q water to a volume of 1000 mL.
5. DNA size marker.
6. 6X Loading buffer: Dissolve 0.05 g of bromophenol blue and 8.0 g of sucrose in 20 mL of Milli-Q water. Aliquot 1-mL amounts and store at 4°C.
7. 0.25 *M* HCl.
8. 0.4 *M* NaOH.
9. GeneScreen Plus (Perkin-Elmer Life Sciences, USA).
10. Vacuum blotter (Bio-Rad, USA).
11. Ultraviolet (UV) transilluminator (UVP, USA).
12. *Myf-3* probe (ATCC 61522).
13. [α-^{32}P] dCTP (Perkin-Elmer Life Sciences, USA).
14. Radiolabeling kit: Rediprime (Amersham Life Science, UK).
15. Hybridization fluid: Rapid Hyb (Amersham Life Science, UK).
16. 20% (w/v) SDS, pH 7.2.
17. 20X SSC: Dissolve 350.6 g of NaCl and 176.4 g of trisodium citrate dihydrate in 1600 mL of Milli-Q water, adjust pH to 7.0, and add Milli-Q water to 2000 mL. Sterilize by autoclaving.
18. High-stringency wash solution 0.1X SSC-0.1% SDS: Dilute 20 mL of 20X SSC and 20 mL of 20% SDS, pH 7.2 in a final volume of 4000 mL.

3. Methods

3.1. DNA Extraction

1. Extract DNA from fresh, solid lymphoid tissue that had been snap-frozen in liquid nitrogen as soon as possible after excision and stored at –80°C, or from the buffy coat layer of peripheral blood. Dice solid tissue (approx 3 mm^3) with a sterile scalpel blade, mix with 5 mL of WCLB, add 10 µL of RNase A, and incubate with mixing at 37°C for 30 min. Add 200 µL of proteinase K and digest overnight at 50°C.
2. Isolate DNA using organic solvents according to standard procedures ***(19)***. Briefly, mix the tissue digest with approx 5 mL of phenol; then, centrifuge to separate DNA in the aqueous upper layer from the phenolic lower layer. A thin layer of denatured protein forms at the interface of the aqueous and phenolic layers. The denatured protein layer must be avoided to prevent contamination of

DNA. Phenol deproteinization of the aqueous layer is repeated and is followed by mixing the DNA-containing aqueous layer with chloroform–isoamyl alcohol. Following centrifugation, the aqueous layer is recovered and DNA is precipitated with an equal volume of chilled isopropyl alcohol ***(19)***. Centrifuge to pellet the DNA; then, drain and dry the DNA at room temperature. Redissolve the DNA in 1X TE buffer to a concentration of approx 200 μg /mL.

3. Quantitate the DNA concentration spectrophotometrically and measure the optical density (OD) at 260 and 280 nm (*see* **Note 2**). Electrophorese 5 μL of DNA in a 0.8% agarose gel to verify that the DNA is of high molecular weight with minimal degradation.

3.2. Southern Blot Analysis

1. In separate digestion mixtures, assemble 10X buffer, BSA (working concentration 100 μg/mL), and water; then, digest 12 μg of DNA to completion with 60 units of *Hpa*II and *Msp*I according to the manufacturer's instructions. Check the completeness of digestion by electrophoresing 5 μL of the digest in a 0.8% agarose gel (*see* **Note 3**).
2. Precipitate digested DNA with chilled isopropanol, dry, and redissolve DNA in 1X TE and 6X loading buffer.
3. Load wells of a 15 × 15-cm 1.8% agarose gel, and electrophorese for 280 V h in recirculated 1X TAE buffer. Load DNA size markers (*see* **Note 4**).
4. Photograph the ethidium bromide-stained gel using UV transillumination. The photographic record of DNA size marker migration is used to estimate the size of hybridized fragments.
5. Nick the DNA by soaking the gel in 0.25*M* HCl with gentle shaking for 15–20 min and the bromophenol blue dye front has just changed from blue to almost yellow. Do not overexpose the gel to 0.25*M* HCl.
6. Rinse the gel in water; then, denature the DNA by soaking in 0.4*M* NaOH with gentle shaking for 30 min.
7. Blot DNA in 0.4*M* NaOH transfer fluid to a positively charged, nylon membrane support using vacuum blotting according to the manufacturer's instructions (*see* **Note 5**).
8. Rinse the membrane in 2X SSC to remove any adherent gel. Drain and dry the membrane on filter paper; then, fix the DNA to the membrane by baking at 65°C overnight.
9. Radiolabel the probe to high specific activity with dCTP ^{32}P using a Rediprime random priming kit according to the manufacturer's instructions (Amersham, UK).
10. Denature the probe; then, hybridize it with membrane-fixed complementary DNA in Rapid Hyb (Amersham, UK) hybridization buffer at 65°C for 1.5–2 h.
11. Remove unbound probe by washing the membrane at 65°C with gentle shaking in three changes of a high-stringency wash solution.
12. Expose X-ray film at –70°C for 1 d or longer using an intensifying screen; then, develop the autoradiograph.

13. The largest hybridizing fragment size, irrespective of density, is used to assign the extent of *Myf-3* methylation.

3.3. Assessment of Myf-3 Methylation Status in LPDs

The extent of DNA methylation of some genes is tissue and age related *(17,18)*. Therefore, when assessing the methylation status of a gene of interest, it is necessary to establish whether the methylation status of the gene under investigation is age or tissue dependent. In a study of *Myf-3* methylation in DNA from patients of different ages who suffered from benign LPDs *(10)*, the level of *Myf-3* methylation did not vary with age or type of lymphoid tissue (*see* **Figs. 3** and **4**).

The accurate interpretation of DNA methylation status also depends on complete restriction enzyme digestion. Digestion can be controlled by including normal peripheral blood DNA, which typically has the same low level of *Myf-3* methylation found in benign lymphoid tissues (*see* **Fig. 2**). Furthermore, digesting DNA with excess amounts of restriction enzyme may also be used to exclude incomplete digestion as a cause of large hybridizing fragments (*see* **Note 6**).

DNA from benign LPDs has a low level of *Myf-3* methylation in which hybridizing fragments larger than 0.8 kb are absent. By contrast, increased methylation of *Myf-3* is found in non-Hodgkin's lymphoma (NHL), in lymphoid leukemia *(10)*, and in a range of other malignant diseases *(12–15)*.

Malignant lymphoid cells frequently have hypermethylated *Myf-3* fragments or a minor increase of *Myf-3* methylation (*see* **Note 1** and **Fig. 5**). Thus, the finding of increased *Myf-3* methylation distinguishes DNA from benign and malignant LPDs (*see* **Note 7**) and, consequently, may be used to determine whether hyperproliferating lymphoid cells are benign or malignant in those cases where standard molecular techniques are uninformative *(10)*. The level of *Myf-3* methylation within categories of malignant lymphoid cells is highly variable and reflects their clinical and histopathologic heterogeneity. The degree of hypermethylation of *Myf-3* is of some value in prognostication because, as indicated in **Fig. 5**, some lymphomas have *Myf-3* methylation levels that correlate with their histopathologic grade of malignancy.

3.4. Methylation Status of Bcl-6 in Benign and Malignant LPDs

With respect to lymphomas, leukemias and other malignancies (*see* **Subheading 3.3.**) it is often considered that hypermethylation of *Myf-3* reflects a downstream molecular genetic event consequential to malignant transformation. Recently, we turned our attention to *Bcl-6*. In contrast to *Myf-3, Bcl-6* is required for the normal development of the lymphoid follicle germinal center. *Bcl-6* is susceptible to somatic mutation *(20)*, and in some types of malignant

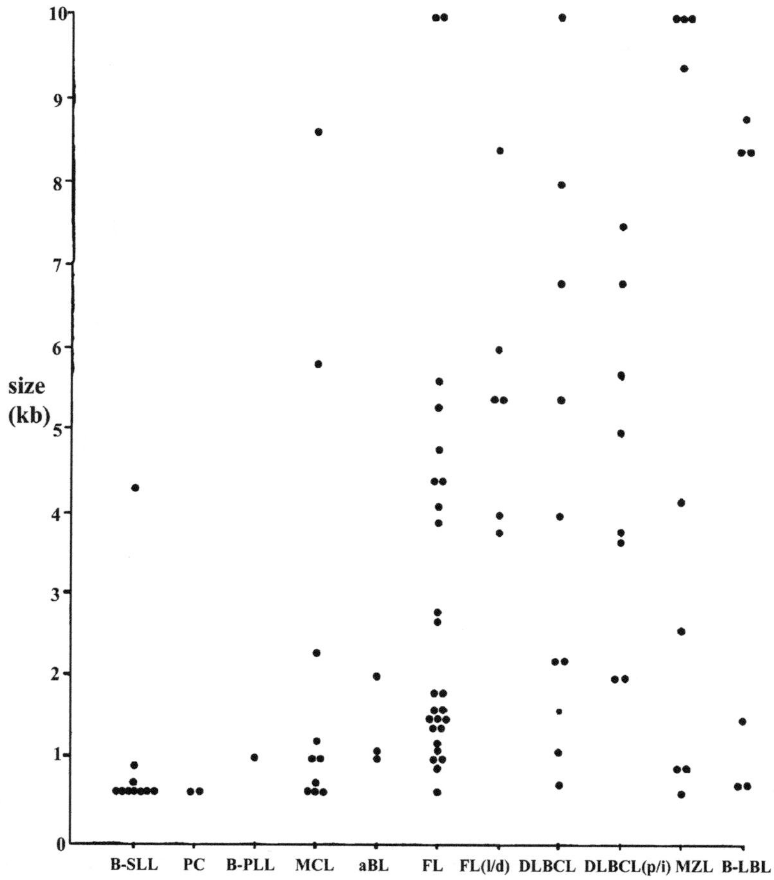

Fig. 5. The distribution of the maximum-sized *Myf-3*-hybridizing fragments in a Southern blot of *Hpa*II-digested DNA from B-cell neoplasms is illustrated. Hypermethylated fragments were absent in some samples; however, the majority of these had a minor increase of methylation that was absent in benign LPDs. FL and DLBCL were subgrouped according to histopathologic criteria that reflected malignancy grade. Those FL that consisted of predominantly large cells with or without diffuse growth were of a higher histopathologic grade of malignancy and frequently had more extensive *Myf-3* methylation than those composed of mainly small cells. Consistent with its low malignancy grade, DNA from B-SLL samples had a uniformly low level of methylation. B-SLL, B-Cell small lymphocytic lymphoma (10); PC, plasma cell myeloma (2); B-PLL, B-cell prolymphocytic leukemia (1); MCL, mantle cell lymphoma (10); aBL, atypical Burkitt lymphoma (3); FL, follicular lymphoma; small cleaved cell, or mixed small and large cell, with follicular growth (26); FL(l/d), follicular lymphoma comprised of predominantly large cells with or without diffuse growth (6); DLBCL, diffuse large B-cell lymphoma, unspecified cytology (9); DLBCL(p/i), diffuse large B-cell lymphoma, pleomorphic or immunoblastic cytology (8); MZL, marginal zone lymphoma, MALT type (7), splenic type (1), nodal type (1); and B-LBL, precursor B-lymphoblastic leukemia/lymphoma (6). The number of samples in each category is indicated in parenthesis. (Reprinted from **ref.** *10* by permission of Nature Publishing Group.)

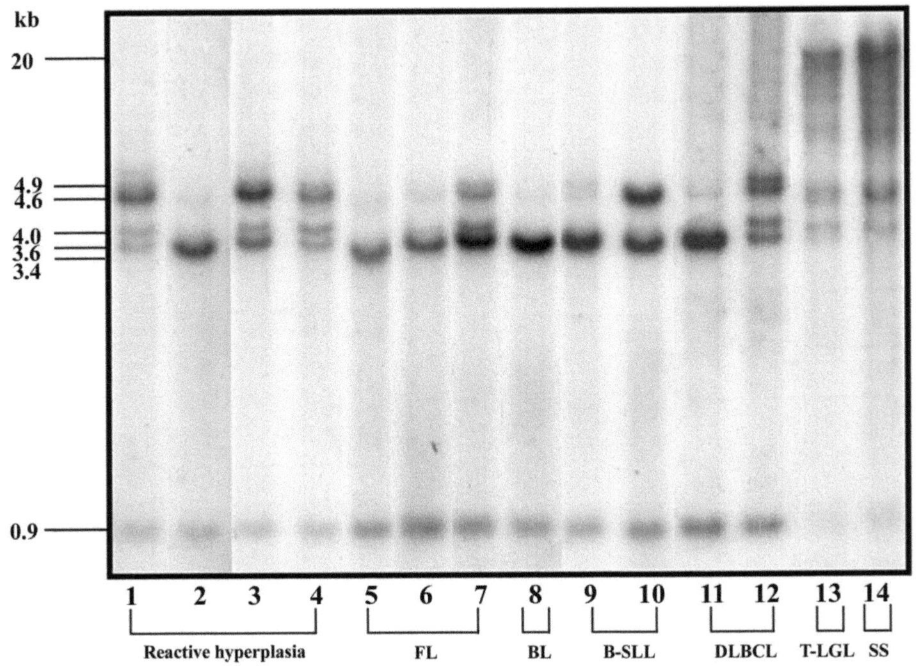

Fig. 6. Southern blot of *Hpa*II- and *Msp*I-digested DNA from benign and malignant LPDs electrophoresed in a 0.8% agarose gel and hybridized to the *Bcl-6 Sac*I 4-kb probe ***(21)***. *Hpa*II-digested DNA from benign LPDs has fragments of approximate size 0.9, 3.6, 4.0, 4.6, and 4.9 kb (lanes 1, 3, and 4). *Msp*I-digested DNA from the sample in lane 1 yields fragments of 0.9 kb and 3.4 kb (lane 2). In contrast to benign LPDs, DNA samples from B-NHL have decreased density of 4.6-kb and 4.9-kb *Hpa*II fragments relative to the 3.6-kb and 4.0-kb *Hpa*II fragments, indicating hypomethylation (*lanes 5–9* and *11*). *Hpa*II fragments from the FL in *lane 5* had the same size as the 3.4-kb and 0.9-kb *Msp*I fragments in *lane 2*, indicating demethylation of all of the *Msp*I sites included in the region bounded by the *Bcl-6* probe. Similar densities of the 3.6 kb and 4.6 kb *Hpa*II fragments from the B-SLL sample in lane 10 might indicate that the two *Bcl-6* gene copies have different sites of methylation. The four hybridizing *Hpa*II-digested DNA fragments having equal density in the DLBCL (*lane 12*) were an unusual finding that might be explained by the cytogenetic finding of tetraploidy. In contrast to samples of B-NHL, *Bcl-6* in DNA from a T-cell large granular lymphocytic leukemia (T-LGL) and Sezary cell leukemia (SS) was markedly hypermethylated (lanes 13 and 14, respectively). *Hpa*II digests: *lanes 1* and *3–14*; *Msp*I digest: *lane 2*. Refer to the Fig. 5 legend for abbreviations.

B-cells, it is a partner gene in reciprocal chromosomal translocation ***(21)***. Because evidence suggests that DNA methylation may influence genomic stability, we have begun to investigate the methylation status of *Bcl-6* in different types of malignant and benign lymphoid cells. Using the same approach that we have used to examine the methylation status of *Myf-3*, a *Bcl-6* 4-kb *Sac*I probe was hybridized to *Hpa*II- and *Msp*I-digested DNA from a series of benign and malignant LPDs. The 4-kb genomic probe hybridizes to the first exon of *Bcl-6* and the 5' flanking sequences included in the breakpoint cluster and hypermutation regions ***(22)***. Preliminary findings, which are included for interest, indicate that, as with *Myf-3*, the methylation status of *Bcl-6* also distinguishes between DNA from benign and malignant LPDs (*see* **Fig. 6**). However, in contrast to the finding of increased *Myf-3* methylation in almost all malignant lymphoid cells, DNA from B-cell non-Hodgkin's lymphoma (B-NHL) was characterized by hypomethylation of *Bcl-6* when compared to the methylation status of *Bcl-6* in DNA from benign LPDs. By contrast, in T-cell lymphomas, *Bcl-6* appears to be hypermethylated, as is *Myf-3*. These findings are inconsistent with the view that *Myf-3* hypermethylation, particularly in malignant LPDs, is consequential to malignant transformation *per se*. Moreover, because evidence suggests that DNA methylation influences genomic stability, it is tempting to speculate that abnormal rearrangements of *Bcl-6* in some B-NHLs is consequential to some form of focal demethylating process unique to cells of B-cell origin. This possibility is consistent with our findings that the same upstream region of *Bcl-6* is generally hypermethylated in malignant T-cell LPDs in which abnormal rearrangements of *Bcl-6* are absent.

Our future work will focus on understanding the complexity of different forms of DNA methylation deregulation and how they may influence or contribute to different molecular genetic pathways leading to malignant transformation of lymphoid cells and lymphoma progression.

4. Notes

1. *Myf-3* methylation status in lymphoid tissues was defined by the size and relative density of *Myf-3*-hybridizing fragments. Hypermethylation was assigned when hybridized fragments were larger than 0.8 kb, a fragment size not found in DNA from benign LPDs. Minor level of methylation change was assigned when there were dense fragments larger than 0.6 kb and up to or including 0.8 kb (these dense fragments were absent in DNA from benign LPDs) and/or 0.4-kb fragments were absent or weakly hybridized compared to the 0.6-kb fragment density. In DNA from the majority of benign LPDs, the density of the 0.4-kb fragment was greater than or similar to the density of the 0.6-kb fragment, whereas in the minority, the 0.6-kb fragment was slightly denser than the 0.4-kb fragment.
2. The OD 260/OD 280 nm ratio should not be less than 1.8 ***(19)***. A ratio lower than 1.8 might indicate contamination of DNA with protein or phenol and this could prevent complete restriction enzyme digestion.
3. Electrophoresed *Msp*I-digested DNA has a wide range of fragment sizes having a

smearlike appearance without a distinct band of high-molecular-weight DNA. By contrast, *Hpa*II-digested DNA frequently has a distinct band of high-molecular-weight DNA in addition to a faint smear of smaller fragments.

4. A combination of *Hin*dIII-digested phage λ DNA and *Msp*I-digested pUC19 DNA has a useful range of DNA size markers (9416–242 bp) for estimating fragment size in a 1.8% agarose gel.
5. Complete DNA transfer is verified by washing the gel thoroughly in water, restaining with ethidium bromide, and viewing the gel with UV transillumination for evidence of residual DNA.
6. Digestion with excess amounts of *Hpa*II may be used to investigate incomplete *Hpa*II digestion as a cause of large hybridizing restriction fragments that might be misinterpreted as representing *Myf-3* hypermethylation. In digests having a range of *Hpa*II amounts, the finding of hybridizing fragments that have a constant size and relative density is supportive of DNA hypermethylation and not of incomplete *Hpa*II digestion.
7. Increased *Myf-3* methylation is not characteristic of DNA from Hodgkin's lymphoma. This might be because the proportion of malignant cells is typically less than 1% in Hodgkin's lymphoma tissue, a proportion that is less than the sensitivity of the Southern blot (5–10%). Alternatively, increased *Myf-3* methylation might not be a feature of the malignant cells of Hodgkin's lymphoma.

References

1. Franchina, M. and Kay, P. H. (2000) Evidence that cytosine residues within 5'-CCTGG-3' pentanucleotides can be methylated in human DNA independently of the methylating system that modifies 5'-CG-3' dinucleotides. *DNA Cell Biol.* **19,** 521–526.
2. Klimasauskas, S., Kumar, S., Roberts, R. J., et al. (1994) *Hha*I methyltransferase flips its target base out of the DNA helix. *Cell* **76,** 357–369.
3. Bestor, T. H. (2000) The DNA methyltransferases of mammals. *Hum. Mol. Genet.* **9,** 2395–2402.
4. Robertson, K. D., Uzvolgyi, E., Liang, G., et al. (1999) The human DNA methyltransferases (DNMTs) 1, 3a and 3b: coordinate mRNA expression in normal tissues and overexpression in tumors. *Nucleic Acids Res.* **27,** 2291–2298.
5. de Bustros, A., Nelkin, B. D., Silverman, A., et al. (1988) The short arm of chromosome 11 is a "hot-spot" for hypermethylation in human neoplasia. *Proc. Natl. Acad. Sci. USA* **85,** 5693–5697.
6. Koi, M., Johnson, L. A., Kalikin, L. M., et al. (1993) Tumor cell growth arrest caused by subchromosomal transferable DNA fragments from chromosome 11. *Science* **260,** 361–364.
7. Oakeley, E. J. (1999) DNA methylation analysis: a review of current methodologies. Pharmacol. Thera. **84,** 389–400.
8. Singer-Sam, J., Grant, M., LeBon, J. M., et al. (1990) Use of *Hpa*II–polymerase chain reaction assay to study DNA methylation in the *Pgk-1* CpG island of mouse

embryos at the time of X-chromosome inactivation. *Mol. Cell. Biol.* **10,** 4987–4989.

9. Herman, J. G., Graff, J. R., Myohanen, S., et al. (1996) Methylation–specific PCR: a novel PCR assay for methylation status of CpG islands. *Proc. Natl. Acad. Sci. USA* **93,** 9821–9826.
10. Taylor, J. M. E., Kay, P. H., and Spagnolo, D. V. (2001) The diagnostic significance of *Myf-3* hypermethylation in malignant lymphoproliferative disorders. *Leukemia* **15,** 583–589.
11. Iacopetta, B. J., Harmon, D. H., Spagnolo, D. V., et al. (1997) Hypermethylation of the *Myf-3* gene in human colorectal cancer. *Anticancer Res.* **17,** 429–432.
12. Shannon, B., Kay, P., House, A., et al. (1999) Hypermethylation of the *Myf-3* gene in colorectal cancers: associations with pathlogical features and with microsatellite instability. *Int. J. Cancer* **84,** 109–113.
13. Hähnel, R., Harvey, J., and Kay, P. H. (1996) Hypermethylation of the myogenic gene *Myf-3* in human breast carcinomas. *Anticancer Res.* **16,** 2111–2116.
14. Cheng, P., Schmutte, C., Cofer, K. F., et al. (1997) Alterations in DNA methylation are early, but not initial, events in ovarian tumorigenesis. *Br. J. Cancer* **75,** 396–402.
15. Rideout, W. M., Eversole-Cine, P., Spruck, C. H., et al. (1994) Progressive increases in the methylation status and heterochromatinisation of the myoD CpG island during oncogenic transformation. *Mol. Cell. Biol.* **14,** 6143–6152.
16. Chen, B., Dias, P., Jenkins, J. J., et al. (1998) Methylation alterations of the *MyoD1* upstream region are predictive of subclassification of human rhabdomyosarcoma. *Am. J. Pathol.* **152,** 1071–1079.
17. Issa, J.-P., Ottaviano, Y. L., Celano, P., et al. (1994) Methylation of the oestrogen receptor CpG island links ageing and neoplasia in human colon. *Nature Genet.* **7,** 536–540.
18. Ahuja, N., Li, Q., Mohan, A. L., et al. (1998) Aging and DNA methylation in colorectal mucosa and cancer. *Cancer Res.* **58,** 5489–5494.
19. Sambrook, J., Fritch, E. F., and Maniatis, T. (1989) *Molecular Cloning: A Laboratory Manual*, 2nd ed., Cold Spring Harbor Laboratory, Cold Spring Harbor, NY.
20. Capello, D., Vitolo, U., Pasqualucci, L., et al. (2000) Distribution and pattern of *BCL-6* mutations throughout the spectrum of B-cell neoplasia. *Blood* **95,** 651–659.
21. Ye, B. H., Rao, P. H., Chaganti, R. S. K., et al. (1993) Cloning of *bcl-6*, the locus involved in chromosome translocations affecting band 3q27 in B-cell lymphoma. *Cancer Res.* **53,** 2732–2735.
22. Ye, B. H., Lista, F., Lo Coco, F., et al. (1993) Alterations of a zinc finger-encoding gene, *BCL-6*, in diffuse large-cell lymphoma. *Science* **262,** 747–750.

19

Quantitative Analysis of PRAME for Detection of Minimal Residual Disease in Leukemia

Maiko Matsushita, Rie Yamazaki, and Yutaka Kawakami

1. Introduction

Preferentially expressed antigen of melanoma (PRAME) was first isolated using cDNA expression cloning techniques as a gene encoding a human melanoma antigen recognized by melanoma reactive cytotoxic T-cells (CTL) *(1)*. This gene codes for a 509-amino-acid protein whose function has not yet been identified. PRAME is expressed in various types of cancer, including melanoma (97%), sarcoma (80%), small-cell lung cancer (70%), renal cell carcinoma (40%), and head and neck cancer (29%) *(1,2)*. PRAME is also found in limited normal tissues, including endometrium and adrenal glands, and found highly expressed in testis.

In our study of Japanese patients, PRAME expression was found in various hematological malignancies, including acute myelogenous leukemia (AML), acute lymphocytic leukemia (ALL), chronic myelogenous leukemia (CML), non-Hodgkin's lymphoma (NHL), and multiple myeloma (MM) *(3)*. In particular, PRAME was frequently expressed in AML M2 (45%), AML M3 (75%), CML BC (50%), and ALL (64%). Expression was less frequent in lymphoma (21%). Interestingly, four of five t(8; 21)-positive AML and five of six t(9; 22)-positive ALL patients evaluated in our study expressed PRAME at a high level. In Japanese patients with CML, PRAME was positive in 23% of chronic phase, 29% of accelerated phase, and 42% of blastic crisis phase, suggesting an increase of the PRAME expression during disease progression. It was also reported that PRAME was highly expressed in 48% of advanced-stage patients with MM *(4)*. These observations suggest that PRAME may be useful for monitoring minimal residual disease (MRD) in various hematological malignancies.

From: *Methods in Molecular Medicine, vol. 97: Molecular Diagnosis of Cancer*
Edited by: J. E. Roulston and J. M. S. Bartlett © Humana Press Inc., Totowa, NJ

Preferentially expressed antigen of melanoma was originally shown to be a target for cytotoxic T-cells, and several epitopes presented by human leukocyte antigen (HLA)-A2 and HLA–A24 have been identified ***(1,5)***. Thus, it is an attractive strategy to apply PRAME-specific immunotherapy for patients with PRAME-positive leukemia in an MRD condition. For example, PRAME-specific CTLs generated from peripheral blood mononuclear cells (PBMC) of patients in complete remission (CR) may be administered to patients with increased PRAME expression detected by polymerase chain reaction (PCR) even without increase of blast counts.

Several tumor-specific genes have been utilized for detection of MRD. Those represent leukemia-specific gene rearrangements, including t(9;22) (q34;q11) ***(6,7)*** and t(8;21) (q22;q22) ***(8)***, as well as gene rearrangement of immunogloblins ***(9)*** and T-cell receptors ***(10)***. Although these markers provided tumor-specific quantitative measuring of leukemic cells, they are available only in limited types of leukemia. In contrast, WT1 (Wilms' tumor 1 gene) shows increased expression in various hematological malignancies and has recently been used to monitor MRD as a genetic marker ***(11)***. Sensitivity of detection for residual leukemia by reverse transcription (RT)-PCR analysis with PRAME and WT1 is similar; however, some of the hematological malignancies do not express WT1, but express PRAME. Particularly, PRAME expression is higher than WT1 in some of ALL and ATL. Thus, the combination of both PRAME and WT1 appears to be a powerful tool for the detection of MRD in hematological malignancies, especially in leukemia without tumor-specific genetic markers.

The real-time PCR method has been used for monitoring MRD using leukemia-specific markers such as the *bcr-abl* fusion gene ***(12)***. This method was proved to be quantitative and less labor-intensive than competitive PCR or limiting dilution assays combined with a single-round or two-step PCR ***(13)***. We have established the real-time PCR method to monitor MRD by quantitative measurement of PRAME expression on peripheral blood (PB) or bone marrow (BM) samples from patients with PRAME-positive leukemia ***(3)***. This technique allows PRAME-positive leukemic cell detection at a sensitivity of 1 in 10^7 cells. Quantitative measuring is possible in over 1 in 10^4 cells. Although weak expression was occasionally observed in normal PB or BM cells, expression levels in healthy samples were 3 log lower than that in leukemia cells; thus, leukemia-associated PRAME expression can be easily distinguished. In our study, the serial analysis of PRAME expression in eight patients with the real-time PCR method revealed a positive correlation between the PRAME expression and clinical status. In particular, relapses were detected in patients by monitoring PRAME expression before being diagnosed by cytology. In this chapter, a protocol of real-time PCR for the quantitative measurement of

PRAME to monitor MRD in patients with hematological malignancies is described.

2. Materials

2.1. Cell Separation

1. Phosphate-buffered saline (PBS): 137 m*M* NaCl, 8.1 m*M* Na_2HPO_4, 2.68 m*M* KCl, 1.47 n*M* KH_2PO_4, pH 7.4.
2. Percoll (Sigma).

2.2. RNA Isolation

All solutions and glasswares should be treated with diethyl pyrocarbonate (DEPC) to remove RNase.

1. GTC: 4*M* guanidine-isothiocyanate, 20 m*M* sodium acetate, pH 5.2, 0.5% *N*-lauroylsarcosine (Sigma). Add 0.1 m*M* dithiothreitol (DTT) immediately before use.
2. CsCl: 5.7*M* CsCl, 0.5 *M* EDTA, DEPC treated (treat solution with DEPC).
3. TES: 10 m*M* Tris-HCl, pH 7.4, 10 m*M* EDTA, 0.1% sodium dodecyl sulfate (SDS) made up with DEPC-treated water.
4. 3*M* Sodium acetate (NaOAc) brought to pH 5.2 with glacial acetic acid (use DEPC-treated water).
5. DEPC-treated water: Add 100 μL of DEPC to 100 mL of water; then, incubate at 37°C for 2 h.
6. 80% Ethanol made up with DEPC-treated water.

2.3. cDNA Synthesis

1. 20 m*M* Random hexamer primers (Worthingen Biochemical, NJ).
2. 5X Reverse-transcriptase buffer: 250 m*M* Tris-HCl, pH 8.3, 375 m*M* KCl, 15 m*M* $MgCl_2$; supplied with Mo-MLV reverse transcriptase (Gibco-BRL, Gaithersburg, MD).
3. Mixture containing 10 m*M* dTTP, dATP, dGTP, and dCTP each (Invitrogen, Groningern, The Netherlands).
4. 0.1*M* DTT (Gibco-BRL, Gaithersburg, MD).
5. 40 U/μL RNase inhibitor (Promega Biotec, WI).
6. 200 U/μL Mo-MLV reverse transcriptase (Gibco-BRL, Gaithersburg, MD).
7. DEPC-treated water (*see* **Subheading 2.2.**).

2.4. Real-Time PCR

1. 10X TaqMan buffer: 500 m*M* KCl, 100 m*M* Tris-HCl, 0.1*M* EDTA, 600 n*M* Passive Reference 1 (*see* **Note 1**), pH 8.3 (PE Biosystems, CA).
2. 25 m*M* $MgCl_2$ (PE Biosystems, CA).
3. dNTPs: 20 m*M* dTTP, 10 m*M* dATP, dGTP, and dCTP each (PE Biosystems, CA).

Table 1
Primers and Probes for PRAME Gene and ß-Actin Gene

Primer/probe	Sequences
PRAME primers	
TaqMan 5'-primer	5'-TCTTCCTACATTTCCCCGGA-3'
TaqMan 3'-primer	5'-GCACTGCAGACTGAGGAACTGA-3'
PRAME probe	
TaqMan probe	5'(FAM)AAGGAAGAGCAGTATATCGCCCAG TTCACC-(TAMRA)-3'
β-actin primers	
TaqMan 5'-primer	5'-TCACCCACACTGTGCCCATCTACGA-3'
TaqMan 3'-primer	5'-CAGCGGAACCGCTCATTGCCAATGG-3'
β-actin probes	
TaqMan probe	5'-(FAM)ATGCCC-X(TAMRA)-3' CCCCCATGCCATCCTGCGTp-3'

4. 1 U/μL AmpErase™ uracil *N*-glycosylase (PE Biosystems).
5. 5 U/μL AmpliTaq Gold DNA polymerase (PE Biosystems).
6. 3 μ*M* PRAME 5'- primer, PRAME 3'-primer, ß-actin 5'-primer, and ß-actin 3'-primer (*see* **Table 1**).
7. 2 μ*M* PRAME probe and ß-actin probe (*see* **Table 1**). These probes are labeled with 5'-reporter dye (FAM) and 3'-quencher dye (TAMRA) (*see* **Note 2**).
8. Reference samples; To obtain standard curves, a serial dilution of the plasmid Vi381 containing PRAME cDNA *(1)* from 1 pg/μL to 0.01 fg/μL was used for the PRAME standard curve, and cDNA synthesized from 2 μg of total RNA of K562 cells were diluted to 1:1 to 1:16 and used for the ß-actin standard curve (*see* **Note 3**).

2.5. Analysis of the Real-Time PCR

ABI Prism 7700 Sequence Detector System (PE Biosystems).

3. Methods

3.1. Cell Separation

1. Dilute PB or BM with PBS at 1:2.
2. Add 10 mL of Percoll to a 50-mL centrifuge tube.
3. Carefully layer 10 mL of diluted blood or BM onto Percoll.
4. Centrifuge at 700*g* for 30 min at room temperature.
5. Remove the top layer (plasma) and transfer mononuclear cells from the next layer to a new tube.
6. Wash the cells twice with 20 mL of PBS at 1000*g* for 10 min.
7. Aspirate and discard remaining fluid.

3.2. RNA Extraction

1. Add 3.5 mL of GTC (guanidine–isothiocyanate) solution to the pellets. Vortex for 1 min. With a 5-mL syringe, rapidly homogenize the cell pellets by passing four times through a 20-gage needle.
2. Put 1.5 mL CsCl into a 13 × 51-mm autoclaved Beckman polyallomer ultracentrifuge tube (Fullerton, CA).
3. Gently layer the GTC lysates on the top of CsCl.
4. Centrifuge the tubes at 150,000*g* for 16 h using a SW55 rotor at 18°C.
5. Aspirate approx 4 mL of the liquid from the top.
6. Pour off the remaining liquid at one time and invert the tubes to drain.
7. Air-dry RNA for 5 min.
8. Cut the bottom part of tubes (1-cm long) with heated razors (*see* **Note 4**).
9. Add 360 µL TES to the pellets. Leave them at room temperature for 10 min. Mix well and transfer to new Eppendorf tubes.
10. Add 40 µL of 3*M* NaOAc, pH 5.2, and 1 mL absolute ethanol and leave at –20°C for more than 30 min.
11. Spin down for 20 min at 10,000*g* at 4°C. Take off all supernatants and wash the pellets with 1 mL of 80% ethanol.
12. Take off all the liquid and air-dry for 10 min.
13. Dissolve the RNA in DEPC-treated water (*see* **Note 5**).

3.3. Preparation of cDNA

1. Add the following reagents to a 0.5-mL Eppendorf tube: 2 µg total RNA, 1 µL random hexamers, and DEPC-treated water up to 12.5 µL of total volume. Incubate at 70 °C for 3 min, followed by quick chill on ice.
2. Add the following reagents to the preceding mixture: 4 µL of 5X reverse transcription buffer, 1 mL of 10 m*M* dNTP mix, 2 µL of 0.1 *M* DTT, and 0.5 µL of 40 U/µL RNase inhibitor.
3. Incubate at 25°C for 5 min. Then, add 1 µL of 200 U/µL reverse transcriptase. Incubate at 25°C for 10 min.
4. Incubate at 42°C for 50 min.
5. Heat up to 70°C for 15 min and then place on ice (*see* **Note 6**).

3.4. Real-Time PCR

1. Prepare a master mix containing 1X TaqMan buffer, 3.5 m*M* $MgCl_2$, 300 n*M* of each primer, 200 n*M* probe, 200 µ*M* dATPs, 200 µ*M* dCTPs, 200 µ*M* dGTPs, 400 µ*M* dUTPs, 0.5 U of AmpErase uracil *N*-glycosylase, and 1.25 U of AmpliTaq Gold DNA polymerase.
2. Aliquot 49 µL of the master mix into reaction tubes. Add 1 µL of cDNA to each tube.
3. Set the tubes in ABI 7700 Sequence Detection System.
4. PCR conditions are 50°C for 2 min, 95°C for 10 min, followed by 60 cycles of 95°C for 15 s plus 60°C for 1 min.

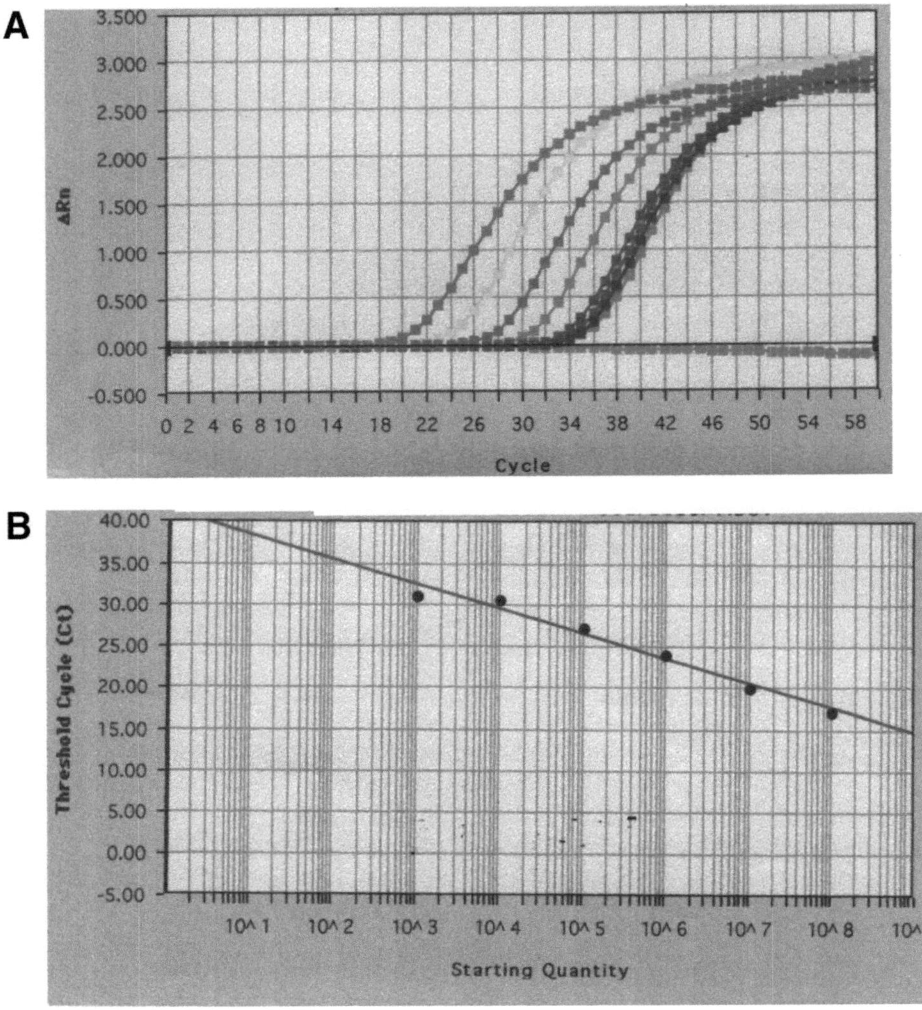

Fig. 1. **(A)** Detection of the PRAME gene by real-time PCR. The PRAME cDNA-containing plasmid Vi381 was serially diluted from 1 pg/μL to 0.01 fg/μL. These templates were amplified with the PRAME-specific primers and fluorescence-labeled probe. Normalized reporter value (R_n) is defined by dividing the emission intensity of the reporter dye by that of Passive Reference 1 in the PCR reaction mixture. The difference of R_n between the target-containing tube and the control tube without template is defined as ΔR_n. The system generates an amplification plot: the numbers of PCR cycles vs ΔR_n. **(B)** C_T (threshold cycle), the cycle number when the fluorescence intensity has reached a detectable value above the background, is proportional to the initial copy number of the target DNA. The standard curve is obtained by plotting C_T vs the initial amount of reference samples.

In every experiment, reference samples should be included for quantification. (*See* **Subheading 2.4.**, **item 8**, and **Note 7**.)

3.5. Analysis

The measurement of reporter fluorescence and data analysis can be performed using the ABI 7700 Sequence Detection System. Briefly, the probe that is designed to locate between forward and reverse primers is labeled with a 5'-reporter dye and a 3'-quencher dye. During PCR cycles, the probe annealed to the target site is cleaved by 5'-nuclease activity of the AmpliTaq Gold DNA polymerase. The separation of the reporter dye from the quencher dye results in an increase of fluorescence of the reporter dye. This process is repeated in every cycle and the increase of fluorescence is directly measured in the closed tube. Normalized reporter value (R_n) is defined by dividing the emission intensity of the reporter dye by that of Passive Reference 1 in the PCR reaction mixture. The difference of R_n between the tube with and without the template is defined as ΔR_n. The system generates an amplification plot: the numbers of PCR cycles versus ΔR_n (see **Fig. 1A**). Subsequently, the cycle number when fluorescence intensity reached to be detectable above the background during the first 3–15 cycles is calculated by computer. This cycle number is called the threshold cycle (C_T), which is proportional to the initial copy numbers of the target DNA. Finally, a standard curve is obtained from the data of reference samples (*see* **Fig. 1B**). The sample data can be plotted on the standard curve (*see* **Note 8**). We performed the real-time PCR analysis for both PRAME and ß-actin (internal control) on the same sample and then calculated the relative PRAME expression as follows:

$$\text{Relative PRAME expression } (U) = \frac{\text{PRAME}_{\text{sample}}}{\text{PRAME}_{\text{plasmid(1 fg/}\mu\text{l)}}}\left(\frac{\beta\text{-actin}_{\text{sample}}}{\beta\text{-actin}_{\text{K562cDNA}}}\right)^{-1}$$

4. Notes

1. Passive Reference 1 is a dye included in the 10X TaqMan buffer and does not participate in the 5'-nuclease PCR. It provides an internal reference to which the reporter dye signal can be normalized. When a PCR system employs two or more reporter dyes, data analysis requires this normalization step.
2. The primers and probe for PRAME was designed using Primer Express software (PE Biosystems). The primers and probe for ß-actin were purchased from PE Biosystems.
3. All of these reference samples should be aliquoted and stored at –20°C.
4. A new razor should be used for each sample to avoid contamination. All of the procedures should be conducted in a laminar-air hood.

5. Because RNA is easily degraded in solution, the reverse transcription-reaction should be performed with samples recently extracted.
6. To avoid contamination, precautions should be taken to avoid cross-contamination of tubes and pipettors. The reagent should be aliquoted.
7. We recommended performing real-time PCR measurements in triplicate.
8. If reference samples do not provide a linear standard curve, check the quality of the reference cDNA by conventional PCR *(3)*.

References

1. Ikeda, H., Lethe, B., Lehmann, F., et al. (1997) Characterization of an antigen that is recognized on a melanoma showing partial HLA loss by CTL expressing an NK inhibitory receptor. *Immunity* **6,** 199–208.
2. Neumann, E., Engelsberg, A., Decker, J., et al. (1998) Heterogeneous expression of the tumor-associated antigens RAGE-1, PRAME, and glycoprotein 75 in human renal cell carcinoma: candidates for T-cell-based immunotherapies? *Cancer Res.* **58,** 4090–4095.
3. Matsushita, M., Ikeda, H., Kizaki, M., et al. (2001) Quantitative monitoring of the PRAME gene for the detection of minimal residual disease in leukemia. *Br. J. Haematol.* **112,** 916–926.
4. van Baren, N., Brasseur, F., Godelaine, D., et al. (1999) Genes encoding tumor-specific antigens are expressed in human myeloma cells. *Blood* **94,** 1156–1164.
5. Kessler, J. H., Beekman, N. J., Bres-Vloemans, S. A., et al. (2001) Efficient identification of novel HLA-A(*)0201-presented cytotoxic T lymphocyte epitopes in the widely expressed tumor antigen PRAME by proteasome-mediated digestion analysis. *J. Exp. Med.* **193,** 73–88.
6. Lin, F., van Rhee, F., Goldman, J. M., et al. (1996) Kinetics of increasing BCR-ABL transcript numbers in chronic myeloid leukemia patients who relapse after bone marrow transplantation. *Blood* **87,** 4473–4478.
7. Lion, T., Gaiger, A., Henn, T., et al. (1995) Use of quantitative polymerase chain reaction to monitor residual disease in chronic myelogenous leukemia during treatment with interferon.*Leukemia* **9,** 1353–1360.
8. Muto, A., Mori, S., Matsushita, H., et al. (1996) Serial quantification of minimal residual disease of t(8;21) acute myelogenous leukemia with RT-competitive PCR assay. *Br. J. Haematol.* **95,** 85–94.
9. Roberts, W. M., Estrov, Z., Ouspenskaia, M. V., et al. (1997) Measurement of residual leukemia during remission in childhood acute lymphoblastic leukemia. *N. Engl. J. Med.* **336,** 317–323.
10. Seriu, T., Hansen-Hagge, T. E., Erz, D. H., et al. (1995) Improved detection of minimal residual leukemia through modifications of polymerase chain reaction analyses based on clonospecific T cell receptor junctions. *Leukemia* **9,** 316–320.
11. Inoue, K., Ogawa, H., Yamagami, T., et al. (1996) Long-term follow-up of minimal residual disease in leukemia patients by monitoring WT1 (Wilms tumor gene) expression levels. *Blood* **88,** 2267–2278.

12. Mensink, E., van de Locht, A., Schattenberg, A., et al. (1998) Quantitation of minimal residual disease in Philadelphia chromosome positive chronic myeloid leukemia patients using real-time quantitative RT-PCR. *Br. J. Haematol.* **102,** 768–774.
13. Dolken, G. (2001) Detection of minimal residual disease. *Adv. Cancer Res.* **82,** 133–185.

20

Determination of Cyclin D1 Expression by Quantitative Real-Time, Reverse-Transcriptase Polymerase Chain Reaction

Karen E. Bijwaard and Jack H. Lichy

1. Introduction

Disorders of the cell cycle regulatory machinery play a key role in the pathogenesis of cancer. The gene encoding the cyclin D1 protein, a regulator of the progression from the G1- to S-phase, is often found disrupted in the cancer cell genome by the processes of chromosome translocation or gene amplification. Regardless of the mechanism, the end result of these genetic alterations is overexpression of the cyclin D1 mRNA and the protein it encodes. Among the tumors in which cyclin D1 overexpression has been observed are carcinomas of the breast *(1,2)*, colon *(3)*, larynx and esophagus *(4,5)*, lung *(6)*, bladder *(7)*, and ovary *(8,9)*, multiple myeloma *(10)*, and parathyroid adenoma *(11)*. However, the detection of overexpression or the specific chromosome translocation responsible for it has found clinical utility primarily in the diagnosis of mantle cell lymphoma, a small lymphocytic lymphoma composed of CD5-positive, CD10-negative B-lymphocytes that can be mistaken histologically for other types of B-cell non-Hodgkin's lymphoma *(12–14)*. The distinction is important because mantle cell lymphomas have a less favorable prognosis and require more aggressive therapy than other, microscopically similar lymphomas *(15)*. Genetically, nearly all mantle cell lymphomas have a characteristic translocation, t(11;14) (q13;q32). The translocation breakpoints on chromosome 11q13 invariably lie near the Cyclin D1 gene at that locus, with about one-third lying within the short segment of DNA designated as the major cluster region. The chromosome 14q32 breakpoint occurs within the immunoglobulin heavy chain (IgH) gene, disrupting that gene adjacent to a J region. The translocation results

From: *Methods in Molecular Medicine, vol. 97: Molecular Diagnosis of Cancer*
Edited by: J. E. Roulston and J. M. S. Bartlett © Humana Press Inc., Totowa, NJ

in activation of the cyclin D1 gene because of its proximity to the transcriptional enhancer of the IgH gene.

Several methods have been described for detecting the specific chromosome translocation as a means for diagnosis of mantle cell lymphoma. Methodologies available for this include classical cytogenetics, fluorescence *in situ* hybridization (FISH), Southern blot analysis of tumor DNA, and polymerase chain reaction (PCR) with primers that span the breakpoint. Each of these methods suffers from significant limitations. Cytogenetic analysis requires dividing tumor cells, which may not be available. FISH, which can be performed on fixed, embedded tissue, has a very high sensitivity (>95%) but requires expensive reagents and specialized technical skills that preclude its use in some medical centers ***(16–19)***. Because of the variability of the chromosome 11 breakpoints, the Southern blot approach to detecting this translocation is cumbersome, requiring multiple probes, and has limited sensitivity, reported to be less than 75% ***(20)***. PCR of the breakpoint region suffers from a lack of sensitivity, because only those translocations involving the major cluster region can be detected ***(21–23)***.

The utility of an assay for overexpression of the cyclin D1 gene results from the very pronounced difference in expesion levels between mantle cell lymphoma and other populations of lymphocytes, both benign and malignant ***(24–27)***. Expression of the gene is essentially undetectable in benign and reactive lymphocytes. In lymphomas other than mantle cell lymphoma, sensitive methods such as reverse transcription (RT)–PCR often detect expression, but at levels significantly less than that seen in mantle cell lymphoma ***(28,29)***. In nonlymphoid tissue, cyclin D1 is normally expressed in the proliferative zones of epithelia of multiple organs, including the skin and gastrointestinal (GI) tract ***(1)***, a fact that must be taken into account when interpreting the results of quantitative expression assays performed on tissue samples. Overexpression of cyclin D1 in tissue specimens can be detected by a variety of methods, including immunohistochemistry ***(30–32)***, Northern blot of tumor RNA ***(25,33)***, and RT-PCR ***(28,29,34)***. Immunohistochemistry has the advantage of identifying the specific cell population that overexpresses cyclin D1, thus avoiding the problem of confusing normal expression in epithelial cells with overexpression in a lymphoma. However, the results of immunohistochemical stains can be equivocal, because of variability in protein expression levels, or falsely negative, because of protein breakdown during the fixation and embedding process ***(35)***. Northern blot analysis requires high-quality RNA, which can be difficult to obtain from surgical specimens. Standard RT-PCR must be performed in at least a semiquantitative manner to distinguish the overexpression seen in mantle cell lymphoma from the low-level expression in other types of lymphoma ***(28)***.

The quantitative real-time RT-PCR protocol presented in this chapter was developed to overcome some of the problems with the above methods ***(29)***. The method involves comparing the results of two multiplex RT-PCR reactions: one containing the test sample and the other containing a control RNA from a mantle cell lymphoma cell line. In each reaction, the real-time fluorescence detection instrument simultaneously monitors amplification of cyclin D1 and a ubiquitously expressed gene, β_2-microglobulin, which is used for standardization. The threshold cycle (C_T) values for each target gene are determined rapidly by the SDS software package provided with the instrument, and the relative expression level of cyclin D1 is expressed as a $\Delta\Delta C_T$ value. For a more detailed discussion of the $\Delta\Delta C_T$ method, the reader is referred to **ref. *36***. This assay offers several advantages over other methods. First, it is rapid and requires no specialized technical skills other than the ability to set up PCR reactions. Second, the assay can be performed on RNA extracted from formalin-fixed, paraffin-embedded tissue as well as from fresh or frozen tissue samples. Third, the use of a control gene from the same sample standardizes the result so that variations in the extent of RNA degradation have little effect on the final result. Finally, the result is quantitative, allowing for the choice of an optimum cutoff value for distinguishing overexpression in mantle cell lymphoma from the lower levels of expression that may be seen in other lymphomas. In our experience, a suitable cutoff value can be chosen such that the assay distinguishes mantle cell lymphoma from benign and reactive lymphoid tissue with close to 100% efficiency.

The protocol detailed in this chapter presents the technique as it is practiced in our laboratory, starting from formalin-fixed, paraffin-embedded (FFPE) tissue. Standard methods of RNA purification from fresh or frozen tissue may be used and, in fact, are preferable, if such material is available. In this procedure, each of the two basic RT-PCR reactions required for the $\Delta\Delta C_T$ calculation is performed in triplicate with two levels of RNA in order to improve accuracy.

2. Materials

2.1. Tissues for Study

This procedure can be applied to any RNA preparation from a human tissue source. In our laboratory, the assay is most frequently performed on paraffin-embedded tissue. To render RNA accessible to PCR, the sample is first deparaffinized with Hemo-DE (a xylene substitute) and then ethanol is added to aid in pelleting of the tissue. The pellet is then washed in ethanol to remove residual Hemo-DE and allowed to air-dry. The dried pellet is digested in buffer containing proteinase K and sodium dodecyl sulfate (SDS), which inhibits endogenous RNases. The RNA is then isolated by organic extraction and isopropanol precipitation ***(37)***.

2.2. Equipment

1. Rotary microtome for paraffin blocks.
2. Thermocycler designed for 0.2 mL PCR tubes.
3. ABI Prism® 7700 Sequence Detection System (TaqMan) (Applied Biosystems, Foster City, CA).
4. Pipets: 0.5–10 μL, 2–20 μL, 10–100 μL, 20–200 μL, 100–1000 μL.
5. Labconco benchtop fume absorber (Model 6900000, Labconco; Kansas City, MO) or chemical hood.
6. Low-speed centrifuge capable of centrifuging microtiter plates.

2.3. Sample Preparation

2.3.1. Sample Preparation From Slides and FFPE Tissue Blocks

1. New single-edged razor blades.
2. Sterile wooden toothpicks.
3. 1.5-mL Nuclease-free microcentrifuge tubes.
4. Microscope.
5. Disposable microtome blades.
6. Sterile gauze pads.
7. Squeeze bottle containing 100% ethanol.
8. Squeeze bottle containing xylenes or xylene substitute (e.g., Hemo-DE [Scientific Safety Solvents, Keller, TX]).

2.3.2. Sample Preparation and RNA Extraction

Listed are the reagents and materials needed for the preparation of samples and RNA extraction (*see* **Note 1**).

1. Extraction (digestion) buffer: 120 m*M* Tris-HCl, pH 7.6, 20 m*M* EDTA, 1% SDS (sodium dodecyl sulfate). Aliquot into 1.5-mL microcentrifuge tubes and store at room temperature.
2. Proteinase K (Gibco/Life Technologies, Grand Island, NY) (ProK). Stock is prepared at 20 mg/mL (in molecular-grade deionized [dH_2O]) and aliquoted into 0.6-mL microcentrifuge tubes. Store at –20°C.
3. TRIzol™ LS (Gibco/Life Technologies). Store at 4°C. Aliquot needed amount (approx 0.8 mL/specimen) into a clean 15-mL polypropylene centrifuge tube just prior to use (*see* **Note 2**).
4. Chloroform (Fisher Scientific, Suwanee, GA). Store at room temperature in a flammable cabinet and aliquot needed amount (0.2 mL/specimen) into a clean, polypropylene centrifuge tube just prior to use.
5. Glycogen, 20 mg/mL (Roche Molecular Bioproducts, Indianapolis, MO), aliquoted into 0.6-mL microcentrifuge tubes and stored at –20°C.
6. Ethanol: Absolute and 75%. Aliquot into 50-mL polypropylene centrifuge tube for short-term use and store at room temperature in a flammable cabinet.
7. Isopropanol (Sigma, St. Louis, MO). Aliquot into 50-mL polypropylene, cen-

trifuge tube for short-term use, and store at room temperature in a flammable cabinet.

8. DEPC (diethyl pyrocarbonate)–treated, molecular-grade (18 MΩ) water (Fisher Scientific) (DEPC–dH_2O), aliquoted into 1.5-mL microcentrifuge tubes and stored at 4°C.
9. Aerosol-barrier pipet tips.
10. 1.5-mL nuclease-free microcentrifuge tubes.
11. Polypropylene centrifuge tubes for aliquoting of reagents (6 mL, 15 mL, 50 mL, etc.).

2.3.3. RT-PCR

1. DEPC–dH_2O (described in **item 8** of **Subheading 2.3.2.**).
2. RT master mix (for cDNA synthesis) is prepared to give a final concentration in the RT reaction of 1X PCR buffer II (50 m*M* KCl, 10 m*M* Tris-HCl, pH 8.3) (Applied Biosystems), 1.5 m*M* $MgCl_2$ (Applied Biosystems), 125 μ*M* each dATP, dCTP, dTTP, and dGTP (Promega, Madison, WI), 0.15 U RNase inhibitor (Gibco/Life Technologies), and 0.01*M* DTT (dithiothreitol, Gibco/Life Technologies). Store at –20°C.
3. Moloney–Murine leukemia virus (MMLV-RT) reverse transcriptase (Gibco/Life Technologies). Stock vial is at a concentration of 200 U/μL. Store at –20°C.
4. Random primers (Gibco/Life Technologies). Stock is adjusted to 0.5 μg/μL with DEPC–dH_2O, aliquoted into 0.6-mL microcentrifuge tubes and stored at –20°C.
5. 2X TaqMan® Universal PCR Master Mix. Store at 4°C (Applied Biosystems).
6. Optical PCR tubes and caps (0.2 mL) (Applied Biosystems).
7. Primers (Integrated DNA Technologies, Coralville, IA) and probes (Integrated DNA Technologies or Applied Biosystems) (5 μ*M* stock). Store at –20°C. Cyclin D1 and β2M primers are each prepared in mixtures such that each primer is present in a concentration of 15 μ*M* (*see* **Table 1**).
8. Tray and retainer assemblies for 0.2-mL optical PCR tubes.

3. Methods

3.1. General Considerations

Care should be taken with the handling and processing of samples because RNA is easily degraded. Optimally, the areas for sample preparation, amplification, and detection should be isolated from each other to minimize the presence of PCR contaminants. Gloves should be worn at all times and the work areas should be kept clean and decontaminated after use with either a 10% bleach solution or ultraviolet light. We typically perform all assay setups in Biosafety Level II hoods, but other types of PCR workstations are available. All chemicals and reagents should be certified as nuclease-free and stored appropriately. Sterile, disposable plasticware should be used whenever possible. Aliquoting of purchased and prepared solutions (immediately prior to

Table 1
Primers and Probes

Primer/probe	Sequence (5'→ 3')
Cyclin D1	
Cycl-304F	CCG TCC ATG CGG AAG ATC
Cycl-389R	ATG GCC AGC GGG AAG AC
Cycl-334TR (probe)	[6–FAM][a] CTT CTG TTC CTC GCA GAC CTC CAG CAT [TAMRA]
β_2-microglobulin	
β2M-246F	TGA CTT TGT CAC AGC CCA AGA TA
β2M-330R	AAT CCA AAT GCG GCA TCT TC
β2M-275R (probe)	[VIC][b] TGA TGC TGC TTA CAT GTC TCG ATC CCA [TAMRA]

[a]6-FAM: 6-carboxy-fluorescein; TAMRA, 6-carboxy-tetramethlyrhodamine.
[b]*See* **Note 3**.

use or aliquoted and then stored) into smaller sterile, polypropylene tubes for single or short-term use aids in preventing contamination of stock solutions.

3.2. Controls

Several types of positive and negative controls are run with each assay as controls for test performance. The data from the positive controls are also used for the $\Delta\Delta C_T$ calculation. Three reactions, which we refer to as the water, lysate, and contamination controls, are run specifically to serve as negative controls.

1. Positive Controls
   a. Positive assay control. The cyclin D1 positive control is a RNA lysate prepared from frozen cells or paraffin-embedded sample of the mantle cell lymphoma (MCL) cell line M02058 (obtained from T. Meeker, M.D., NCI, NIH, Bethesda, MD) or a known overexpressing patient sample. The amplified cyclin D1 product is 86 bp and the β2M product is 85 bp. The amounts of cyclin D1 template added per assay (50 ng and 1 ng) are at levels to give adequate amplification near that of the unknown samples (*see* **Note 4**).
   b. Amplification control. Paraffin-embedded tissues may contain inhibitors of PCR or fixatives that severely compromise nucleic acid integrity. In addition to serving as a basis for standardization of the results, the amplification of β_2-microglobulin in the test sample serves as a control to demonstrate the presence of amplifiable nucleic acid in the sample.
2. Negative assay controls. A negative control is used to control for each step in the test system: lysate preparation, reagent mix preparation, and carryover contamination from sample to sample in the assay setup procedure:

a. Water control. A PCR reaction mix containing water as the sample tested is set up first in the RT-PCR run, before samples, to assess the purity of the assay reagents.
b. Lysate control. A lysate (no RNA template) prepared in parallel with samples should give no detectable band, indicating that the tube was not contaminated with RNA during lysate preparation.
c. Contamination control. A negative control RT-PCR reaction containing water as the sample tested is again set up last in the RT-PCR run, after the positive control. This reaction assesses the overall quality of the assay setup procedure in avoiding carryover contamination from a positive to an adjacent negative sample.

3.3. Sample Preparation

3.3.1. Isolation of Tissue From Slides

1. Scrape entire section or desired portion off slides using a new razor blade for each case (*see* **Note 5**).
2. Transfer scraped sections into a new, labeled 1.5-mL microcentrifuge tube with a new sterilized toothpick. Cap tube.

3.3.2. Isolation of Tissue From FFPE Tissue Blocks

1. Clean microtome with a gauze pad wetted with a small amount of Hemo-DE. Wipe down clamp assembly and stage area to remove any residual paraffin and tissue. Repeat procedure with a fresh gauze pad wetted with absolute ethanol. Allow area to air-dry (*see* **Note 5**).
2. Place new disposable microtome blade in knife clamp assembly and tighten.
3. Adjust block position until a complete section of tissue is achieved. Carefully cut six 6–μm sections from the block and transfer all six sections to a new, labeled 1.5-mL microcentrifuge tube using the sterilized toothpicks. Close tube.
4. Repeat **steps 1–3** for each block.

3.4. RNA Isolation

3.4.1. Deparaffinization and Sample Digestion

1. Prepare tubes plus an additional empty tube to act as a control for sample preparation and extraction (lysate control).
2. Decant a sufficient amount (at least 1 mL of Hemo-DE and 1.5 mL absolute ethanol per specimen) of Hemo-DE and absolute ethanol from stock bottles into a labeled sterile conical tube.
3. Add 800 μL of Hemo-DE to each tube containing six 6–μm sections of tissue plus the lysate control tube. Vortex for 5 s. Add 400 μL of ethanol. Vortex tubes for 5 s. Centrifuge at full speed for 5 min. If residual paraffin is visible, repeat this step (*see* **Note 6**).
4. Decant the liquid carefully into a waste container and add 800 μL of absolute

ethanol. Vortex tubes for 5 s. Centrifuge at full speed for 5 min. Decant the liquid.
5. Dry pellet in 55°C oven for approx 5 min or air-dry for at least 15 min at room temperature inverted over a clean Kimwipe.
6. Determine total amount of extraction buffer needed (250 μL/sample). Remove ProK stock from freezer (–20°C) and thaw. Tap tube to mix. Add 45 μL ProK to 1.5 mL extraction buffer and mix.
7. Add extraction buffer (250 μL) to specimen tubes and vortex a few seconds at slow speed (setting 2–3). Place samples in a 55°C water bath for 4 h to overnight.

3.4.2. RNA Extraction

1. Pulse-spin tubes to remove any condensate from the tube caps.
2. Aliquot sufficient TRIzol LS and chloroform into individual centrifuge tubes.
3. Add 750 μL TRIzol LS to each sample tube. Vortex at medium speed to mix thoroughly. Incubate 5–10 min at room temperature. Pulse-spin to remove residual liquid from cap.
4. Add 200 μL chloroform to each tube and shake vigorously by hand for 15–20 s. Incubate at room temperature 5–10 min (*see* **Note 7**).
5. Centrifuge at 12,000*g* for 10 min.
6. Transfer upper aqueous layer to a fresh 1.5-mL microcentrifuge tube containing 1.5 μL glycogen (30 μg). Add 500 μL isopropanol and mix by inversion. Incubate on ice for at least 10 min.
7. Collect precipitate by centrifugation at 12,000*g* for 10 min.
8. Wash pellet with 1.0 mL of 75% ethanol, centrifuge at 9000*g* for 5 min. Decant supernatant.
9. Collect residual liquid at the bottom of the tube by centrifuging for a few seconds. Remove liquid with a pipet. Allow any remaining liquid to evaporate by leaving the tube inverted on a Kimwipe for 10–15 min or in a 55°C oven for approx 5 min. Add 40 μL of DEPC-treated water and incubate in a 55°C water bath for approx 10 min to resuspend RNA. Mix gently by tapping bottom of tube and store at –70°C until use.

3.5. RT-PCR

3.5.1. cDNA Synthesis

All samples (including positive and negative controls) are amplified in triplicate (*see* **Note 8**). Samples and positive controls are also tested at two levels of template. Patient samples are tested at 1 and 5 μL of template. An 8 × 12 grid map serves as a map for the assay setup and tube contents (*see* **Table 2**).

1. Determine the number of samples to be assayed (two levels of each patient lysate, a water control, one lysate control, two positive controls, and a contamination control) plus two additional samples to allow for errors in pipetting or pipet calibration. (*N* = number of samples + 2.)
2. Fill out a setup map with sample identifications and locations on the plate.

Table 2
Sample 8 × 12 Grid Map Corresponding to a 96-Well Tray

	1	2	3	4	5	6	7	8	9	10	11	12
A		dH_2O			Lysate			Sample 1 1 μL			Sample 1 5 μL	
B		Sample 2 1 μL			Sample 1 5 μL			M02058 +C 1 ng			M02058 +C 50 ng	
C		dH_2O										
D												
E												
F												
G												
H												

3. Place optical tubes in the sample rack with the sample tray according to the setup map. Attach the retainer to secure the tubes.
4. Remove the needed amount of RT-master mix and random primers and allow to thaw. Remove MMLV-RT from the freezer and store on ice. Determine the amount of master mix needed (4.25 μL × *N*) and aliquot into a 0.6- or 1.5-mL microcentrifuge tube.
5. Add 0.5 μL × *N* random primers and 0.25 μL × *N* MMLV-RT to tube containing RT master mix. Mix gently by tapping bottom of the tube and keep chilled until use.
6. Add 5 μL of DEPC–dH_2O to the water control tubes and 4 μL to the lysate control tubes, 1X sample tubes, and positive control tubes.
7. Add 5 μL of RT mix to each tube. Cap tubes with optical strip caps (*see* **Note 9**).
8. Add 1 μL of negative control lysate to the negative lysate control tubes. Cap tubes with optical strip caps.
9. Add 1 and 5 μL of sample RNA to the respective sample tubes. Cap tubes with optical strip caps.
10. Add 1 μL of 50 and 1 ng/μL M02058 RNA (respectively) to the positive control tubes. Cap tubes with optical strip caps.
11. Add 5 μL of DEPC–dH_2O to the contamination control tubes. Cap tubes with optical strip caps.
12. Place tray in the thermocycler and run the RT method with volume set at 10 μL. The RT method consists of three hold cycles: 60 s at 37°C; 5 s at 95°C; soak at 4°C.

3.5.2. Amplification and Detection

1. Prepare sufficient PCR mix for *N* samples (40 μL × *N*). 11 μL × *N* DEPC–dH_2O, 25 μL × *N* 2X TaqMan Universal PCR master mix, 1 μL × *N* each primer mix, and probes. Mix well by inversion or low-speed vortexing. Keep chilled until use (*see* **Note 9**).
2. Remove tray from thermocycler. Spin plate for 3–5 min at 200*g* if condensation is apparent on caps.

3. Remove caps one row at a time. Add 40 µL of PCR mix to each tube and recap row.
4. Spin plate for 5 min at 200*g* to remove air bubbles and get all components to the bottom of the tube.

3.5.3. Real-Time PCR Analysis

This section and the next are written as instructions to an operator sitting in front of the computer operating the ABI 7700 (*see* **Notes 10** and **11**).

1. Place plate in ABI 7700 and close dust cover.
2. Double-click on the TaqMan (Sequence Detection) icon on the desktop.
3. From the Title bar, choose File → New Plate. Check the information in the New Plate Box. Make sure the settings are as follows:
   Plate Type: Single Reporter
   Instrument: 7700 Sequence Detector
   Run: Real Time
   Click → OK
4. From the Title bar, choose Edit → Preferences and verify that the reaction volume is at 50 µL. Enter User name. Choose Setup → Thermocycler conditions. Verify that the reaction volume is at 50 µL and the cycles box is set at 40.
5. Click on the "Sample Type" scroll bar in the left corner. Scroll to "Sample Type Setup." Click on the "Add" button and scroll down to the bottom of the list. Type "NTC" in the left box. Identify it as "No Template Control" in the sample type box. Choose a color to assign to each NTC sample in the third box from the left. Under "Reporter Type," scroll down to VIC™. Repeat for UNKN (Unknown). Click OK.
6. Fill in Setup view map so that it corresponds to the plate. Use NTC for the water and contamination controls and UNKN for the lysate control, patient samples, and positive controls. In the Sample Name field, identify each sample, including the amount of template added. Assign the replicate value as 3 (each sample is in triplicate).
7. Click on Dye Layer pop-up menu and scroll down to VIC. This will give you a blank screen.
8. Choose Setup → Sample Type Palette. The Sample palette box will appear. Block off the wells that correspond to the NTC wells on the FAM layer on the new screen. Click "Update" in the box, and the wells that were blocked off should be identified with the color chosen in **step 5**. Repeat for UNKN wells. All wells should correspond to that of the FAM layer (*see* **Notes 12** and **13**).
9. Save file. Toggle screen to the "Show Analysis" and click the red "Run" button.

3.5.4. Data Analysis

1. On the Title bar, choose: Analysis → Analyze (*see* **Note 14**). A screen displaying the amplification curves of the run will be displayed.
2. In Threshold Cycle calculations box → Suggest → Update calculations.

Table 3
Sample Calculation to Determine $\Delta\Delta C_T$ Values for Cyclin D1 Expression

Triplicate ID	(A) Avg. cyclin D1 C_T value	(B) Avg. β2M C_T value	(C) ΔC_T	(D) Avg. ΔC_T	(E) $\Delta\Delta C_T$
Water	40	40	NA	NA	NA
Lysate	40	40	NA	NA	NA
Sample 1 (1 μL)	25.26	19.5	5.76	6.00	5.7
Sample 1 (5 μL)	26.60	19.83	6.23		
Sample 2 (1 μL)	26.04	22.86	3.18	3.13	2.83
Sample 2 (5 μL)	25.51	22.43	3.08		
M02058 (50 ng)	20.93	20.48	0.45	0.30	—
M02058 (1 ng)	25.50	25.35	0.15		
Water	40	40	NA	NA	NA

3. Go to the Reporter scrolldown menu and scroll down to VIC. Repeat **step 2**.
4. Check NTC C_T values for both FAM and VIC. If C_T value for FAM reporter is <40 even though the amplification curve shows no product formation, then adjust the threshold line in plot until the FAM C_T value is 40. Click on → Update calculations. Adjust VIC threshold to that of the FAM layer and → Update calculations.
5. Choose: File → Export → Results. Name file to be exported the same as the TaqMan run. Click → OK.
6. Close out of Spectral Analysis software.
7. Import results into Excel using Excel Import Wizard. Print spreadsheet.
8. Average the C_T values for each sample. Enter values for the average C_T for cyclin D1 in column A (*see* **Table 3**) and the average C_T for β2M in column B. Subtract the value of column B from column A to determine the ΔC_T value and enter the value in column C (A – B = C). Sample amplification curves for both cyclin D1 and β2M for each example in **Table 3** are presented in **Fig. 1**.
9. Average the ΔC_T values for each level of template for both the samples and the M02058 control. Enter the resulting values in column D.
10. Subtract the Avg. ΔC_T of the M02058 control from the Avg. ΔC_T of each sample to determine $\Delta\Delta C_T$. Enter the value in column E.

3.5.5. Results

The distribution of $\Delta\Delta C_T$ values obtained based on tumor or sample type (e.g., MCL, non-MCL, reactive lymph node, etc.) will indicate the assay's clinical utility in distinguishing specimens that show cyclin D1 overexpression from those that do not. Cutoff values, which should be set based on a validation study by each individual laboratory, can be determined by plotting a distribu-

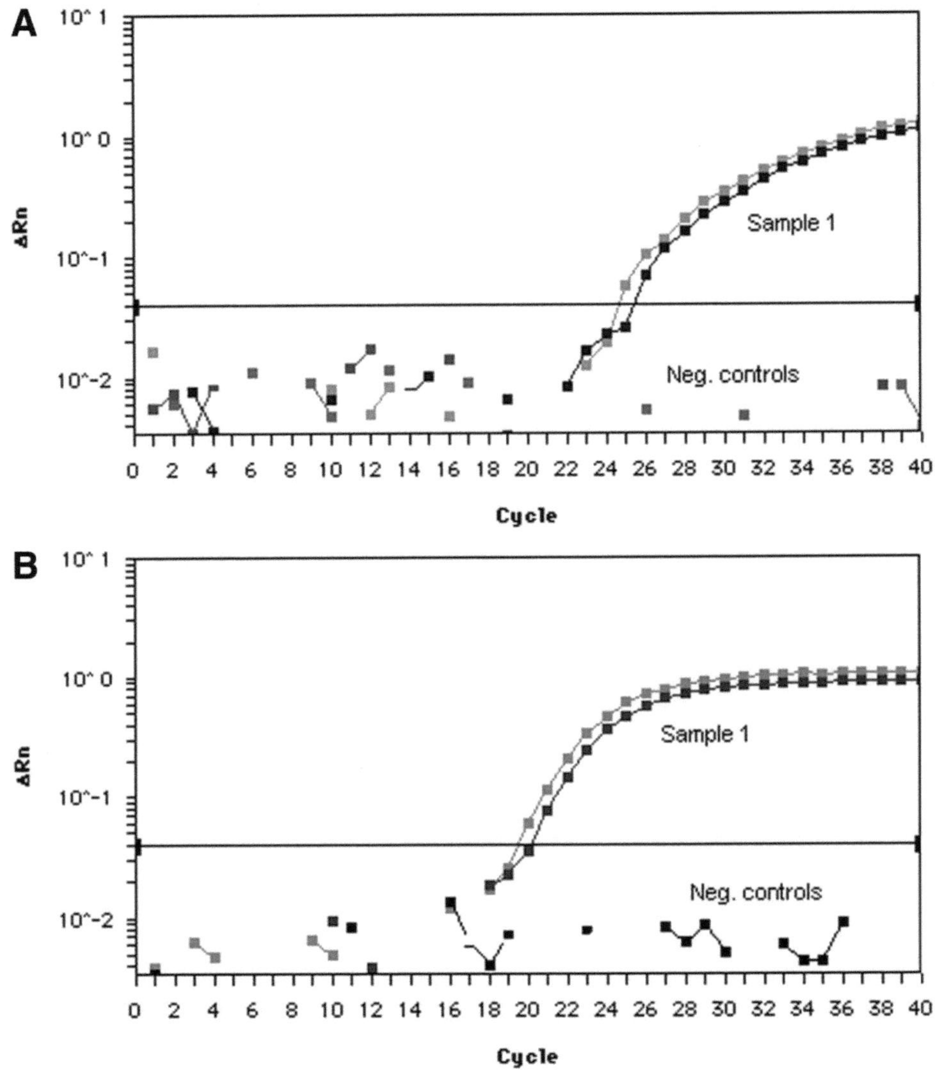

Fig. 1. Amplification curves for the samples shown in **Table 3**. **(A, C, E)** Cyclin D1 amplification curves for samples 1 and 2 and M02058, respectively. **(B, D, F)** β2M amplification curves for samples 1 and 2 and M02058, respectively. Grey boxes in (A–D) represent the 5-μL triplicate levels of template and black boxes represent the 1-μL triplicate levels of template. (E, F) Gray boxes represent the 50-ng triplicate level and the black boxes represent the 1-ng triplicate level of the M02058 template.

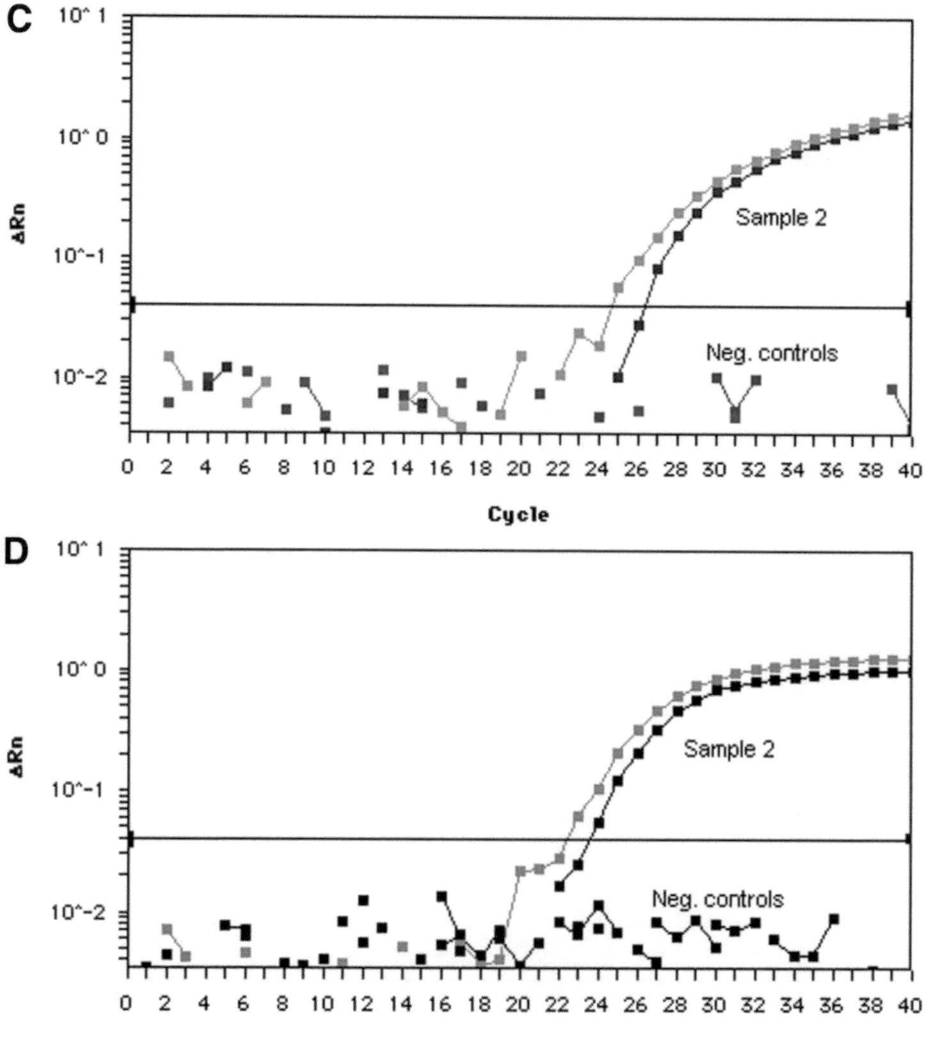

Fig. 1. *(continued)*

tion of $\Delta\Delta C_T$ values relative to tumor or sample diagnosis. In our laboratory however, a cutoff $\Delta\Delta C_T$ value of 4 resulted in a sensitivity and specificity of 100%. All of the MCL cases tested were determined to be positive for cyclin D1 overexpression ($\Delta\Delta C_T < 4$), whereas none of the other types of lymphoma or reactive lymph node demonstrated $\Delta\Delta C_T$ values less than 4. Two non-MCL samples yielded $\Delta\Delta C_T$ values between 4 and 5. Immunohistochemical staining of these specimens for cyclin D1 demonstrated positive staining of epithelial cells but not tumor within these specimens, an observation consistent with the

E

F

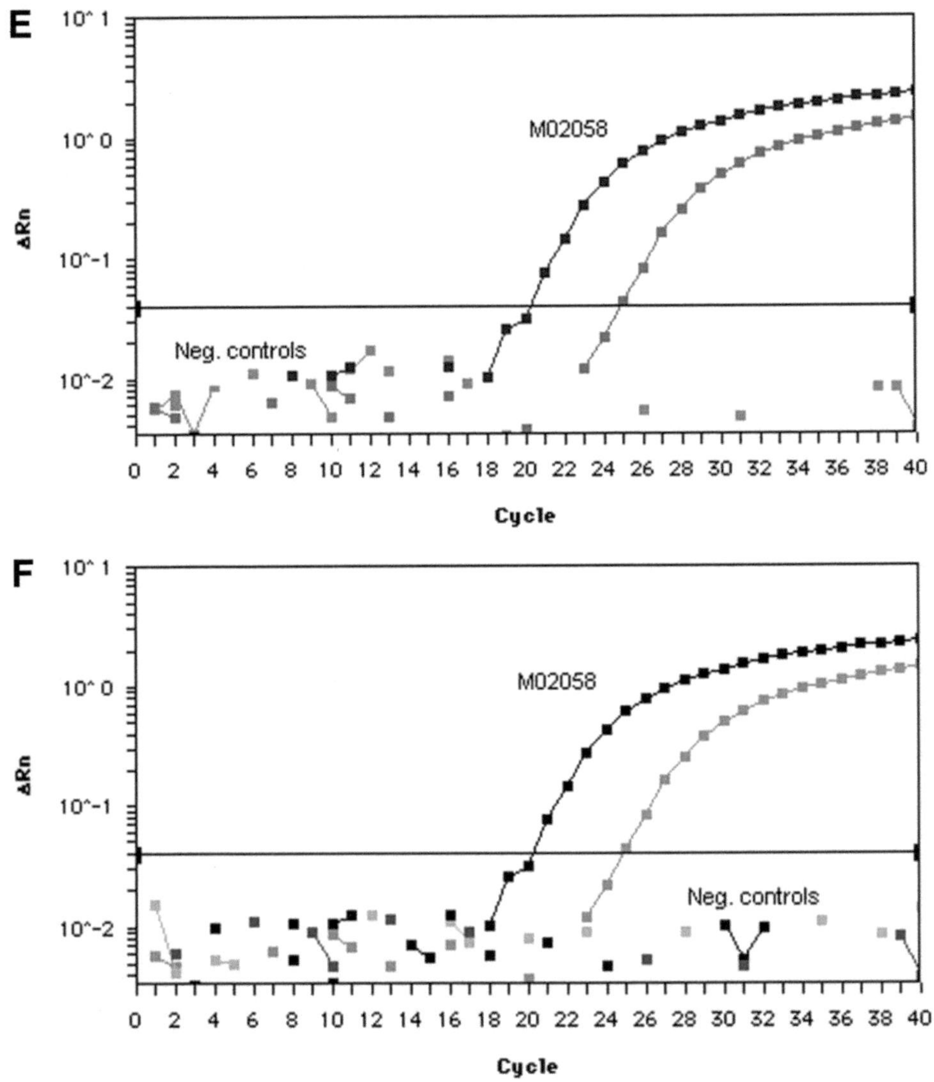

Fig. 1. *(continued)*

known pattern of cyclin D1 expression. Because the presence of epithelial cells in a specimen may result in $\Delta\Delta C_T$ values within this range regardless of expression levels in the associated lymphoid lesion, such values are reported as indeterminate for cyclin D1 overexpression (*see* **Note 15**).

Results for this assay can be reported out only if the β2M result is positive. In our laboratory, we have designated that a cutoff value of $C_T < 38$ (for both levels of template) indicates the presence of amplifiable RNA. If only one level of template has a C_T < 38, the assay is repeated and the level of template adjusted up or down accordingly. $\Delta\Delta C_T$ values of less than 4 are indicative of elevated levels (overexpression) of cyclin D1. $\Delta\Delta C_T$ values of greater than or equal to 4 but less than 5 are considered Indeterminate and $\Delta\Delta C_T$ values of greater than 5 are considered to be nonoverexpressing for cyclin D1.

4. Notes

1. All reagents should be biotechnology/molecular grade or certified as nuclease-free (DNase/RNase) and proteinase-free. Reagents should be diluted or resuspended in sterile molecular-grade (18 MΩ) water.
2. TRIzol LS, xylenes, xylene substitutes, and chloroform are highly flammable, toxic, and reactive solutions. TRIzol LS should be stored in a refrigerator designed for storage of flammable substances. Proper personal protective equipment should be worn at all times when working with hazardous materials. Refer to each chemical's Material Safety Data Sheet (MSDS) for more information. Always work in a well-ventilated area. Although Hemo-DE is not as noxious as xylene, long exposure in a poorly ventilated area can cause severe headaches and occasionally nausea.
3. VIC™ fluorescent dye is proprietary to Applied Biosystems and can only be purchased from that company. Dual-labeled probes, labeled with 6-Fam and TET reporter dyes, however, can be purchased from several reputable suppliers.
4. Any MCL cell line can be used as a positive control. Cell lines are generally preferable because they are easily renewable, provide consistent results, and do not require re-evaluation of reporting criteria. Cell lines can also be grown up in large quantities and the cells frozen (at –70°C) as cell pellets or fixed and embedded in paraffin for long-term storage. If cell pellets are prepared, resuspend thawed pellet in 250 μL of Dulbecco's phosphate-buffered saline (D-PBS) and extract RNA as indicated in **Subheading 3.** or, alternatively, the pellets can be resuspended in 250 μL of D-PBS and then frozen at –70°C (stable for greater than 5 yr).
5. Used razor and microtome blades, toothpicks, glass slides, and gauze pads should be considered to be biohazardous and disposed of in accordance with each facility's hazardous waste regulations. Hemo-DE- and ethanol-wetted gauze pads can be allowed to evaporate in a chemical hood prior to disposal to diminish hazardous exposure to chemical fumes and flammable hazards.
6. Residual paraffin will appear as a nearly pure white precipitate, generally pelletting above the tissue. If the addition of fresh Hemo-DE does not dissolve the residual paraffin, heat the tube gently in a 55–70°C dry bath for 3–5 min until dissolved. Pulse-spin to remove residual liquid from the tube caps and add ethanol and proceed as directed.
7. Avoid vortexing samples to minimize shearing of RNA.
8. Samples are tested in triplicate at each level to control for pipetting error and to

aid in the final analysis of each sample. If one of the three results is inconsistent with the other two, it can be disregarded from the calculations.

9. For full 96-well plates, a multichannel pipet and disposable sterile reagent trays are useful for both decreasing repetitive stress and keeping track of the setup procedure during the addition of master mix to the reaction tubes. Increase *N* in all calculations by 4.
10. The "→" in **Subheadings 3.5.3.** and **3.5.4.** indicates the selection that is chosen for that particular step.
11. In 2000–2001, Applied Biosystems converted their computer systems to Windows NT from Macintosh. **Subheadings 3.5.3.** and **3.5.4.** are based on the Macintosh version of the software. The Windows NT version may differ in some details from those described here.
12. When adding a second dye layer this way, only block off wells containing the same type of sample (e.g., NTC, UNKN, etc.) at a time.
13. ABI recommends having the "Use Spectral Components for Real Time" function on. This is an enhancement of the multicomponent algorithm used to improve the spectral resolution for multireporter applications. To check if this function is on, go to: Instrument (on the Title bar) → Diagnostics → Advanced options → Miscellaneous Options to see if the function is chosen. If not, click on the box and then click OK.
14. There is a glitch in the Sequence Detection software (version 1.6.3) that occasionally will not allow the data to be analyzed or the run to be saved if it was saved prior to starting the run. If this occurs, check the file in the SDS Runs folder on the hard drive that corresponds to the run to make sure that data were collected. The file should be greater than 1 MB. Close out of the run and open a new plate. Re-enter well identifiers and save file. From the File menu on the Title bar choose Import → Import → LabView Format Raw Data. A window will appear for the file to import. On the hard drive, go to the SDS Runs*f* file that corresponded with the run → OK. Toggle screen to the "Show Analysis" and analyze plate as described.
15. Isolation of tissue from slide sections is most helpful when there is only a small area of involved tissue (micro dissection), the involved area is surrounded by areas of epithelium or large blood vessels, which can product false positive results due to endogenous expression of cyclin D1 by epithelial and endothelial tissue, or unstained slides are the only available material. Microdissection of the involved area can be aided by placing the unstained slide over an hemoxylin and eosin-stained section on which the desired area has been marked with a permanent marker, so that only the desired area can be isolated using a clean razor blade or toothpick. The microdissected tissue is then placed in the microcentrifuge tube and processed as described in **Subheading 3.4.1**.

References

1. Bartkova, J., Lukas, J., Strauss, M., et al. (1994) Cell cycle-related variation and tissue-restricted expression of human Cyclin D1 protein. *J. Pathol.* **172(3),** 237–245.
2. Vos, C. B., Ter Haar, N. T., Peterse, J. L., et al. (1999) Cyclin D1 gene amplification and overexpression are present in ductal carcinoma in situ of the breast. *J. Pathol.* **187(3),** 279–284.
3. Bartkova, J., Lukas, J., Strauss, M., et al. (1994) The prad-1/Cyclin D1 oncogene product accumulates aberrantly in a subset of colorectal carcinomas. *Int. J. Cancer* **58(4),** 568–573.
4. Jares, P., Fernandez, P. L., Campo, E., et al. (1994) Prad-1/Cyclin D1 gene amplification correlates with messenger RNA overexpression and tumor progression in human laryngeal carcinomas. *Cancer Res.* **54(17),** 4813–4817.
5. Shinozaki, H., Ozawa, S., Ando, N., et al. (1996) Cyclin D1 amplification as a new predictive classification for squamous cell carcinoma of the esophagus, adding gene information. *Clin. Cancer Res.* **2(7),** 1155–1161.
6. Reissmann, P. T., Koga, H., Figlin, R. A., et al. (1999) Amplification and overexpression of the Cyclin D1 and epidermal growth factor receptor genes in non-small-cell lung cancer. Lung cancer study group. *J. Cancer Res. Clin. Oncol.* **125(2),** 61–70.
7. Tut, V. M., Braithwaite, K. L., Angus, B., et al. (2001) Cyclin D1 expression in transitional cell carcinoma of the bladder: correlation with p53, waf1, prb and ki67. *Br. J. Cancer* **84(2),** 270–275.
8. Zukerberg, L. R., Yang, W. I., Gadd, M., et al. (1995) Cyclin D1 (prad1) protein expression in breast cancer: approximately one-third of infiltrating mammary carcinomas show overexpression of the Cyclin D1 oncogene. *Mod. Pathol.* **8(5),** 560–567.
9. Barbieri, F., Cagnoli, M., Ragni, N., et al. (1997) Expression of Cyclin D1 correlates with malignancy in human ovarian tumours. *Br. J. Cancer* **75(9),** 1263–1268.
10. Chesi, M., Bergsagel, P. L., Brents, L. A., et al. (1996) Dysregulation of Cyclin D1 by translocation into an IgH gamma switch region in two multiple myeloma cell lines. [see comments]. *Blood* **88(2),** 674–681.
11. Motokura, T. and Arnold, A. (1993) Cyclin D and oncogenesis. *Curr. Opin. Genet. Dev.* **3(1),** 5–10.
12. Campo, E., Raffeld, M., and Jaffe, E. S. (1999) Mantle-cell lymphoma. *Semin. Hematol.* **36(2),** 115–127.
13. Garcia-Conde, J. and Cabanillas, F. (1996) Mantle cell lymphoma: a lymphoproliferative disorder associated with aberrant function of the cell cycle. *Leukemia* **10(Suppl 2),** s78–s83.
14. Kurtin, P. J. (1998) Mantle cell lymphoma. *Adv. Anat. Pathol.* **5(6),** 376–398.
15. Pittaluga, S., Wlodarska, I., Stul, M. S., et al. (1995) Mantle cell lymphoma: a clinicopathological study of 55 cases. *Histopathology* **26(1),** 17–24.
16. Avet-Loiseau, H., Garand, R., Gaillard, F., et al. (1998) Detection of t(11;14)

using interphase molecular cytogenetics in mantle cell lymphoma and atypical chronic lymphocytic leukemia. *Genes Chromosomes Cancer* **23(2),** 175–182.

17. Remstein, E. D., Kurtin, P. J., Buno, I., et al. (2000) Diagnostic utility of fluorescence in situ hybridization in mantle-cell lymphoma. *Br. J. Haematol.* **110(4),** 856–862.
18. Coignet, L. J., Schuuring, E., Kibbelaar, R. E., et al. (1996) Detection of 11q13 rearrangements in hematologic neoplasias by double-color fluorescence in situ hybridization. *Blood* **87(4),** 1512–1519.
19. Li, J. Y., Gaillard, F., Moreau, A., et al. (1999) Detection of translocation t(11;14)(q13;q32) in mantle cell lymphoma by fluorescence *in situ* hybridization. *Am. J. Pathol.* **154(5),** 1449–1452.
20. Williams, M. E., Swerdlow, S. H., Rosenberg, C. L., et al. (1993) Chromosome 11 translocation breakpoints at the prad1/Cyclin D1 gene locus in centrocytic lymphoma. *Leukemia* **7(2),** 241–245.
21. Rimokh, R., Berger, F., Delsol, G., et al. (1994) Detection of the chromosomal translocation t(11;14) by polymerase chain reaction in mantle cell lymphomas. *Blood* **83(7),** 1871–1875.
22. Luthra, R., Hai, S., and Pugh, W. C. (1995) Polymerase chain reaction detection of the t(11;14) translocation involving the bcl-1 major translocation cluster in mantle cell lymphoma. *Diagn. Mol. Pathol.* **4(1),** 4–7.
23. Pinyol, M., Campo, E., Nadal, A., et al. (1996) Detection of the bcl-1 rearrangement at the major translocation cluster in frozen and paraffin-embedded tissues of mantle cell lymphomas by polymerase chain reaction. *Am. J. Clin. Pathol.* **105(5),** 532–547.
24. Bergsagel, P. L., Nardini, E., Brents, L., et al. (1997) IgH translocations in multiple myeloma: a nearly universal event that rarely involves c-myc. *Curr. Topics Microbiol. Immunol.* **224,** 283–287.
25. Bosch, F., Jares, P., Campo, E., et al. (1994) Prad-1/Cyclin D1 gene overexpression in chronic lymphoproliferative disorders: a highly specific marker of mantle cell lymphoma. *Blood* **84(8),** 2726–2732.
26. de Boer, C. J., Schuuring, E., Dreef, E., et al. (1995) Cyclin D1 protein analysis in the diagnosis of mantle cell lymphoma. *Blood* **86(7),** 2715–2723.
27. Zukerberg, L. R., Yang, W. I., Arnold, A., et al. (1995) Cyclin D1 expression in non-Hodgkin's lymphomas. Detection by immunohistochemistry. *Am. J. Clin. Pathol.* **103(6),** 756–760.
28. Aguilera, N. S., Bijwaard, K. E., Duncan, B., et al. (1998) Differential expression of Cyclin D1 in mantle cell lymphoma and other non-Hodgkin's lymphomas. *Am. J. Pathol.* **153(6),** 1969–1976.
29. Bijwaard, K. E., Aguilera, N. S., Monczak, Y., et al. (2001) Quantitative real-time reverse transcription-PCR assay for Cyclin D1 expression: utility in the diagnosis of mantle cell lymphoma. *Clin. Chem.* **47(2),** 195–201.
30. Alkan, S., Schnitzer, B., Thompson, J. L., et al. (1995) Cyclin D1 protein expression in mantle cell lymphoma. *Ann. Oncol.* **6(6),** 567–570.
31. Banno, S., Yoshikawa, K., Nakamura, S., et al. (1994) Monoclonal antibody

against prad1/Cyclin D1 stains nuclei of tumor cells with translocation or amplification at bcl-1 locus. *Jpn. J. Cancer Res.* **85(9),** 918–926.

32. Vasef, M. A., Medeiros, L. J., Koo, C., et al. (1997) Cyclin d1 immunohistochemical staining is useful in distinguishing mantle cell lymphoma from other low-grade B-cell neoplasms in bone marrow. *Am. J. Clin. Pathol.* **108(3),** 302–307.
33. de Boer, C. J., van Krieken, J. H., Kluin-Nelemans, H. C., et al. (1995) Cyclin d1 messenger rna overexpression as a marker for mantle cell lymphoma. *Oncogene* **10(9),** 1833–1840.
34. Medeiros, L. J., Hai, S., Thomazy, V. A., et al. (2002) Real-time RT-PCR assay for quantifying Cyclin D1 MRNA in B-cell non-Hodgkin's lymphomas. *Mod. Pathol.* **15(5),** 556–564.
35. Chan, J. K., Miller, K. D., Munson, P., et al. (1999) Immunostaining for Cyclin D1 and the diagnosis of mantle cell lymphoma: is there a reliable method? *Histopathology* **34(3),** 266–270.
36. Applied Biosystems. (1997) *User Bulletin #2: Relative Quantitation of Gene Expression.* ABI prism 7700 sequence detection system, PE Applied Biosystems, Foster City, CA.
37. Krafft, A. E., Duncan, B. W., Bijwaard, K. E., et al. (1997) Optimization of the isolation and amplification of RNA from formalin-fixed, paraffin-embedded tissue: The Armed Forces Institute of Pathology experience and literature review. *Mol. Diagn.* **2(3),** 217–230.

21

Detection of Telomerase hTERT Gene Expression and Its Splice Variants by RT-PCR

W. Nicol Keith and Stacey F. Hoare

1. Introduction

The finite growth potential of normal cells is termed "cellular senescence" and its regulation appears to involve specialized DNA structures known as telomeres that exist at the ends of all eukaryotic chromosomes ***(1)***. Human telomeres consist of tandem nucleotide repeats of 6 bp, TTAGGG. They act as protective caps, stabilizing the chromosomes and preventing their degradation and aberrant recombination during cell division. However, they also have the potential to act as a molecular counting mechanism, marking the number of cell divisions. As chromosomes are replicated during cell division, approx 50 bp of telomeric material are lost because of incomplete replication of the lagging strand, termed "the end-replication problem." In the telomeric clock model, after a certain number of cell divisions, the telomere becomes truncated to a critical level, generating a signal that results in cessation of cell division and senescence ***(1–3)***.

Cells that have an unlimited replicative capacity such as male germ cells and the majority of human cancers, are able to circumvent the end-replication problem through the activity of an enzyme called telomerase, which is capable of adding telomeric repeat sequence back on the ends of telomeres ***(1,2)***. Telomerase is a ribonucleoprotein reverse transcriptase and its activity can be reconstituted in vitro by two essential components, the RNA subunit, h*TR* (which acts as the template for the addition of new telomeric repeats), and the catalytic protein component h*TERT* ***(1)***. The expression of telomerase is strictly regulated in normal human cells. During development, telomerase expression is extinguished after embryonic differentiation in most cells. Notable excep-

From: *Methods in Molecular Medicine, vol. 97: Molecular Diagnosis of Cancer*
Edited by: J. E. Roulston and J. M. S. Bartlett © Humana Press Inc., Totowa, NJ

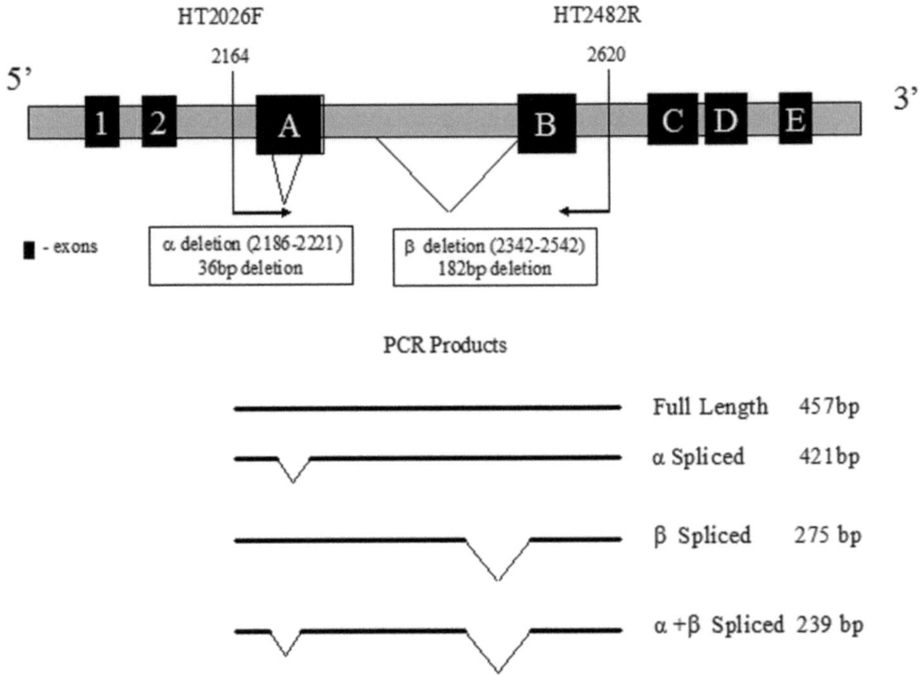

Fig. 1. Structure of hTERT RNA showing sites for the α and β deletions. The primers used to amplify the splice variant region are superimposed on the hTERT sequence. The hTERT gene sequence used has the GenBank accession number AF015950.

tions are male germ cells, lymphocytes, and stem cell populations such as basal keratinocytes that maintain their proliferative capacity in adult life ***(1,2)***.

Extensive evidence from expression studies suggests that hTR and hTERT are regulated on a transcriptional level and that this regulation is a major deterministic factor governing the activation of telomerase activity in normal and cancer cells ***(1)***. Interestingly, however, posttranscriptional mechanisms play a role in regulating telomerase activity ***(3,4)***. Kilian et al. identified several splice variants of the hTERT transcript that are expected to be inactive as a result of truncations or mutations in domains essential for catalytic activity ***(5)***. Of particular interest, one variant called hTERTα contains a deletion in the conserved reverse-transcriptase (RT) motif A and has been characterized as a dominant-negative inhibitor of hTERT activity in cell lines ***(3,6–9)***. Thus, alternative splicing enables multiple proteins to be formed, with different functions from a single gene ***(4)***. This allows a posttranscriptional mechanism of gene regulation, as it can reduce telomerase activity without reducing hTERT transcription. It is the wild-type or full-length (α+β+) variant that is closely associated with telomerase activity ***(3,7)***. It is possible that under certain external influ-

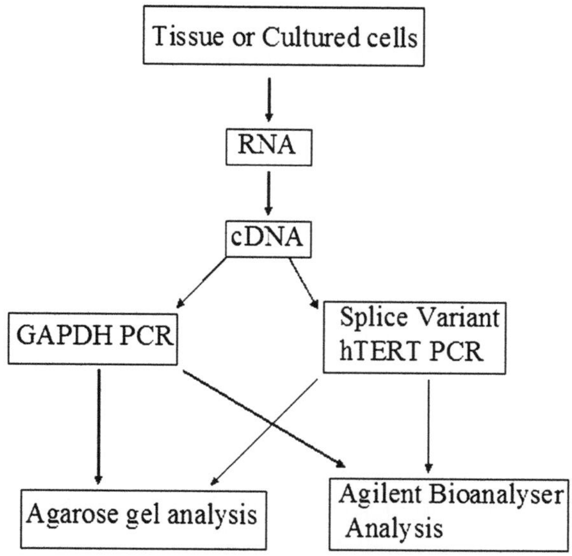

Fig. 2. Schematic diagram of the RT-PCR methodology.

ences, the hTERT gene can be induced to change the pattern of the splice variants. Several studies have begun to examine more precisely the role that alternative splicing might play in the regulation of telomerase activity in various tissues ***(10–18)***.

The hTERT gene contains four insertion sites and two deletion sites (*see* **Fig. 1**) ***(5,19)***. All of the insertion sites cause a truncated nonfunctional protein to be formed, as they disrupt the RT domain. The β deletion (182 bp) also causes a nonfunctional protein to be formed, whereas the α deletion (36 bp) causes an in-frame mutation, which can act in a dominant-negative fashion on enzyme activity ***(6,8)***. Because these two deletions are close together, they may be studied with one set of polymerase chain reaction (PCR) primers in a single reaction. In addition, the number of molecules of hTERT mRNA in tumor cells varies between 1 and 30 and so RT-PCR is the best way to study this expression as it involves an amplification step ***(6–8)***.

Figure 2 shows a schematic diagram of the RT-PCR methodology. RNA is extracted from tissues or cultured cells, reverse-transcribed to make cDNA, which is then used as the template in the PCR reactions. The primers were designed to span the region where the α and β deletions occur ***(5,6)***. This can generate four different PCR products according to the splice variants present (*see* **Fig. 1**). These can then be analyzed on a gel to see the banding pattern or on the Agilent Bioanalyser (Agilent Technologies, http://we.home.agilent.com/), which gives the size and quantity of each of the variants. The internal control PCR (GAPDH) is amplified in a separate tube, giving a relative rather than an

Table 1
Summary of Pattern and Frequency of HTERT Splice Variants in Cancer Cell Lines in Tissue Culture

Splice variant		PCR product size (bp)	Activity	Relative amount expressed in cell lines
Wild type	$\alpha+\beta+$	457	Functional	5%
α deletion	$\alpha-\beta+$	421	Dominant negative	<1%
β deletion	$\alpha+\beta-$	275	Nonfunctional	80–90%
$\alpha + \beta$ deletion	$\alpha-\beta-$	239	Nonfunctional	5–15%

absolute measurement of gene expression. Generally, the cell lines produce the same pattern of splice variants (*see* **Table 1**) ***(7)***. Therefore, possibly there is a common splicing pattern in diverse tumor types, at least in culture. The presence of the full-length variant in tissue samples would indicate the likelihood of telomerase activity and might be a useful aid to predict cancer progression. There is the potential also for cancer therapy in ways to influence the production of the nonfunctional variants or, even more useful, the dominant-negative variant, rather than the full-length variant ***(3,9,20)***.

2. Materials

2.1. RNA Extraction From Cultured Cells

1. P.E. buffer (1X PBS, 1 m*M* EDTA, pH 7.3).
2. 2.5% (w/v) Trypsin (10X stock) 0.85% NaCl, dilute 1:10 P.E. buffer for working solution (Invitrogen).
3. Phosphate-buffered saline (PBS) (1X PBS), pH 7.3 (Oxoid).
4. 15-mL Falcon tubes.
5. Centrifuge (capable of 2000*g* and cooled to 4°C).
6. Microcentrifuge.
7. RNase Zap® (Ambion).
8. Diethyl pyrocarbonate (DEPC)-treated Eppendorfs (*see* **Note 1**).
9. DEPC water (*see* **Note 1**).
10. 70% Ethanol (v/v)–DEPC-treated water (*see* **Note 1**).
11. NucleoSpin RNA® II Kit Macherey (Nagel) (*see* **Note 2**). Contains RA1 buffer, RA2 buffer, MDM buffer, RA3 buffer, RNase-free DNase I (keep at –20°C), DNase reaction buffer, RNase-free water. NucleoSpin RNA columns, NucleoSpin filter units, collecting tubes, and RNase-free 1.5-mL Eppendorfs.
12. β-Mercaptoethanol (Sigma).
13. 2-mL Syringe and 20 gage needle.
14. Spectrophotometer.

2.2. cDNA Synthesis

1. GeneAmp® RNA core kit (Applied Biosystems, store at –20°C). Contains RNase free water, 10X reverse transcriptase buffer, 25 m*M* Magnesium Chloride, Random Hexamers (50 μ*M*), (or use oligo dT's [50 μ*M*]), RNase inhibitor (20 U/μL) and Multiscribe Reverse transcriptase enzme (50 U/μL).
2. dNTP's (Geneamp® dNTP blend 10 m*M*; Applied Biosystems, store at –20°C).
3. DEPC treated 0.5 mL Eppendorf tubes.
4. RNase free water.
5. Template tamer hood (optional). Equivalent to a class 1 flow hood, but dedicated to PCR (LabCaire systems).
6. UV Crosslinker (Stratagene, optional).

2.3. GAPDH PCR

Control for integrity of cDNA.

1. PCR Core kit (Qiagen), store at –20°C. Contains 10X buffer (Tris-HCl, KCl, $(NH_4)_2SO_4$, 15 m*M* $MgCl_2$, pH 8.7, at 20°C), dNTP's (10 m*M* each), *Taq* polymerase enzyme (5 U/μL).
2. GAPDH control primers (20 μ*M* each [Clontech], keep at –20°C)
   5' primer: 5' TGA AGG TCG GAG TCA ACG GAT TTG GT 3'
   3' primer: 3' CAT GTG GGC CAT GAG GTC CAC CAC 3'
3. Sterile water (Braun or autoclaved).
4. Sterile 0.5-mL and 1.5-mL Eppendorfs.
5. Template tamer hood (optional) equivalent to a Class 1 flow hood, but dedicated to PCR (LabCaire Systems).
6. Ultraviolet (UV) crosslinker (optional) (Stratagene).

2.4. Splice Variant PCR

1. Hotstar *Taq* PCR kit (Qiagen), keep at –20°C, contains 10X PCR buffer, Hotstar *Taq* DNA polymerase (5 U/μL).
2. dNTP mix (10 m*M* each [Qiagen or Roche], keep at –20°C).
3. 250 μ*M* HT2026F stock forward primer: 5' GCCTGAGCTGTACTTTGTCAA 3' (keep at –20°C).
4. 250 μ*M* HT2482R stock of reverse primer 5' CGCAAACAGCTTGTTCTCC ATGTC 3' (keep at – 20°C).
5. 0.5-mL and 1.5-mL Sterile Eppendorf tubes.
6. Sterile water (Braun or autoclaved).
7. Template tamer hood (optional, LabCaire Systems).
8. UV crosslinker (optional) (Stratagene).

2.5. Preparing a Gel

1. Agarose.
2. Tris-HCl (0.45*M*); borate (0.45*M*); EDTA (0.01*M*) (5X TBE), pH 8.3 (Amresco).

3. Distilled water.
4. Flat-bed gel electrophoresis apparatus and power pack (e.g., Bio-Rad).
5. Microwave.
6. Ethidium bromide (0.5 mg/mL).
7. Loading dye: water, glycerol (30%, v/v), bromophenol blue (0.25%, w/v); and xylene cyanol (0.25%, w/v).
8. DNA markers between 100 bp and 1 kb (i.e., 100 bp and/or λ *Hin*d III marker (Invitrogen).
9. Gel photographing system.

2.6. Agilent Bioanalyser

1. DNA 1000 CHIP kit (store at 4°C) (Agilent Technologies), contains DNA 1000 chip, ladder, markers, gel matrix, dye concentrate, and syringe.
2. 1.5-mL Eppendorf tubes.
3. Microcentrifuge.
4. Adapted vortexer (Agilent Technologies).
5. Agilent 2100 Bioanalyzer (Agilent Technologies).
6. Chip priming station (Agilent Technologies).

3. Methods

3.1. RNA Extraction From Cells (see Notes 3 and 4)

1. Grow cells of interest to near confluence in 75-cm^2 flasks.
2. Rinse cells in 5 mL P.E. buffer and discard buffer.
3. Add 2 mL diluted trypsin (i.e., 0.25%, w/v) for 5 min at 37°C (times may vary for different cell lines).
4. Add 3 mL PBS at room temperature and transfer cell suspension to a 15-mL Falcon tube.
5. Spin at 1420*g* for 5 min at room temperature.
6. Remove supernatant by decanting and discard.
7. Add 2 mL PBS and resuspend pellet by gentle agitation.
8. Spin down again at 1420*g* for 5 min at room temperature.
9. Remove supernatant by decanting and discard.
10. In a DEPC-treated Eppendorf tube, make up (350 μL RA1 buffer + 1 μL of β-mercaptoethanol; Nucleospin II kit; *see* **Notes 2** and **4**) per sample (make up fresh each time).
11. Add this to the pellet and vortex to mix.
12. If more than 1×10^6 cells are present, then pass through a 20-gage needle with a 2-mL syringe 5–10 times; if not, go to **step 14**.
13. Add cell lysate to a filter column and spin at 10,400*g* for 1 min in a microcentrifuge, collecting in a DEPC-treated Eppendorf. Continue with protocol.
14. Add 350 μL of 70% ethanol (*see* **Note 1**) and then vortex.
15. Apply sample to Nucleospin II column in collecting tube, including precipitate.

16. Spin at 8000*g* for 1 min at room temperature, collect and discard eluate, and then add 350 μL MDM buffer to column.
17. Spin the column at 10,400*g* for 1 min at room temperature, collect, and discard eluate.
18. In a DEPC-treated Eppendorf, add 90 μL DNase reaction buffer + 10 μL DNase I per sample (*see* **Note 5**).
19. Apply 95 μL of this solution to the column, leave at room temperature for 15 min, and then add 200 μL RA2 buffer to the same column.
20. Spin at 8000*g* for 1 min at room temperature and then place column in a fresh collecting tube and add 600 μL RA3 buffer. Spin at 8000*g* for 1 min at room temperature.
21. Collect and discard eluate.
22. Add 250 μL RA3 buffer to column, and spin at 10,400*g* for 2 min.
23. Collect and discard eluate.
24. Place column in a 1.5-mL (RNAse-free) Eppendorf.
25. Add 60 μL RNAse-free water.
26. Spin at 10,400*g* for 1 min. Collect and *retain* eluate.
27. Read RNA concentration and ratio on a spectrophotometer (*see* **Note 6**).
28. Store RNA at –70°C (*see* **Note 7**).

3.2. cDNA Synthesis

1. Use 1 μL of RNA for each 40-μL reaction (protocol in cDNA synthesis kit for 250 ng in 10-μL reaction).
2. Make up master mix for number of samples (*see* **Note 8**) and include a no RNA template (negative control). Also, make up a master mix with no reverse transcription enzyme as a control for each sample (*see* **Notes 9** and **10**). Make up master mix in template tamer hood if possible (*see* **Notes 11** and **12** and **Tables 2** and **3**).
3. Aliquot out 40 μL of the master mix– the amount of RNA for 1 μg into the separate tubes, UV irradiate (*see* **Note 13**), and then add 1 μg RNA to each tube for both +RT and –RT mixes.
4. Place in PCR machine and run on program: 25°C for 10 min (primer annealing), 48°C for 30 min (enzyme extension), 95°C for 5 min (reverse transcriptase inactivation).
5. Store cDNA at –20°C until ready to perform PCR.

3.3. GAPDH PCR (see **Notes 14** and **15**)

1. Thaw out PCR reagents and then keep on ice (*see* **Note 16**).
2. Make up master mix for number of samples and include a no template (negative) control for a 25 μL volume (*see* **Note 8** and **Table 4**).
3. Mix and aliquot out 24 μL master mix to sterile 0.5 mL Eppendorf tubes and then UV irradiate (*see* **Note 13**).
4. Add 1 μL of the sample cDNA to separate tubes (one per sample) and then put in the PCR block.

Table 2
Reaction Mixture With Reverse Transcriptase Enzyme

Reagent	Volume (μL) per reaction
RNase-free water	15.4–RNA volume
10X Reverse transcriptase buffer	4
25-m*M* Magnesium chloride	8.8
dNTPs (10 m*M*)	8
Random hexamers (50 μ*M*)	2
RNase inhibitor (20 U/μL)	0.8
Multiscribe reverse transcriptase (50 U/μL)	1
Final volume	40 (including RNA)

Table 3
Reaction Mixture for Negative Control (–Reverse Transcriptase Enzyme)

Reagent	Volume (μL) per reaction
RNase-free water	16.4–RNA volume
10X reverse transcriptase buffer	4
25-m*M* Magnesium chloride	8.8
dNTPs (10 m*M*)	8
Random hexamers (50 μ*M*)	2
RNase inhibitor (20 U/μL)	0.8
Final volume	40 (including RNA)

Table 4
Reaction Mixture for GAPDH PCR

Reagent	Volume (μL) per reaction
ddH_2O	20.8–cDNA volume
10X Buffer	2.5
dNTPs (10 m*M*)	0.5
5' GAPDH primer (20 μ*M*)	0.5
3' GAPDH primer (20 μ*M*)	0.5
Taq polymerase enzyme (5 U/μL)	0.2
Final volume	25 (including cDNA)

Table 5
Reaction Mixture for hTERT Splice Variant PCR

Reagent	Volume (μL) per reaction
ddH_2O	39.8–cDNA volume
10X Buffer	5
dNTPs (10 m*M*)	1
HT2026F primer (25 μ*M*)	2
HT2482R primer (25 μ*M*)	2
HotStar *Taq* polymerase enzyme (5 U/μL)	0.2
Final volume	50 (including cDNA)

5. Run on program: 94°C for 45 s, 60°C for 45 s, 72°C for 2 min for 30 cycles, then 72°C for 10 min.
6. PCR products can then be run on an agarose gel or the Agilent Bioanalyzer used to check for concentration and integrity of cDNA (*see* **Note 17**).

3.4. Splice Variant PCR

1. Thaw out PCR reagents and keep on ice.
2. Dilute primers to a working concentration of 25 μ*M* (25 μL stock primer + 225 μL sterile water; *see* **Note 18**) in template tamer hood if possible (*see* **Note 11**).
3. Make up a master mix in a sterile Eppendorf for the number of samples and include a no template control and a positive control (if possible); make up in a 50-μL volume for each sample (*see* **Table 5** and **Notes 8** and **16**).
4. Make up master mix on ice and keep on ice throughout (*see* **Note 19**).
5. Aliquot out master mix (50 μL of cDNA) into 0.5-mL Eppendorf tubes and then UV irradiate (*see* **Note 13**).
6. Add 1–2 μL cDNA to tubes (still kept on ice).
7. Then, put tubes in PCR block.
8. Run on program: 94°C for 15 min (initiates enzyme), 95ºC for 30 s, 64°C for 45 s; 72°C for 45 s × 40 cycles, 72°C for 5 min.
9. Analyze PCR products either by gel electrophoresis or the Agilent Bioanalyzer (*see* **Note 17**).

3.5. Preparing and Running an Agarose Gel (see Notes 20–22)

1. Make up TBE buffer to 0.5X TBE (*see* **Note 20**).
2. Prepare a 1.5% (w/v) agarose gel for splice variant PCR or 0.8% gel for GAPDH PCR.
3. Weigh out 1.5 g agarose (for splice variant PCR products) or 0.8 g agarose (for GAPDH PCR products) in a conical flask and add 100 mL of 0.5X TBE buffer.
4. Put in a microwave and heat until dissolved; leave to cool slightly.

5. Add 100 μL ethidium bromide to a final concentration of 0.5 μg/mL in 100 mL; swirl to mix (*see* **Note 21**).
6. Make up casting tray with comb and tape.
7. Pour out agarose into casting tray and leave to set.
8. Take out comb and put gel into gel tank.
9. Add 0.5X TBE buffer until the gel is covered.
10. Mix 2 μL loading dye + 10 μL PCR sample, for splice variant PCR, and 1 μL loading dye + 5 μL PCR sample for GAPDH PCR (*see* **Note 22**).
11. Load this into the wells of the gel.
12. Load a ladder on either side of samples such as λ *Hin*dIII and 100 bp ladder.
13. Run gel at 100–150 V for about 1 h.
14. Then photograph gel, the bands should appear between 250 bp and 500 bp for the splice variants and 983 bp for the GAPDH.

3.6. Agilent Bioanalyser Analysis (*see* **Note 17**)

1. Take out DNA 1000 kit from refrigerator and allow to come up to room temperature (20–30 min).
2. Switch on Agilent Bioanalyser machine.
3. Make up gel matrix by adding 25 μL DNA dye to gel matrix vial, vortex, and then apply to filter column and spin at 2240*g* for 15 min.
4. Take out DNA 1000 chip and put on the chip priming station.
5. Pipet 9 μL of the gel–dye mix into the well marked **G** and depress syringe for 1 min, then release; the syringe should come back up quite quickly.
6. Check that no bubbles are present in capillaries.
7. Pipet 9 μL gel–dye mix into the other wells marked **G**.
8. Pipet 5 μL of the gel–dye mix into the ladder well.
9. Pipet 5 μL of the DNA 1000 markers into each of the 12 sample wells.
10. Pipet 1 μL of the ladder into the ladder well.
11. Pipet 1 μL of each sample into the other wells, adding water to any not used.
12. Place chip in adapted vortexer and vortex for 1 min.
13. Place chip in the Agilent 2100 Bioanalyzer and run the DNA 1000 program.
14. Samples are read individually and the size and concentration of each band shown in a table as well as producing a virtual gel image of the bands.

4. Notes

1. Diethyl pyrocarbonate (DEPC) treatment of solutions and tubes. To make DEPC water, add 1 mL DEPC to 1 L of water (so at 0.1%); leave overnight at 37–42°C. Then, autoclave; this inactivates the DEPC. For DEPC-treated Eppendorfs, place in a beaker, add water and DEPC, steep overnight, tip off water the next day, and autoclave. The 70% ethanol should be made up with DEPC-treated water.
2. We use the Nucleospin II kit because it is easy to use and produces good quality RNA, but there are plenty of other methods for RNA extraction.
3. RNA is more labile than DNA and is very prone to degradation by ribonucleases, which present in the environment. These ribonucleases are very difficult to inac-

tivate. Therefore, special care must be taken to avoid contamination with environmental RNAses while extracting RNA.

4. We have a designated bench for RNA use, but it is swabbed down with RNase Wipes® (Ambion) or RNase Zap® (Ambion) before it is used and the pipets and racks also, then rinsed in the DEPC-treated water. It is also important to regularly change gloves while making RNA to avoid contamination.
5. This protocol includes a DNase enzyme treatment, which gets rid of any contaminating DNA; this should be included in any RNA extraction.
6. RNA concentration can be read on a spectrophotometer; A_{260} of 1 is equivalent to 40 µg RNA/mL, and the ratio of purity A_{260}/A_{280} should fall between 1.7 and 2.1 if of good quality. DNA will also be read at this wavelength.
7. To minimize RNA degradation, it is recommended that RNA be stored at –70°C. Once thawed, keep on ice; then, put away shortly after use.
8. The master mix volume should be made up with an extra tube amount to ensure sufficient reagents for all samples.
9. It is a good idea to prepare a duplicate reaction for each sample minus the reverse transcription enzyme, as this acts as a control for DNA contamination in the PCR.
10. Use a set of pipets that has not been in contact with any DNA, to minimize the chances of contamination, and DEPC-treated Eppendorfs.
11. The Template tamer hood is useful to minimize the aerosol contamination while setting up the cDNA synthesis or PCR, because it has positive pressure. It also has a built in UV irradiation feature, so all tips, pipets, and tubes can be irradiated before use.
12. It is a good idea to have a separate PCR setup station from which the PCR products are run on gels, as well as two sets of dedicated pipets for PCR—a non-DNA set and a DNA set.
13. The UV crosslinker is useful for crosslinking any contaminating DNA after aliquoting out the master mix into the separate tubes. Again, this minimizes any DNA contamination while setting up the reaction.
14. An internal control such as GAPDH should be carried out to check for integrity and quantity of cDNA made.
15. Although, for the splice variant PCR, contaminating DNA will not interfere with the results, it is good practice to check for contaminating DNA by running the no reverse transcriptase enzyme controls on the internal control PCR.
16. Care should be taken to minimize cross-contamination by changing gloves regularly and UV-irradiating solutions and tubes before the addition of cDNA. A no DNA (negative) control should always be run, and if a band is present, discount results. If possible, a positive control should also be included to check the efficiency of the PCR reaction.
17. The Agilent Bioanalyser is a machine that is able to give you a size and quantity of your PCR bands using only 1 µL of PCR product. It presents this in the form of a virtual gel, a table, or electropherograms. It is particularly useful for the splice variant PCR, as it quantifies each band.
18. Stocks of splice variant primers come lyophilized. These are made up in ddH_2O

to be at 250 μ*M*. Aliquots are made to a working concentration of 25 μ*M*. This minimizes the potential for contaminating stock solutions.

19. When using HotStar *Taq* enzyme, the tubes should be kept on ice as much as possible.
20. Tris-borate EDTA (TBE) buffer is made up to a stock of 5X, and then diluted 1:10, so make a 0.5X TBE running stock.
21. Ethidium bromide stock at 0.5 mg/mL, dilute so at 0.5 μg/mL made up in 0.5X TBE (i.e., 100 μL in 100 mL). We tend to only add ethidium bromide to our gel and not to the buffer, as it is a COSSH 3 chemical. It should be disposed of and handled with caution, note that during electrophoresis, it will migrate into the buffer chamber.
22. Because the dye front of xylene cyanol runs at the same point as the splice variant bands, it is better to eliminate this from the gel-loading dye.

References

1. Keith, W. N., Evans, T. R. J., and Glasspool, R. M. (2001) Telomerase and cancer: time to move from a promising target to a clinical reality. *J. Pathol.* **195,** 404–414.
2. Keith, W. N., Bilsland, A., Evans, T. R. J., et al. (2002) Telomerase-directed molecular therapeutics. *Exp. Rev. Mol. Med.*; http://www.expertreviews.org/02004507h.
3. Aisner, D. L., Wright, W. E., and Shay, J. W. (2002) Telomerase regulation: not just flipping the switch. *Curr. Opin. Genet. Dev.* **12,** 80–85.
4. Caceres, J. F. and Kornblihtt, A. R. (2002) Alternative splicing: multiple control mechanisms and involvement in human disease. *Trends Genet.* **18,** 186–193.
5. Kilian, A., Bowtell, D. D., Abud, H. E., et al. (1997) Isolation of a candidate human telomerase catalytic subunit gene, which reveals complex splicing patterns in different cell types. *Hum. Mol. Genet.* **6,** 2011–2019.
6. Colgin, L. M., Wilkinson, C., Englezou, A., et al. (2000) The hTERTalpha splice variant is a dominant negative inhibitor of telomerase activity. *Neoplasia* **2,** 426–432.
7. Yi, X., Shay, J. W., and Wright, W. E. (2001) Quantitation of telomerase components and hTERT mRNA splicing patterns in immortal human cells. *Nucleic Acids Res.* **29,** 4818–4825.
8. Yi, X., White, D. M., Aisner, D. L., et al. (2000) An alternate splicing variant of the human telomerase catalytic subunit inhibits telomerase activity. *Neoplasia* **2,** 433–440.
9. Kyo, S. and Inoue, M. (2002) Complex regulatory mechanisms of telomerase activity in normal and cancer cells: how can we apply them for cancer therapy? *Oncogene* **21,** 688–697.
10. Cerezo, A., Kalthoff, H., Schuermann, M., et al. (2002) Dual regulation of telomerase activity through c-Myc-dependent inhibition and alternative splicing of hTERT. *J. Cell Sci.* **115,** 1305–1312.

11. Ding, Z., Green, A. G., Yang, X., et al. (2002) Retinoic acid inhibits telomerase activity and downregulates expression but does not affect splicing of hTERT: correlation with cell growth rate inhibition in an in vitro cervical carcinogenesis/multidrug-resistance model. *Exp. Cell Res.* **272,** 185–191.
12. Kim, Y. W., Hur, S. Y., Kim, T. E., et al. (2001) Protein kinase C modulates telomerase activity in human cervical cancer cells. *Exp. Mol. Med.* **33,** 156–163.
13. Kotoula, V., Hytiroglou, P., Pyrpasopoulou, A., et al. (2002) Expression of human telomerase reverse transcriptase in regenerative and precancerous lesions of cirrhotic livers. *Liver* **22,** 57–69.
14. Krams, M., Claviez, A., Heidorn, K., et al. (2001) Regulation of telomerase activity by alternate splicing of human telomerase reverse transcriptase mRNA in a subset of neuroblastomas. *Am. J. Pathol.* **159,** 1925–1932.
15. Ulaner, G. A., Hu, J. F., Vu, T. H., et al. (1998) Telomerase activity in human development is regulated by human telomerase reverse transcriptase (hTERT) transcription and by alternate splicing of hTERT transcripts. *Cancer Res.* **58,** 4168–4172.
16. Ulaner, G. A., Hu, J. F., Vu, T. H., et al. (2001) Tissue-specific alternate splicing of human telomerase reverse transcriptase (hTERT) influences telomere lengths during human development. *Int. J. Cancer* **91,** 644–649.
17. Ulaner, G. A., Hu, J. F., Vu, T. H., et al. (2000) Regulation of telomerase by alternate splicing of human telomerase reverse transcriptase (hTERT) in normal and neoplastic ovary, endometrium and myometrium. *Int. J. Cancer* **85,** 330–335.
18. Yokoyama, Y., Wan, X., Takahashi, Y., et al. (2001) Alternatively spliced variant deleting exons 7 and 8 of the human telomerase reverse transcriptase gene is dominantly expressed in the uterus. *Mol. Hum. Reprod.* **7,** 853–857.
19. Wick, M., Zubov, D., and Hagen, G. (1999) Genomic organization and promoter characterization of the gene encoding the human telomerase reverse transcriptase (hTERT). *Gene* **232,** 97–106.
20. Mercatante, D. and Kole R. (2000) Modification of alternative splicing pathways as a potential approach to chemotherapy. *Pharmacol. Ther.* **85,** 237–243.

22

Detection of Telomerase Enzyme Activity by TRAP Assay

W. Nicol Keith and Aileen J. Monaghan

1. Introduction

The telomeric repeat amplification protocol (TRAP) assay, first published by Kim et al. in 1994 ***(1)***, is used to detect telomerase activity. The scope of the technique is far reaching and has implications for telomere, telomerase, aging, and cancer research ***(2,3)***. In particular, it has revolutionized our understanding of the cancerous cell and its route to escaping senescence or programmed cell death.

Telomerase is a ribonucleoprotein ***(4,5)*** that, using its RNA component as a template, adds TTAGGG repeats to the 3' end of eukaryotic chromosomes. Telomerase is generally not expressed in somatic cells ***(6)***. In these cells, the chromosomes shorten with each cell division as a result of the end-replication problem. This shortening leads to chromosome instability and senescence or cell death. In contrast, germline cells need to protect their genetic information, and telomerase enables these cells to circumvent the end-replication problem and maintain the length of their telomeres. In addition, 85–90% of tumors abnormally express telomerase ***(7)***. This confers the capacity for unlimited growth upon the cell and enables the cell to escape senescence.

Thus, the development of this very sensitive technique has provided us with an outstanding marker of progression toward malignancy. The technique is based on the ability of telomerase to add the telomeric repeats described to the telomerase substrate (TS) primer (*see* **Fig. 1**). This extended primer is then amplified in the polymerase chain reaction (PCR) stage. Technical limitations of the original assay threaten to undermine its importance, however with false-positive and false-negative results, leading to some confusion. This method seeks to highlight some of the recent technical advances ***(8–10)*** that overcome some of these limitations, providing a much sturdier assay. In particular, the

From: *Methods in Molecular Medicine, vol. 97: Molecular Diagnosis of Cancer*
Edited by: J. E. Roulston and J. M. S. Bartlett © Humana Press Inc., Totowa, NJ

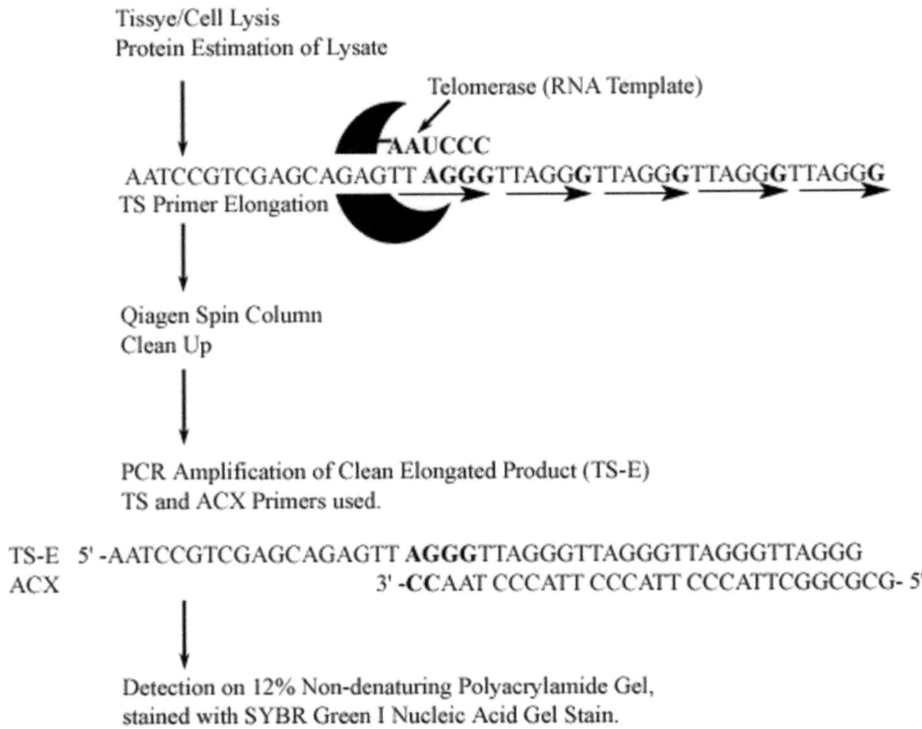

Fig. 1. Overview of the modified TRAP assay. Lysis of the sample and protein estimation are followed by the TRAP assay. The first stage is extension of the TS primer by telomerase present in the sample lysate. This is followed by cleanup of the extended product, before polymerase chain reaction amplification using the TS and ACX alternative complementary primer, and, finally, detection on an acrylamide gel.

addition of the "cleanup" step ***(11)*** after primer elongation is an exciting step forward to allow inclusion of a broader range of clinical samples. These samples would previously have been discounted from any study because of a lack of amplified product after PCR. This is the result of inhibitors of *Taq* DNA polymerase ***(12)*** present in many tissues. These can be removed easily prior to PCR using this simple step.

2. Materials

2.1. Sample Preparation and Lysis

1. Sample washing: Phosphate-buffered saline (PBS).
2. Lysis buffer: 10 m*M* Tris-HCl (pH 7.5), 1 m*M* $MgCl_2$, 1 m*M* ethylene glycol–*bis*(β-aminoethylether-)–*N,N,N',N''*-tetraacetic acid (EGTA), 0.5% (v/v) of 3-([3-cholamidopropyl]-dimethylammonio)-1-propanesulfonate (CHAPS), 10% (v/v)

glycerol, 5 m*M* β-mercaptoethanol, 0.1 m*M* phenylmethyl sulfonyl fluoride (PMSF), diethyl pyrocarbonate (DEPC)-treated double-distilled water (ddH_2O), RNase inhibitor (Perkin Elemer).

3. Mix all constituents except PMSF and β-mercaptoethanol (these maintain their activity for only a short time after addition to the lysis buffer) and filter-sterilize lysis buffer (Millipore Steriflip GP 0.22 μm sterile filter). Aliquot lysis buffer in volumes of 2–3 mL per sterile tube and store at 4°C. Add PMSF and β-mercaptoethanol to an aliquot immediately prior to use to concentrations detailed in **step 2**.

2.2. Protein Estimation

1. 5 mg/mL Bovine serum albumin (BSA).
2. 0.15*M* NaCl.
3. 95% (v/v) ethanol.
4. 85% (w/v) phosphoric acid.
5. ddH_2O.
6. Coomassie brilliant blue solution: In a 1 L volumetric flask, dissolve 100 mg Coomassie brilliant blue G250 in 50 mL of 95% (v/v) ethanol. Add 100 mL of 85% (w/v) phosphoric acid and bring to volume with ddH_2O. Filter through Whatman no. 1 filter paper and store at 4°C.

2.3. Expanded TRAP Assay

1. Lysis buffer.
2. RNase inhibitor (PerkinElmer) 160 U/mL lysis buffer.
3. 1X Reaction buffer: 20 m*M* Tris-HCl (pH 8.3), 1.5 m*M* $MgCl_2$, 63 m*M* KCl, 0.1 mg/mL BSA, 1 m*M* EGTA. Make a 10X batch of this and then store liquots at –20°C.
4. Elongation buffer (final concentration in a 50-μL reaction): 1X reaction buffer, 50 μ*M* dNTPs (Invitrogen), ddH_2O, 0.1 μg TS primer 5' AATCCGTCG AGCAGAGTT 3' (custom-made high-performance liquid chromatographic [HPLC] grade; Sigma Genosys).
5. Qiagen nucleotide removal kit, 100% ethanol.
6. 0.1 μg TS primer 5' AATCCGTCGAGCAGAGTT 3', 0.1 μg of ACX primer (alternative complementary primer) (*see* **Notes 1** and **2**), 5' GCGCGGC [TTACCC]3TAACC 3' (both primers custom-made HPLC grade, Sigma Genosys).
7. 2 U recombinant *Taq* DNA polymerase (Invitrogen).
8. ITAS (internal telomerase amplification standard), 15 ag (*see* **Note 3**).
9. Mineral oil or heated lid PCR block.

2.4. Detection of Telomerase Activity

1. Nondenaturing polyacrylamide gel (final concentrations): 12% (w/v), acrylamide/bisacrylamide ratio 19:1 (Severn Biotech Ltd).
2. 10% (v/v) ammonium persulfate (APS) (its possible to make a batch of this and store aliquots at –20°C).

3. 1% (v/v) *N,N,N',N''*-tetramethylethylenediamine (TEMED). (*Note:* Acrylamide is neurotoxic; therefore, caution should be exercised to avoid any skin contact.)
4. Sample loading buffer: Novex Hi-Density TBE Sample Buffer (Invitrogen).
5. DNA molecular weight markers V and VIII (Roche), or similar, giving band sizes which would be between 30 and 200 bp.
6. Running buffer: 0.5X Tris-borate EDTA (0.045*M* Tris-borate, 0.001*M* EDTA), pH 8.2.
7. Stain: 10,000X SYBR Green I Nucleic Acid Gel Stain (Invitrogen).

2.5. Controls

1. Positive control: telomerase positive cell lysate (e.g., GLC4).
2. Negative control: Each sample should be run in duplicate and one replicate (of 0.2 μg) heat inactivated. Lysis buffer should also be assayed.
3. Internal telomerase amplification standard (ITAS) (*see* **Note 3**).

2.6. Equipment

1. Refrigerated microcentrifuge.
2. Millipore Steriflip GP 0.22-μm sterile filter.
3. 1.5-mL Microcentrifuge tubes.
4. Spectrophotometer (capable of measuring absorbance in the ultraviolet–visible range).
5. 1-cm path-length microcuvet.
6. DNase- and RNase-free 0.5-mL and 0.2-mL tubes.
7. Aerosol-resistant tips.
8. Thermocycler (with heated lid).
9. Two completely separate sets of Gilson pipets for pre-PCR and post-PCR.
10. Vertical electrophoresis system: XCell Sure Lock (Invitrogen).

3. Methods

The telomerase enzyme has an RNA component in addition to the protein component; it is therefore imperative that RNase contamination be prevented. It is essential to wear gloves at all steps of the protocol; use ultrapure, preferably DEPC-treated water for all solutions; aliquot reagents into a volume sufficient for one experiment and bin any remainder; use aerosol-resistant tips at all times. It is good practice to keep separate work areas for all three stages of the assay—in particular, the pre- and post-PCR stages. It is crucial to have two completely separate sets of Gilson pipets for pre- and post-PCR in order to prevent false positives and cross-contamination.Control reagents are also essential and give a measure of the efficacy of the assay (*see* **Notes 3–5**).

3.1. Sample Preparation

3.1.1. Tissues

1. Surgical specimens should be flash-frozen (*see* **Note 6**) in liquid nitrogen immediately after removal and stored in liquid nitrogen until lysis. Tissue stored cor-

Table 1
Calculation for Lysis Buffer and RNase Inhibitor

Lysis buffer (μL) per sample	200
RNase inhibitor (U/μL)	20
NEED	160 U/mL lysis buffer = 16 U/100 μL lysis buffer = 32 U/200 μL lysis buffer
Volume of RNase inhibitor required (μL)	32/20 × (n + 3)
Volume (+/+) lysis buffer required (μL)	200 × (n + 3)

Abbr: n = number of samples in experiment (*see* **Note 9**).

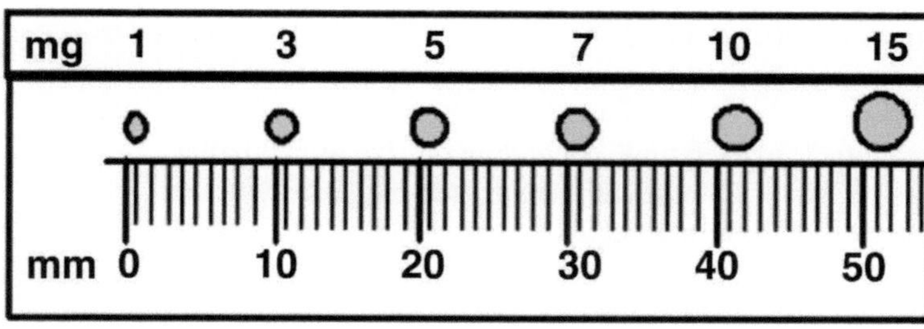

Fig. 2. Estimation of tissue size. In order to use the correct amount of lysis buffer, estimate the size of the biopsy using the chart. If the biopsy is larger than 10 mg, the sample can be frozen solid on dry ice and shattered into smaller fragments using a pestle and mortar. Any equipment used should be treated with Rnase Zap (Ambion).

rectly in liquid nitrogen even for several years can be used for extraction of the telomerase enzyme.

2. Add enough ice-cold PBS to cover the sample (100–500 μL) immediately prior to lysis. Gently wash the tissue sample and then discard PBS.
3. Make up lysis buffer with RNase inhibitor (*see* **Note 7**) to 160 U/mL lysis buffer (*see* **Table 1** and **Notes 8** and **9**) *(13)*.
4. Add 200 μL of lysis buffer with RNase inhibitor to approx 5–10 mg (*see* **Fig. 2**) of tissue.
5. Incubate on ice for 25 min. Vortex vigorously at regular intervals to agitate and disrupt the tissue sample during incubation.
6. Centrifuge for 20 min at 20,000*g* and 4°C.
7. Transfer the supernatant (approx 180 μL) carefully to a fresh tube, removing 45 μL of lysate for protein determination.
8. Flash-freeze (*see* **Note 6**) both aliquots and store at –80°C.

3.1.2. Cells

1. Cells should be trypsinized, pelleted, and washed in ice-cold PBS.

Table 2
Elongation Master Mix

Component	(μL)
2 m*M* dNTPs	1.25
TS primer (0.05 μg/uL)	2
10X RB	5
dH_2O	31.75
Total	40
Final volume including sample	50

2. Cells are pelleted at 10,000*g*, 4°C for 1 min and all PBS aspirated from cell pellet using a fine needle.
3. With pellets on ice, add between 100 and 200 μL lysis buffer with RNase inhibitor (*see* **Note 7**) to each tube, depending on size of cell pellet.
4. Incubate on ice for 25 min with intermittent vigorous vortexing.
5. Pellet at 4°C for 20 min at 20,000*g*.
6. Transfer the supernatant (approx 180 μL) carefully to a fresh tube, removing 45 μL lysate for protein determination.
7. Flash-freeze (*see* **Note 6**) both aliquots and store at –80°C.

3.2. Protein Estimation by Bradford Method (see Note 10) *(14)*

1. Standards: Place duplicate aliquots of 0.5 mg/mL BSA (5, 10, 15, and 20 μL) into eight 1.5-mL tubes and dilute each to 100 μL with 0.15 *M* NaCl.
2. Into two more tubes, place 100 μL each of 0.15 *M* NaCl (these are blanks).
3. Test samples: Place duplicate aliquots of each test extract into 15-mL tubes using 5–10 μL of extract. Dilute each to 100 μL with 0.15*M* NaCl.
4. Add 1 mL Coomassie brilliant blue solution and vortex. Stand for 2 min at room temperature.
5. Determine the sample absorbance at 595 nm (A_{595}) using a 1-cm path-length microcuvet. Make a standard curve using the BSA samples and plot absorbance at 595 nm against protein concentration.
6. Determine the absorbance for the unknown and use the standard curve to determine the concentration of protein in the unknown. If the unknown protein concentration is too high, dilute the protein, assay a smaller amount of the unknown, or generate another standard curve in a higher concentration range.

3.3. Expanded TRAP Assay

3.3.1. Telomerase-Mediated Primer Extension

1. Make up lysis buffer with RNase inhibitor at 160 U/mL lysis buffer as described (*see* **Table 1**). This extra lysis buffer is used for dilution of samples.

Table 3
PCR Master Mix

Component	(μL)
2 m*M* dNTPs	1.25
TS primer (0.05 μg/uL)	2
ACX primer (0.05 μg/uL)	2
10X RB	5
Taq DNA polymerase (5 U/μL)	0.4
ITAS (15 ag/μL)	1.5
Total	12.15
Final volume including sample	approx 50

Note: *See* **Notes 1** and **2**.

2. On ice, make appropriate dilutions of sample lysate, in lysis buffer with RNase inhibitor, to give 2 and 0.2 μg total protein in a 10-μL volume.
3. Make up elongation buffer (*see* **Table 2**) for $n + 3$ samples immediately prior to use.
4. Add 40 μL elongation buffer per sample and incubate at room temperature for 30 min to facilitate telomerase elongation of TS primer.

*3.3.2. Cleanup of Elongated Product (*see **Note 11**)*: QIAquick Nucleotide Removal Kit Protocol (Qiagen)*

1. Add 10 vol of buffer PN to 1 vol of the sample from **step 4** of **Subheading 3.3.1.** and mix (i.e., add 500 μL buffer PN to 50 μL elongation reaction).
2. Place a QIAquick spin column in a provided 2-mL collection tube.
3. To bind DNA, apply the sample to the QIAquick column and centrifuge for 1 min at 3500*g*.
4. Discard the flowthrough and place QIAquick column back into the same tube.
5. Add ethanol (96–100%) to buffer PE before use (see bottle label for volume).
6. To wash QIAquick column, add 750 μL of Buffer PE and centrifuge for 1 min at 3500*g*.
7. Discard the eluate and place the QIAquick column back in the same tube. Centrifuge for an additional 1 min at 10,000*g* (approx 13,000 rpm) (*see* **Note 12**).
8. Place the QIAquick column in a clean 1.5-mL microcentrifuge tube.
9. To elute DNA, add 40 μL ddH_2O (*see* **Notes 13** and **14**) to the center of the QIAquick membrane and let the column stand for 1 min. Centrifuge the column for 1 min at 10,000*g* (approx 13,000 rpm).

3.3.3. PCR Amplification

1. Make up PCR master mix (*see* **Table 3**) for $n + 3$ samples and aliquot to 0.2-mL PCR tubes (*see* **Notes 1** and **15**). ITAS is used in attogram (ag) amounts. This is 10^{-18} g.

Table 4
Acrylamide Gel Mix

Component	Final concentration (mL)
Mix A	
30% (w/v) Acylamide/1.579% Bisacrylamide	12% (w/v) Acylamide (20)
10X TBE	0.5X TBE (2.5)
dH_2O	Make up to 50 mL final volume (27.5)
Mix B	
10% APS	1% APS (500)
1% TEMED	0.1% TEMED (50)

Note: *See* **Note 11**.

2. Add eluted sample from "cleanup" stage (*see* **Subheading 3.3.2.**).
3. Overlay sample with mineral oil.
4. Transfer samples to thermal cycler and amplify telomerase products as follows: 85°C for 10 min, and 31 cycles of 94°C for 30 s, 50°C for 30 s, and 72°C for 90 s.
5. Amplified samples can be stored at 4°C for several days or at –20°C over longer periods.

3.4. Detection of Telomerase Activity (see *Note 16)*

1. Mix 20 mL of acrylamides, 2.5 mL of TBE, and 27.5 mL ddH_2O (*see* **Notes 17** and **18**) (*see* **Table 4**), and filter-sterilize using the Millipore Steriflip GP 0.22-μm filter or similar.
2. Add 500 μL APS and 50 μL TEMED (*see* **Table 4**, Mix B) and pour gel immediately, remembering to insert gel comb.
3. After polymerization, remove comb. Wells should then be rinsed with running buffer prior to addition of samples, to remove APS and TEMED residues. Run gel without samples for 15 min to equilibrate the ion concentration across the gel.
4. Five microliters of PCR sample should be mixed with 2.5 μL of sample loading buffer (Invitrogen) and samples run out alongside Roche marker V and VIII (1 μg of each), the GLC4 positive control, and a heat-inactivated and/or lysis buffer negative control.
5. Gels are run at 200 V for approx 2 h in 0.5X TBE running buffer or until the xylene cyanol front reaches the bottom of the gel.
6. Gels are stained in 1X SYBR Green (Invitrogen) diluted in 0.5X TBE running buffer, for approx 20 min.
7. Gels are viewed on the transilluminator with a 3-s exposure time.
8. Samples are graded positive or negative in relation to the GLC4 controls for each particular assay (see **Note 4** and **Fig. 3**).

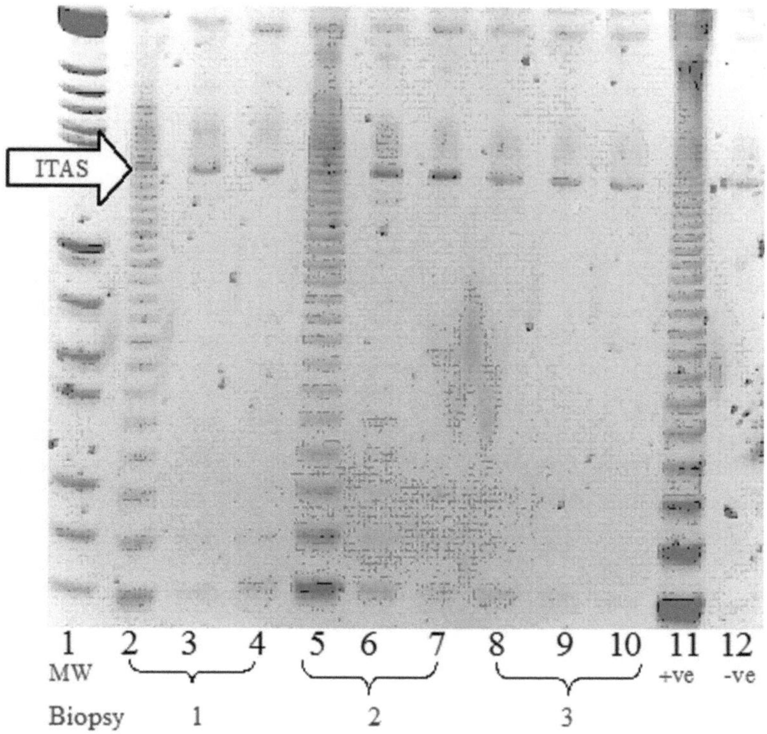

Fig. 3. Typical appearance of TRAP assay products. Results are from three separate biopsies, each has been assayed at 2 μg of protein, 0.2 μg and 0.2 μg heat-inactivated. The heat-inactivated sample provides a negative control for each biopsy. Biopsies 1 and 2 are positive for telomerase. They show the typical ladder of telomeric repeats without the random variation in band intensity that would signal a false positive from primer dimers. Biopsy 3 is negative for telomerase. Also shown are a positive and negative control (*lanes 11* and *12*) for the whole assay.

4. Notes

1. The ACX primer is used, as it is much more resistant to primer dimer artifact formation as compared with the original CX primer and so combat false-positive results. Very rarely, primer dimer artifacts may form with primers TS and ACX; however, these do not produce the renowned 6-bp TRAP ladder and are easily distinguishable.
2. The ACX primer is also an anchored primer. Because it does not produce primer dimers in the manner of the original CX primer, it is possible to add the ACX primer directly to the master mix without the need for wax beads.
3. Control reagents are essential as always, to give a measure of the efficacy of the assay. ITAS was developed by Wright et al. ***(10)*** and provides an external quality control check. It is a myogenin cDNA fragment containing the TS and ACX

primer sequences and is, therefore, amplified during the PCR stage of the assay to a 150-bp product. Consequently, ITAS amplification is completely independent of telomerase and is imperative because it is dependent solely on an active *Taq* enzyme. Inhibitors of *Taq* DNA polymerase can hamper the PCR amplification stage. ITAS amplification shows true telomerase status of a sample.

4. Positive control: An aliquit of a GLC4 cell lysate or other telomerase positive cell line should be run with every assay as a positive control. The number of cell equivalents assayed can be used as a measure of the sensitivity of the assay.
5. Negative control: Each sample should have an additional aliquot of 0.2 μg of protein, heat inactivated at 85°C for 10 min which is assayes alongside the active sample in order to rule out a false positive. Lysis biffer should also be assayed as a negative control.
6. Flash-freezing of tissue samples is done by placing a biopsy in liquid nitrogen. This is done immediately after removal to protect the enzyme from degradation. A quick freeze of supernatant can be done on dry ice, but liquid-nitrogen use is essential to protect freshly harvested biopsies.
7. The addition of RNase inhibitor to lysis buffer is crucial, particularly in clinical samples of the gastrointestinal (GI) tract, to protect telomerase from endogenously expressed RNases. This simple step can easily counter false-negative results.
8. A modification of the original lysis buffer has also been reported ***(13)***. The addition of 1% NP-40 and 0.25 m*M* deoxycholic acid to the lysis buffer constituents facilitates enhanced extraction efficiency and would allow re-extraction from a cell pellet. Although we have not found this modification necessary, it would be of particular use if very small quantities of sample (biopsy or cells) were to be assayed.
9. When generating a master mix, it is always advisable to make up excess to cover pipetting errors. If n is the number of samples in the assay (e.g., 24 samples in the assay so $n = 24$), make up master mix for $n + 3 = 27$ samples.
10. The Bradford or Lowry method should be used for protein estimation of the lysate. The Bisinchoninic Acid (BCA) Protein Assay should be avoided because of the incompatibility of several lysis buffer components with the assay constituents.
11. It has been noted by ourselves and others ***(11,12)*** that clinical samples (in particular, those originating from the GI tract) may contain inhibitors of *Taq* DNA polymerase. This consequently hinders the PCR stage of the assay and thus generates false negatives. Dilution of samples to counter this is possible, but not always beneficial. The use of the QIAquick Nucleotide Removal Kit is a quick and easy step to clean up the elongated product with minimal loss of sample.
12. It is essential to discard the flowthrough before the additional configuration step in order to remove residual ethanol completely from the column.
13. Ensure that the ddH_2O is dispensed dirctly onto the AIAquick membrane for complete elution of bound DNA.
14. Elution efficiency from the QIAquick column is dependent on pH. The maxi-

mum elution efficiency is achieved between pH 7.0 and 8.5. When using water, make sure that the pH value is within this range.

15. The 10 min incubation at 85°C denatures telomerase present in the sample, in order that PCR amplification is restricted to the elongated product of the 30 min room temperature incubation.
16. This method describes variations on the TRAP assay itself. Our detection method remains simple but reliable; quantification of a semiquantitative assay is often difficult to qualify. Two promising new and highly sensitive methods of quantification are the Hybridization Protection Assay (HPA) ***(15)*** and Enzymatic Luminometric Inorganic Pyrophosphate Detection Assay (ELIDA) ***(16)***. Both of these are nonradioactive.
17. Acrylamide is highly neurotoxic; therefore, caution should be exercised to avoid any skin contact. It is better to use an acrylamide solution as described here or wear a face mask to avoid inhaling the powdered form.
18. We have consistently used the X-Cell Sure Lock System (Invitrogen) for casting and running of acrylamide gels. The availability of disposable plastic casting cassettes for this system overcomes many technical problems concerning the set up, casting, and aftercare of glass plates.

References

1. Kim, N. W., Piatyszek, M. A., Prowse, K. R., et al. (1994) Specific association of human telomerase activity with immortal cells and cancer. *Science* **266,** 2011–2015.
2. Shay, J. W. and Wright, W. E. (1996) The reactivation of telomerase activity in cancer progression. *Trends Genet.* **12,** 129–131.
3. Bodnar, A. G., Ouellette, M., Frolkis, M., et al. (1998) Extension of life-span by introduction of telomerase into normal human cells. *Science* **279,** 349–352.
4. Morin, G. B. (1989) The human telomere terminal transferase enzyme is a ribonucleoprotein that synthesizes TTAGGG repeats. *Cell* **59,** 521–529.
5. Blackburn, E. H. (1991) Structure and function of telomeres. *Nature* **350,** 569–573.
6. Damm, K., Hemmann, U., Garin-Chesa, P., et al. (2001) A highly selective telomerase inhibitor limiting human cancer cell proliferation. *EMBO J.* **20,** 6958–6968.
7. Shay, J. W. and Bacchetti, S. (1997) A survey of telomerase activity in human cancer. *Eur. J. Cancer* **33,** 787–791.
8. Kim, N. W. and Wu, F. (1997) Advances in quantification and characterization of telomerase activity by the telomeric repeat amplification protocol (TRAP). *Nucleic Acids Res.* **25,** 2595–2597.
9. Krupp, G., Kuhne, K., Tamm, S., et al. (1997) Molecular basis of artifacts in the detection of telomerase activity and a modified primer for a more robust "TRAP" assay. *Nucleic Acids Res.* **25,** 919–921.
10. Wright, W. E., Shay, J. W., and Piatyszek, M. A. (1995) Modifications of a

telomeric repeat amplification protocol (TRAP) result in increased reliability, linearity and sensitivity. *Nucleic Acids Res.* **23,** 3794–3795.

11. Bachor, C., Bachor, O. A., and Boukamp, P. (1999) Telomerase is active in normal gastrointestinal mucosa and not up-regulated in precancerous lesions. *J. Cancer Res. Clin. Oncol.* **125,** 453–460.
12. Nakamura, Y., Tahara, E., Tahara, H., et al. (1999) Quantitative reevaluation of telomerase activity in cancerous and noncancerous gastrointestinal tissues. *Mol. Carcinog.* **26,** 312–320.
13. Norton, J. C., Holt, S. E., Wright, W. E., et al. (1998) Enhanced detection of human telomerase activity. *DNA Cell Biol.* **17,** 217–219.
14. Bradford, M. M. (1976) A rapid and sensitive method for the quantitation of microgram quantities of protein utilizing the principle of protein-dye binding. *Anal. Biochem.* **72,** 248–254.
15. Hirose, M., Abe-Hashimoto, J., Ogura, K.,et al. (1997) A rapid, useful and quantitative method to measure telomerase activity by hybridization protection assay connected with a telomeric repeat amplification protocol. *J. Cancer Res. Clin. Oncol.* **123,** 337–344.
16. Xu, S., He, M., Yu, H., et al. (2001) A quantitative method to measure telomerase activity by bioluminescence connected with telomeric repeat amplification protocol. *Anal. Biochem.* **299,** 188–193.

23

Identification of *TP53* Mutations in Human Cancers Using Oligonucleotide Microarrays

Wen-Hsiang Wen and Michael F. Press

1. Introduction

1.1. Significance and Implication of p53 Mutation and Its Detection

TP53 mutations are the most common genetic alterations in human malignancies. Since it was first discovered in 1989, more than 1700 different *TP53* mutations have been described at more than 310 distinct resides. According to the most recent updated (September 2002) *TP53* mutation database (www.iarc.fr/p53), more than 17,689 somatic mutations and 225 germline mutations have been reported ***(1)***. Detection of *TP53* mutations have the following implications: (1) *TP53* mutations cause inactivation of p53 protein, (2) different *TP53* mutations are associated with different mechanisms causing the mutation, spontaneous mutations versus chemical carcinogen-induced mutations, and (3) *TP53* mutations have been correlated with clinical stage and patient survival and are considered a potential prognostic indicator in some cancers. *TP53* is a sensor of genomic stress and is involved in cell cycle control, angiogenesis, apoptosis, and DNA repair pathways. Therefore, detection of *TP53* mutations can provide a basis for understanding interactions of other genes with p53.

1.2. History and Current Demand for Efficient p53 Mutation Detection

Since 1989, most *TP53* mutations were identified by methods such as single-strand conformational polymorphism (SSCP) and DNA sequencing. Other methods such as denaturing gradient gel electrophoresis (DGGE), dideoxy fingerprinting (ddF), heteroduplex analysis, and cleavage methods ***(2)*** have also been used. In general, these traditional gel-based sequencing methods are rela-

From: *Methods in Molecular Medicine, vol. 97: Molecular Diagnosis of Cancer*
Edited by: J. E. Roulston and J. M. S. Bartlett © Humana Press Inc., Totowa, NJ

tively time-consuming and labor intensive, especially for analyzing the entire coding sequence from exons 2–11. Therefore, a high-throughput, low-cost, and accurate method is needed for screening large numbers of clinical samples. In addition, most tumor DNA samples are a mixture of carcinoma cell DNA and normal cellular DNA from the interstitial tissues (heterogenous cell population). Therefore, a sensitive method that can detect a low percentage of mutant alleles is also desirable.

1.3. Oligonucleotide Microarray in Genomic Research and Expression Study

Methods based on the hybridization of test DNA or RNA with multiple, defined oligonucleotides or cDNA probes attached to a solid glass or nylon matrix have been developed and are referred to as "oligonucleotide microarrays," "DNA microarrays," or "gene chips." By analyzing different hybridization patterns or levels between control and test DNA or RNA, oligonucleotide microarrays have been used for the analysis of various known genes, such as those encoding p53, breast cancer susceptibility, type 1 (*BRCA1*), ataxia–telangiectasia (*ATM*), cystic fibrosis transmembrane conductance regulator, HIV reverse transcriptase and protease, and cytochrome P450 ***(3–5)***.

1.4. Oligonucleotide Microarray Used in p53 Mutation Detection

Three different array-based approaches have been developed or are under development for the study of *TP53* mutations. These include (1) GeneChip® p53 assay developed by Affymetrix, (2) APEX (arrayed primer extension) on the array, (3) multiplex polymerase chain reaction (PCR)/ligase detection reaction (PCR/LDR) on array. In this chapter, we will focus on the usage of GeneChip p53 assays.

1.4.1. GeneChip p53 Assay

The GeneChip p53 assay developed by Affymetrix is based on the hybridization of labeled target nucleic acid to a chip followed by fluorescence detection. It allows rapid sequence variation analysis of exons 2–11 of the human p53 gene, including the flanking intron sequences of the splice junctions. Probes on the array are arranged in both standard tiling and redundant tiling arrangements (*see* **Subheading 3.1.**).

Genomic DNA from tissue or cells is amplified by a single multiplex PCR. The amplified target is then fragmented with DNase I and end labeled with terminal deoxynucleotidyl transferase and fluoresceinated dideoxy-AMP. The fragmented, labeled target DNA is then hybridized to the array. This is followed by washing and scanning of the microarray.

The hybridization pattern and intensity of the hybridization signals is then determined by laser scanner and analyzed by software based on a mixture detection algorithm. Mutations are detected based on differences in hybridization pattern and intensities between reference and target DNA. The algorithm also assigns a score for each site containing a mutation based on the sum of mixture variables calculated from all corresponding probe sets, including probe sets for both sense and antisense strands and both tiling formats. The higher the score for a probe set contributing to a given base, the higher the likelihood for the base to be mutated. Mutations that occurred in codons with redundantly tiled nucleotides, in addition to the standard tiling, usually have the highest confidence score. These scores were higher because of the increased number of probes available to calculate the average intensity from each probe cell.

Using this approach, several studies have shown a high sensitivity and specificity of oligonucleotide microarray analysis for detection of single-base substitutions and single-basepair deletion mutations and compared detection of these same mutations with conventional manual DNA sequencing methods *(6–8)*. However, oligonucleotide microarray analysis is less sensitive in the detection of multiple basepair deletions or insertions because it is not designed to do so. The results of previous studies also indicate a small advantage to adding DNA sequencing for the detection of multiple-base deletion/insertion/ frame-shift mutations (*see* **Table 1**). The occurrence of multiple-basepair deletions and/or insertions is estimated to be approx 12% of the *TP53* mutations in the database, depending on tumor type (www.iarc.fr/p53). In its current format, the GeneChip p53 assay is ideal for screening mutations of single-base substitution, such as missense, nonsense, and splice junction mutations. Those samples that were detected as wild type could be subjected to further analysis to exclude possible multiple-basepair deletions or insertions.

1.4.2. Arrayed Primer Extension on Microarray

Arrayed primer extension (APEX) is based on incorporation of four dye terminators into oligonucleotide primers with a DNA polymerase *(9)*. A DNA sample is amplified by PCR, fragmented enzymatically, and annealed to an array of immobilized primers, which promote sites for template-dependent DNA polymerase extension reactions using four unique fluorescently labeled dideoxy nucleotides (ddNTPs) as substrate. Each base is probed with two primers: one for the sense strand and one for the antisense strand. Because all four dye terminators (ddNTPs) are present in the primer extension reaction, oligonucleotides are extended by a complementary nucleotide.

Those ddNTP-labeled primers are evanescently excited and the induced fluorescence is imaged by a charge-coupled device (CCD) camera. Compared

Table 1
Comparison of p53 Mutations Detected by Oligonucleotide Microarray and Conventional DNA Sequence Analysis

	Type of cancer	No. of tumors studied	Total no. of mutations identified	Same mutations identified by both methods	Same cases wild type by both methods	Mutations missed by DNA sequencing	Mutations missed by microarray	Sensitivity of microarray	Specificity of microarray
Ahrendt et al., 1999 *(7)*	Lung	100	57 (in 56 tumors)	31	43	15 (mutation type NA)	11 (10 tumors: 5 frame shift, 6 missense)	81%	98%
Wen et al., 2000 *(6)*	Ovary	108	77	57	31	14 (9 missense, 3 nonsense, 2 splice site)	6 (5 frame shift, 1 missense)	92%	100%
Lu et al., 2002 *(8)*	Bladder	140	79	62	61	8 (2 missense, 2 nonsense, 4 splice site)	9 (5 del/ins, 4 point mutation)	89%	100%

to wild-type DNA, mutant DNA might not anneal to some of the primers (such as deletion and insertion) or anneal at different nucleotide positions (such as some missense mutations), leading to a loss or change in signal at a designated site on the array. This corresponding change in the color code of the primer sites helps to identify the mutation.

Using this approach, two studies have attempted to analyze *TP53* by fabricating a DNA chip comprising complementary primers according to the human wild-type *TP53* sequence. One study has developed a prototype array for exon 7 using 37 probes (up to 18mers) and has demonstrated its ability to detect substitution mutations, single-basepair deletion mutations, and single-basepair insertion mutations ***(10)***. Tonisson et al. have developed an array containing exons 2–9 together with flanking splice sites and introns 5 and 8 from both strands (total 1218 bases). Each base in *TP53* is identified by two unique 25mer oligonucleotides: one for the sense strand and one for the antisense strand ***(9)***. One hundred normal DNA and 11 tumor DNA samples have been evaluated for a single nucleotide polymorphism at exon 4 *(Arg72Pro)* and mutations. Temporal temperature gradient gel electrophoresis (TTGE) followed by direct sequencing has also been used for analysis of the mutations in those 11 tumors. Ten mutations were identified by both approaches in these 11 tumor DNA samples, including a 2-bp insertion. In one tumor DNA, APEX and sequence analysis have detected different basepair changes in the same codon. In addition, APEX has detected one mutation missed by conventional DNA sequence analysis. APEX-based *TP53* sequencing in this study showed promising results in a limited number of tumor samples.

1.4.3. Multiplex PCR/LDR on Universal Microarray

The third array-based approach is based on multiplex PCR/LDR followed by hybridization on a universal zip code array ***(11)***. The current array contains 98 different nongenomic zip-code sequence (24mers) with similar melting temperatures (T_m) and no homology with human genes (no cross-hybridization). Each addressed nucleotide is assigned with paired oligonucleotides (primers) as follows: (1) a common primer with a 3' end containing nongenomic 24-base sequences that are complementary to the 24-base zip-code sequences present at known locations on the microarray surface for attachment to the array surface and (2) mutation-specific primers with a 3' base complementary to the mutation of interest and a corresponding label at the 5' end.

Following a multiplex PCR amplification of the regions of interest, a thermostable ligase is added. Ligation occurs only when the sequence at the junction between the paired oligonucleotides is exactly complementary to the template sequence. In the absence of mutation, no ligation occurs and no fluorescent-labeled probe is associated with the oligonucleotide.

In the presence of a mutation, the sequence change brings the corresponding mutation-specific primer next to the template and ligation occurs. After ligation, each LDR product contains a fluorescent label on one end and a zip-code complement on the other end. Analysis of PCR/LDR products is achieved by hybridization to the Universal DNA microarray using a zip-code sequence attached to a ligation oligonucleotide. Because the hybridization sequences are independent of the target gene and have similar thermodynamic properties, the hybridization is carried out at constant temperature and higher stringency to reach even hybridization than microarrays with built-in probes of wide sequence variation and T_m. In addition, mutation detection and hybridization to the array surface is carried out as separate events, this might avoid some of the problems associated with direct hybridization between target and probe. So far, universal microarrays have been tested for detection of mutations in p53, VHL, K-ras, APC, BRCA1, and BRCA 2 for a limited number of cases. The current LDR/Universal Array for p53 is for some of the known mutations in exons 5–8.

1.4.4. "Ideal" Approach for p53 Mutation Detection

Thus, all three oligonucleotide microarrays were able to demonstrate their sensitivity to discriminate low-abundance mutation(s) from heterogenous cell populations or pooled samples ***(9,11,12)***. However, in their current formats, only the GeneChip p53 assay developed by Affymetrix has complete coverage of all coding sequences and all splice junctions and has the potential to detect all possible substitution mutations in addition to approx 300 frequent mutations reported from the database. The GeneChip has been tested in studies containing substantial numbers of cases that are compared with a second (or third) method of sequence evaluation ***(6–8)***. This approach has proven to be an efficient and practical tool in the laboratory, although additional refinements are needed.

On the other hand, both APEX and Universal Array have the potential to address genes other than p53 and detection of small deletion/insertion mutations and some frame-shift mutations. They are also alternate approaches for resequencing or screening a known/specific mutation or polymorphism of interest. However, more samples will need to be evaluated to demonstrate their overall sensitivity and specificity regarding detection of p53 mutations, especially deletion/insertion mutations.

In conclusion, for general p53 mutation detection in a large number of samples, we continue to recommend using the Affymetrix GeneChip p53 assay for initial assessment. Depending on the purpose of the study, those cases with no mutation detected or an ambiguous result by the GeneChip p53 assay might be subjected to a secondary method such as automated DNA sequencing for identification of mutations not consistently recognized by the GeneChip p53 assay, including especially multiple-basepair deletion or insertion mutations. Other methods, such as mutation-specific oligonucleotide hybridization, have also been used previously for confirmation of mutations with satisfactory results *(7)*. Oligonucleotide microarray analyses are still under development and future improvements are expected on all array-based methods for genomic screening, including evaluation of *TP53*.

The following materials and methods are used in the GeneChip p53 assay.

2. Materials

2.1. GeneChip p53 Probe Array

See **Subheading 3.1.**

2.2. Target Preparation

2.2.1. Extract DNA From Tissue

1. DNeasy Tissue Kit (QIAGEN, cat. no. 69504).
2. Ethanol.
3. Water, molecular biology grade.

2.2.2. Amplification of Extracted Genomic DNA

1. p53 Primer Set and GeneChip p53 reference DNA, supplied as components of Affymetrix, GeneChip p53 Reagent Kit (P/N 900132).
2. AmpliTaq Gold™ set (Perkin Elmer, cat. no. N808-0241). This includes AmpliTaq Gold polymerase, 10X PCR buffer II, and 25 m*M* $MgCl_2$. The 10X buffer II and 25 m*M* $MgCl_2$ are used for preparartion of 4X PCR reagent used in PCR master mix.
3. 100 m*M* dNTPs set (Invitrogen cat. no. 10297018).
4. Preparation of 4X PCR reagent: For a total of 12.5 mL 4X PCR reagent, add 5 mL of 10X PCR buffer II with 5 mL of 25 m*M* $MgCl_2$ and 100 µL of each dNTP (100 m*M* for each of dA, dC, dG, dT) and 2.1 mL of water. Then, aliquot to 50 microcentrifuge tubes, store at –20°C. Each tube containing 250 µL of 4X PCR reagent will be good for 10 PCR reactions (*see* **Subheading 3.2.2.**).
5. Water, molecular biology grade.
6. Agarose gel.
7. DNA 50-bp ladder (Invitrogen, cat. no. 10416-014).

2.2.3. Fragmentation of the DNA Amplicons

The following four reagents will be mixed for preparation of fragmentation working mix described in **Subheading 3.2.3.**

1. GeneChip Fragmentation Reagent (DNase I in 10 m*M*/L Tris-HCl [pH 7.5], 10

mM/L $CaCl_2$, 10 mM/L $MgCl_2$, 50% glycerol), supplied as a component of the GeneChip p53 Reagent Kit (Affymetrix, cat. no. P/N 900132).

2. 0.5M EDTA (Ambion, cat. no. 9261).
3. Calf intestine alkaline phosphatase (1 U/μL) (Promega, cat. no. 1821).
4. 400 mM Tris-acetate (10X TAE), pH 8.2 (Ambion, cat. no. 9869).

2.2.4. Labeling the Fragmented DNA Amplicons

1. Fluorescein-N^6-dideoxy-ATP (Dupont/NEN, cat. no. P/N NEL503).
2. 5X terminal transferase reaction buffer (Promega, cat. no. P/N M1871).
3. Terminal transferase (Promega, cat. no. P/N M1871).

2.2.5. Preparing the Hybridization Target

1. 20X SSPE (3M NaCl, 0.2M NaH_2 PO_4, 0.02M EDTA) (Sigma, cat. no. P/N S2015).
2. Triton X-100 (Sigma, cat. no. P/N T 9284).
3. Control oligonucleotide F1, supplied as a component of the GeneChip p53 Reagent Kit (Affymetrix, cat. no. P/N 9001324).
4. 20 mg/mL Acetylated Bovine Serum Albumin (BSA) (Sigma, cat. no. P/N B 8894).
5. Water, molecular biology grade.

2.3. Target Hybridization

1. Genechip Fluid station (Affymetrix)
2. GeneChip p53 probe array (Affymetrix, cat. no. P/N500398).
3. Wash buffers (3X SSPE, 0.005% Triton X-100).
4. 20X SSPE (Sigma, cat. no. P/N S2015).
5. Triton X-100 (Sigma, cat. no. P/N T 9284).

2.4. Probe Array Scan

GeneArray scanner (Hewlett-Packard, cat. no. HP G2500A).

2.5. Data Analysis and Interpretation

GeneChip workstation and Affymetrix Microarray Suite.

3. Methods

3.1. GeneChip p53 Probe Array Design

1. Oligonucleotide microarrays are manufactured using photolithographic methods and combinatorial chemistry.
2. In the context of the p53 GeneChip, the synthesis cycles are repeated until oligonucleotides of approx 18 bases in length are constructed. Approximately 65,000 different oligonucleotide probes are synthesized on a 1.2-cm × 1.2-cm area (grid) consisting of 256 cells in each dimension.

3. Each probe cell (50 µm × 50 µm) is arranged and constructed to accommodate 10^7 copies of each oligonucleotide (probe).
4. These probes are designed to interrogate each base of exons 2–11 of the human *TP53* coding sequence and +2/–2 splice sites in a standard tiling format as well as a redundant tiling format for both sense and antisense strands.
5. The first format, standard tiling, contains probes with each of the 4 possible base substitution positions and deletions located at the 12th base from the 3' end. Each probe set represents A, C, G, T, a one-bp deletion, and an empty cell for background subtraction. Five probes per sense and antisense directions are arranged for each nucleotide position.
6. The second format, redundant tiling, is designed to interrogate over 300 common mutations reported more than once in the *TP53* database ***(13)***, with the exception of deletions or insertions greater than 1 bp. Each redundantly tiled mutation has 12 probes (6 sense, 6 antisense) designed to interrogate the mismatch. The substitution position is placed at different locations on the probe for maximum hybridization and discrimination of the mutant target.

3.2. Target Preparation

3.2.1. Extract DNA From Tissue

Reliable results have been obtained using QIAGEN DNA Easy Tissue Kit. The genomic DNA may also be extracted from samples using other standard laboratory techniques.

1. For the DNA Easy Tissue Kit, follow the manufacturer's guidelines.
2. Elute DNA in 10 m*M* Tris-HCl, pH 9.0.
3. Determine the concentration of DNA by absorbance at 260 nm.
4. Dilute the DNA with 10 m*M* Tris-HCl, pH 9.0, to a final concentration of 50 ng/µL.
5. Store the DNA at 4°C.

3.2.2. Amplifying Extracted Genomic DNA

The genomic DNA is amplified with PCR using the GeneChip p53 Primer Set and AmpliTaq Gold. The coding regions of the human *TP53* gene are amplified as 10 separate amplicons in a single multiplex PCR reaction.

1. Preparation of PCR master mix: Each 50 µL of PCR master mix contains 25 µL of 4X PCR reagent, 5 µL of p53 primer set, 2 µL of AmpliTaq Gold, and 18 µL of water.
2. Add 100–250 ng of extracted sample DNA (5–50 µL suggested) and add water (4–50 µL suggested) to a total volume of 50 µL. The total volume of the PCR is 100 µL, including 50 µL of PCR master mix.
3. Run a positive control reaction by adding 5 µL of GeneChip p53 Reference DNA and 45 µL water to 50 µL PCR master mix in a reaction tube.

4. Run a negative control reaction by adding 50 μL of water to 50 μL PCR master mix in a reaction tube.
5. Therefore, apart from the DNA, each PCR reaction contains 10 U of AmpliTaq Gold, PCR buffer II, 2.5 mmol/L $MgCl_2$, 5 μL of the primer set, and 0.2 mmol/L of each dNTP. The reaction is carried out in a final volume of 100 μL.
6. The PCR cycles are as follows: 95°C for 10 min, followed by 35 cycles at 95°C for 30 s, 60°C for 30 s, and 72°C for 45 s, with a final extension step at 72°C for 10 min.
7. Gel analysis: Load at least 5 μL of each PCR product with loading buffer in 4X agarose gel for better separation of bands. Run gel in 1X TBE for 50–90 min and stain with ethidium bromide for visualization of bands.

3.2.3. Fragmentation of the PCR Product

1. Prepare the fragmentation working mix for 10 reactions. The working mix must be prepared fresh and any remainder should be discarded after use. For a total volume of 50 μL of working mix (used for 10 samples), 1 μL of fragmentation reagent, 1 μL of EDTA (20 m*M*), 25 μL of alkaline phosphatase (1 U/μL), and 23 μL of Tris-acetate (10 m*M*).
2. Add 5 μL of the working mix prepared in **step 1** to 45 μL of the PCR product for a total reaction volume of 50 μL.
3. Store the remaining 50 μL of each PCR at 4°C for future use.
4. Put the fragmentation reaction tubes into a PCR thermal cycler: incubation at 25°C for 15 min, followed by heat inactivation at 95°C for 10 min, followed by 4°C.

3.2.4. Labeling the Fragmented DNA Amplicons

1. Preparation of labeling master mix: For every single sample (case), mix 20 μL of TdTase buffer (5X) with 28 μL water, 1 μL of fluorescein-N^6-dideoxy-ATP (1 m*M*) and 1 μL of terminal transferase (25 U/μL) to a total volume of 50 μL.
2. For each sample (case), 50 μL of the fragmented DNA is mixed with 50 μL of labeling master mix and incubated at 37°C for 45 min, followed by heat inactivation at 95°C for 10 min.

3.2.5. Preparing the Hybridization Target

1. Combine the following components in every 400 μL of hybridization master mix: 250 μL of hybridization concentrate (12X SSPE + Triton), 50 μL of acetylated BSA (20 mg/mL), 10 μL of control oligonucleotide F1 (100 n*M*) and 90 μL of water.
2. Aliquot 400 μL of the hybridization master mix to microcentrifuge tubes.
3. Retrieve the labeling reaction tubes from the thermal cycler.
4. Hybridization target (500 μL) = 100 μL labeling reactions + 400 μL of the hybridization master mix. Mix the tubes thoroughly. The hybridization target samples may be stored at –20°C protected from light for up to 4 wk. Avoid repeated freezing and thawing.

3.3. Target Hybridization

1. As described in **Subheading 3.2.5.**, the fluorscein-labeled sample is hybridized to the chip in a volume of 0.5 mL containing 6X SSPE buffer, 0.05% Triton X-100, 1 mg of acetylated BSA, 2 nmol/L control oligonucleotide.
2. The hybridization is carried out in an oven at 45°C for 30 min. The chip is then washed with wash buffer A (3X SSPE, and Triton X-100 0.0005%).

3.4. Probe Array Scan

The probe array is ready to be scanned after the hybridization and wash protocols are complete. The hybridized probe array is scanned using the GeneArray Scanner 50 or the HP GeneArray scanner (Hewlett-Packard, cat. no. HP G2500A). Scans take approx 4 min producing a data image file (*.DAT). As a quality assurance step, a control oligonucleotide is added to each sample during hybridization to examine the signal intensity and proper alignment of the probe array after the scan. Prior to the collection of image data, the scanner confirms the correct position and alignment of the chip by focusing on a series of defined positions. The scanner is controlled by the Affymetrix Microarray Suite. Refer to the Affymetrix Microarray Suite user's guide and online help and GeneArray Scanner user's guide for more information on scanning.

1. Choose Scanner from the Run menu. Alternatively, click the Start Scan icon in the Affymetrix Microarray Suite tool bar.
2. Choose the experiment name corresponding to the probe array to be scanned.
3. Load the probe array to the scanner.
4. Start the Scan.

3.5. Data Analysis and Interpretation

Data are generated and analyzed using an Affymetrix Microarray Suite in the following order:

1. EXP→DAT: After scanning the probe array, the resulting image data created are stored on the hard drive of the GeneChip workstation as a .DAT file with the name of the scanned experiment (EXP).
2. CEL: The data of calculated average intensity are assigned an X/Y-coordinate position and stored as a .CEL file.
3. CHP: The software then applies the selected probe array algorithm to compare the cell intensities and determine a base call at each position. A report with a summary of nucleotide changes in the sample is automatically displayed as a .CHP file in the Sequence Analysis window of the Affymetrix Microarray Suite. The .CHP file has the same name as the .EXP, .DAT, and .CEL files.
4. The hybridization intensities of the probes hybridized to the sample DNA are calculated by the software and compared with those hybridized to a reference DNA. The intensity patterns diverging from the reference are identified and sites

containing mutant bases are displayed. Refer to the Affymetrix Microarray Suite user's guide and online help for information on analyzing the data.

4. Notes

1. There might be some difficulty in amplifying products larger than 200 bp using genomic DNA extracted from formalin-fixed, paraffin-embedded tissue because of the fixation agent used. This is more common in exon 4 and exon 5, resulting in a loss of PCR products or products of low yield on the gel. In this case, it may be necessary to repeat the amplification.
2. The fragmentation working mix must be prepared fresh and any remainder should be discarded after use.
3. One study suggests regarding each chip position as a separate entity with its own noise and threshold characteristics. When using probe-specific cutoffs, it might be advisable to increase the specificity and decrease the sensitivity of the microarray *(12)*.
4. Modification of hybridization oven has been suggested to provide constant agitation of the chip to achieve more uniform staining *(12)*.
5. Assigning a different lower threshold for frame-shift mutations might lead to identification of some single-basepair deletions *(7)*.

Acknowledgment

The authors would like to gratefully acknowledge the assistance of Ms. Ivonne Villalobos in the preparation of this manuscript.

References

1. Olivier, M., Eeles, R., Hollstein, M., et al. (2002) The IARC TP53 database: new online mutation analysis and recommendations to users. *Hum. Mutat.* **19(6),** 607–614.
2. Cotton, R. (1997) Slowly but surely towards better scanning for mutations. *Trends Genet.* **13,** 43–46.
3. Southern, E. M. (1996) DNA Chips: analysing sequence by hybridization to oligonucleotides on a large scale. *Trends Genet.* **12,** 110–115.
4. Wallace, R. (1997) DNA on a chip:serving up the genome for diagnostics and research. *Mol. Med. Today* **3,** 384–389.
5. Lipshutz, R., Fodor, S., Gingeras, T., et al. (1999) High density synthetic oligonucleotide arrays. *Nature Genet.* **21(Suppl.),** 20–24.
6. Wen, W.-H., Bernstein, L., Lescallett, J., et al. (2000) Comparison of TP53 mutations identified by oligonucleotide microarray and conventional DNA sequence analysis. *Cancer Res.* **60,** 2716–2722.
7. Ahrendt, S., Halachmi, S., Chow, J., et al. (1999) Rapid p53 sequence analysis in primary lung cancer using an oligonucleotide probe array. *Proc. Natl. Acad. Sci. USA* **96,** 7382–7387.
8. Lu, M., Wikman, F., Orntoft, T., et al. (2002) Impact of alterations affecting the

p53 pathway in bladder cancer on clinical outcome, assessed by conventional and array-based methods. *Clin. Cancer Res.* **8(1),** 171–179.

9. Tonisson, N., Zernant, J., Kurg, A., et al. (2002) Evaluating the arrayed primer extension resequencing assay of TP53 tumor suppressor gene. *Proc. Natl. Acad. Sci. USA* **99(8),** 5503–5508.
10. Shumaker, J., Tollet, J., Filbin, K., et al. (2001) APEX disease gene resequencing: mutations in exon 7 of the p53 tumor suppressor gene. *Bioorg. Med. Chem.* **9(9),** 2269–2278.
11. Favis, R. and Barany, F. (2000) Mutation detection in K-ras, BRCA1, BRCA2, and p53 using PCR/LDR and a universal DNA microarray. *Ann. NY Acad. Sci.* **906,** 39–43.
12. Wikman, F., Lu, M., Thykjaer, T., et al. (2000) Evaluation of the performance of a p53 sequencing microarray chip using 140 previously sequenced bladder tumor samples. *Clin. Chem.* **46(10),** 1555–1561.
13. Beroud, C., Verdier, F., and Soussi, T. (1996) p53 gene mutation: software and database. *Nucleic Acid Res.* **24,** 147–150.

24

Detection of *K-ras* Mutations by a Microelectronic DNA Chip

Evelyne Lopez-Crapez, Thierry Livache, Patrice Caillat, and Daniela Zsoldos

1. Introduction

The increased knowledge of the human genome, thanks to its sequencing and to the accumulation of data that ensue from it, prompts the characterization of disease-causing genes. Especially because of the continuing expansion of cancer-related gene discovery, oncobiology is a discipline that is undergoing rapid change. Detection of point mutations in oncogenes or tumor suppressor genes associated with the multistep process of oncogenesis could be of value in patient management. These potential molecular tumor markers are essential not only for the diagnosis, prognosis, or the follow-up of the disease but also for the management of therapy *(1,2)*. Particularly, the *K-ras* protooncogene is altered, by point mutations within codons estimated to be critical for the biological activity of the protein (codons 12, 13, or 61), in a wide variety of tumors *(3)*. The incidence of these mutations can reach 95% in pancreatic carcinoma *(4)* and occurs in 40–60% of colorectal cancers, where they are associated with the progression from adenoma to carcinoma *(5)*. The detection of *K-ras* mutations enables the understanding of cancer biology and pathogenesis with, for example, a role in the mucinous differentiation pathway *(6)*. Alterations involving this oncogene may be of clinical importance because they can provide information for early diagnosis and clinical outcome. Their analysis within the tumor makes them of prognostic value (risk of relapse, mortality) *(7)*. Moreover, activation of the *K-ras* gene has been detected not only in the tumor but also in the stools *(8)* of patients with colorectal cancer. Where lymph nodes are concerned, *K-ras* mutation analysis permits a good classification that is useful

From: *Methods in Molecular Medicine, vol. 97: Molecular Diagnosis of Cancer*
Edited by: J. E. Roulston and J. M. S. Bartlett © Humana Press Inc., Totowa, NJ

for decision-making in adjuvant therapy *(9)*. Finally, search for mutations in serum *(10)* would be useful for diagnosis, postoperative checkup, as well as the early detection of recurrence.

The potential of these molecular data in the clinical field have led to the emergence of a demand for systems able to analyze several parameters from a single biological sample. The idea of using arrays for genotyping has been in existence for many years, and early arrays were two-dimensional spots of DNA targets on nylon or nitrocellulose membranes *(11)*. Now, oligonucleotide microarrays displaying numerous probes packed into a small area and allowing a reduction of both sample volumes and biological material have been developed *(12,13)*. Different supports have been used, such as glass *(14,15)*, polypropylene sheets *(16)*, polyacrylamide gel pads *(17)*, and silicon *(18)*. The precise location of oligonucleotides can be achieved through photochemistry *(19)*, micromecanical devices *(20)*, or electrosynthesis *(21–23)*.

At the moment, the microarray format is preferentially used for expression assays. Mutation detection techniques testing for known mutations include allele-specific polymerase chain reaction (PCR) *(24)*, primer-introduced restriction analysis *(25)*, 5' nuclease assay *(26)*, minisequencing *(27)*, allele-specific oligonucleotide ligation (ASO) *(28)*, and oligonucleotide ligation assay (OLA) *(29)*. Nevertheless, the last three techniques are the more adaptable to the microarray format. The prime considerations in any approach to mutation detection are sensitivity (the proportions of mutations that can be detected) and specificity (the proportion of false negatives). Moreover, cost per analysis and throughput are also important factors.

In order to fulfill some of the above criteria, we have developed a new silicon device based on electrocopolymerization of 5'-pyrrole-labeled oligonucleotides and pyrrole. Then, the potentialities of this methodology have been evaluated through the detection of *K-ras* mutations according to the ASO principle in DNA from human colorectal carcinomas.

2. Materials

2.1. Electroaddressed Oligonucleotide Silicon Chip

The Apibio Compagny designs, manufactures, and commercializes the MICAM® biochip based on probe coupling by electrocopolymerization of pyrrole (*see* **Note 1**).

2.2. Oligonucleotides

All of the oligonucleotides used in the assay are from Genset (France): eight 5'biotin-labeled synthetic targets:

t-W 5'Bio-CCT ACG CCA CCA GCT CCA AC 3' wild-type RAS

Table 1
K-ras Codon 12 Sequence on Selected Cell Lines

Cell line	K-ras codon 12 sequence	Amino acid
SW620	GTT	Val
MIA PaCa-2	TGT	Cys
SW1116	GCT	Ala
LS 174T	GAT	Asp
LNCaP	GGT	Gly

t-M1	5'Bio-CCT ACG CCA C**T**A GCT CCA AC 3'	
t-M2	5'Bio-CCT ACG CCA C**G**A GCT CCA AC 3'	
t-M3	5'Bio-CCT ACG CCA C**A**A GCT CCA AC 3'	
t-M4	5'Bio-CCT ACG CCA **T**CA GCT CCA AC 3'	
t-M5	5'Bio-CCT ACG CCA **G**CA GCT CCA AC 3'	
t-M6	5'Bio-CCT ACG CCA **A**CA GCT CCA AC 3'	
t-PC	5'Bio-TAG CTG TAT CGT CAA GGC A 3'	Control primer without mutation region

one 5'phosphate-labeled primer P-ras1 (5' Phophate-GGC CTG CTG AAA ATG ACT GAA TAT 3') and one 5'biotin-labeled primer Bio-ras2 (5' Biotin-TGT TGG ATC ATA TTC GTC CAC AAA ATG 3').

2.3. Biological Material

1. Cell lines displaying the wild-type (LNCaP) or a mutated *K-ras* codon 12 sequence (SW 620, MIA PaCa-2, SW 1116, LS 174T) are purchased from the American Type Culture Collection (*see* **Table 1** and **Note 2**).
2. Tissue samples are obtained during surgery from patients with colorectal cancer (CRLC Val d'Aurelle, Montpellier, France) (*see* **Note 3**).

2.4. Generation of the Target From Genomic Extracted DNA

1. *Taq* DNA polymerase and 10X *Taq* buffer (Invitrogen, France).
2. 100 m*M* dNTP solutions (Amersham-Parmacia Biotech, France).
3. 6400 U/mL λ exonuclease (New England Biolabs, MA).
4. Gradient T apparatus (Biometra, Germany).
5. DNA 1000 kit and BioAnalyzer 2100 (Agilent, France).
6. RNAse- and DNAse-free water (Sigma, France).

2.5. Specific Hybridization of the Target

1. 20X SSC, pH 7.0: Dissolve 175.3 g NaCl and 88.2 g sodium citrate in 800 mL distilled water, pH to 7.0 with 10 *M* NaOH; make up to 1 L with distilled water and autoclave.

2. 50X Denhart's solution: Dissolve 5 g of Ficoll (Type 400, Amersham–Pharmacia–Biotech), 5 g of polyvinyl pyrrolidone, and 5 g of bovine serum albumin (BSA) (Fraction V, Sigma) in 500 mL distilled water. Filter and store at –20°C.
3. 3*M* Tetramethyl ammonium chloride.
4. 1*M* Tris-HCl, pH 7.4.
5. 0.5*M* EDTA.
6. 10 g/L sodium dodecyl sulfate (SDS).
7. 10 mg/mL Salmon sperm DNA.
8. 1X Hybridization buffer: 1.8*M* tetramethyl ammonium chloride, 50 m*M* Tris-HCl, pH 7.4, 2 m*M* EDTA, 1 g/L SDS, 5X Denhart's solution, 10 μg/mL salmon sperm DNA. Prepare hybridization and washing buffers using the concentrated starting solutions above.
9. 1X Washing buffer A: 2X SSC, 1 g/L SDS.
10. 1X Washing buffer B: 5X SSC, 1 g/L SDS.
11. Temperature-controlled incubator.

2.6. Acquisition and Analysis of Signals

1. Phosphate-buffered saline (PBS) tablets (Sigma, France): Dissolve 1 PBS tablet in 100 mL of distilled water to obtain 20 m*M* phosphate buffer, 5.4 m*M* KCl, pH 7.4, 274 m*M* NaCl.
2. 4 *M* NaCl.
3. Tween-20.
4. Prepare 1X detection buffer by using the dissolved tablets and the concentrated buffers. 1X detection buffer: 10 m*M* phosphate buffer, 2.7 m*M* KCl, 500 m*M* NaCl, and 0.05% Tween-20.
5. Streptavidin-R-phycoerythrin (1 mg/mL) (Molecular Probes, OR). Prepare a 50 μg/mL solution in detection buffer.
6. 0.1*N* NaOH.
7. Epifluorescence microscope equipped with a 100-W mercury lamp (BH2, Olympus, France).
8. Chilled charge-coupled device (CCD) camera (HAMAMATSU, France).
9. Image analysis software (Morphostar, Imstar, France).

3. Methods

3.1. DNA Extraction

Prepare high-molecular-weight DNA from cell lines and biopsies by standard proteinase K digestion and phenol–chloroform extraction (*see* **Note 4**).

3.2. Generation of the Targets

1. In a 500-μL PCR reaction tube, mix 250 ng of extracted DNA (cell line, patient sample), 2 U of *Taq* DNA polymerase, and 12 pmol of each amplification primer (P-ras1 and Bio-ras2). Add dNTP solutions to obtain a 200 μ*M* final concentra-

tion and 5 μL of 10X *Taq* buffer. Immediately transfer the 50-μL reaction volume in a Gradient T system and perform 32 cycles of amplification (*see* **Note 5**).

2. Check the specificity of amplicons by analyzing 1 μL of product with the DNA 1000 kit and the BioAnalyzer 2100.
3. Generate single-strand DNA by digesting 20 μL of PCR product with 5 U of λ exonclease at 37°C for 30 min. Then, inactive the enzyme by incubating the reaction at 80°C for 10 min. Both reactions are performed consecutively on the Gradient T apparatus.

3.3. Specific Hybridization of the Targets

1. Carry out hybridization reactions in the microreaction chamber of the chip created by the packaging (4 × 5 × 1 mm).
2. Before the first use rehydrate the MICAM biochip at room temperature first with 20 μL of RNAse-DNAse-free water and then with 20 μL of hybridization buffer for 5 min each in the hybridization chamber.
3. After this step, it is important to prevent complete dessication of the silicon surface. Therefore, elimination of the buffers are performed by dripping the biochip on Kimwipes® Lite.
4. Perform hybridation in the 1X hybridation buffer with 4 μL of single-strand DNA (patients and cell lines studies) or 5 fmol of 5'biotinylated complementary synthetic oligonucleotide target. Add the 20-μL mix from **step 2** in the hybridization chamber and cover with a glass cover (14 mm in diameter).
5. Put the biochip in a closed Petri dish containing a humid paper and carry out the reaction for 30 min at 50°C in a temperature-controlled incubator.
6. After the incubation, remove the biochip from the Petri dish and wash with 500 μL of 1X washing buffer A at room temperature. Then, add 30 μL of 1X washing buffer B and incubate at 50°C for 3 min. Discard the buffer and drip on Kimwipes Lite.

3.4. Revelation of Perfect Duplexes

1. During the revelation step, it is neccessary to prevent direct illumination of the label: streptavidin-R-phycoerythrin.
2. Rinse the biochip with 200 μL of detection buffer.
3. Incubate the biochip for 3 min with 20 μL of detection buffer.
4. Add 20 μL of streptavidin-R-phycoerythrin in the reaction chamber, cover with a glass coverslip, and incubate in the dark at room temperature for 10 min.
5. After completion of the incubation, rinse the biochip with 500 μL of detection buffer.

3.5. Acquisition and Analysis of Signals

1. Apply 20 μL of detection buffer in the reaction chamber and check that the mixture covers the entire active surface. Place a coverslip, taking care to prevent the introduction of an air bubble and transfer rapidly to the image analysis station.

2. Identify in white light the position of the 128 electrodes.
3. Use a 10× objective to see all of the electrodes at the same time.
4. Use the specific phycoerythrin filters for correct excitation and emission wavelengths.
5. Illuminate the biochip and accumulate photons for 1 s.
6. Using the Morphostar software design and annotate, directly on the captured image, a mask containing 128 regions of interest; each region of interest corresponds strictly to the area of one electrode.
7. For each electrode, record the mean and the mode of fluorescent signals.
8. After analysis, regenerate the biochip by incubating the active surface with 20 μL of 0.1*M* NaOH for 1 min at room temperature.
9. Rinse several times with RNAse- and DNAse-free water.
10. Completely dessicate the active surface with argon.
11. Place the biochip in a sterile tube containing argon and store at 4°C until the next use.

4. Results and Discussion

In the course of the diagnosis of mutations, the ASO principle based on the prevention of hybridization by a single-base pair mismatch has been widely used ***(30,31)***. First, this approach relied on attached DNA and the membrane was the solid support. Now, the need for both microanalysis devices and multiparametric assays has prompted the emergence of oligonucleotide array formats. These types of support are theoretically compatible with ASO; nevertheless, because this approach requires experimental hybridization and wash stringencies, features like the quality of the surface-bound oligomer and the type of linkage between the oligonucleotide and the solid support are critical.

We have developed a new silicon oligomer array and applied it to the detection of *K-ras* gene mutations according to the ASO method.

4.1. Features of the Silicon Chip

The chip (*see* **Fig. 1A**) is a 10-mm^2 active multiplexed device containing 128 octogonal microelectrodes with 9 gold inputs/outputs. The 50-μm-wide microelectrodes are arranged in a rectangular matrix of 8 rows and 16 columns. Each electrode has its own unique address and could be selected individually. The silicon chip is integrated in a package (*see* **Fig. 1B**) compatible with both the electrocopolymerization step and the biological reactions. Concerning the geometry of the packaging, the T-shaped chip is easy to handle, and the micreaction chamber created is suitable for both the hybridization and detection steps. The amount of hybridizable oligonucleotides linked to the support is estimated to be 200 fmol/mm^2 ***(23)***. The copolymerization on the surface of gold electrodes results in the formation of an insoluble, homogeneous, thin film (20 nm thick) with a high chemical stability. In contrast with *in situ*

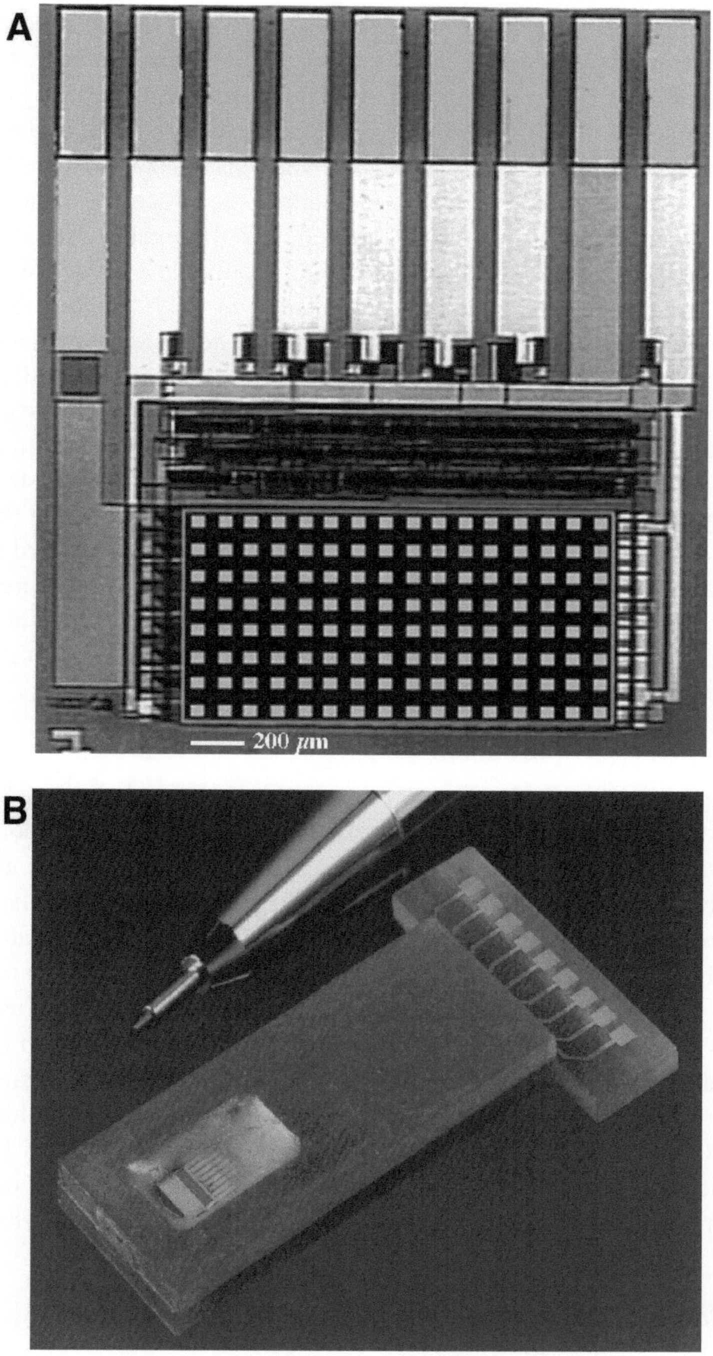

Fig. 1. **(A)** White-light-illuminated image of the multiplexed silicon chip; **(B)** view of a packaged chip.

synthesis strategies *(15)*, the developed postsynthesis grafting process allows the purification of pyrrole-labeled oligonucleotides before the addressing step, thus producing well-defined copolymers. Then, because the grafting process is integrated onto the chip, this technology is very flexible and the replacement of an oligonucleotide sequence by another is very easy. Thanks to the limitation of the film surface to the electrode, the addressing process was achieved by sequentially switching the different electrodes. With regard to the duration of the process, the synthesis of electroconjugated polymers is very fast because the oxidation of the monomer is accomplished in only one step. Moreover, cross-contamination during the successive copolymerizations are avoided by a washing step of the electrochemical cell and the electrode matrix, allowing the obtention of electrodes bearing only one specific oligonucleotide sequence.

The features of this covalent immobilization makes it possible to carry out hybridization and washing steps under high temperatures and salt stringencies (necessary when the ASO principle is used) without any alteration of the grafted oligonucleotides. These experimental conditions are neutral toward the polymer film and have no side effects on the packaging compounds. Moreover, the stability of the ODN–polypyrrole surface is also compatible with NaOH, and a regeneration of the ODN chip after a complete run (hybridization, washing, and detection) is possible without significant loss of signal.

4.2. A Dedicated K-ras Silicon Chip

In order to determine the *K-ras* codon 12 sequence, a dedicated *K-ras* silicon chip was designed (*see* **Fig. 2**) with a set of eight oligonucleotides (*see* **Table 2**) addressed to eight different gold microelectrodes. Seven allele-specific oligonucleotides displaying the wild-type (WT) or the six allelic versions of the *K-ras* codon 12 sequence were designed. The potential mismatched base is located in the middle of the oligonucleotide, as this is the least stable position for a base pair mismatch and the oligonucleotides are as short as possible (14 bases). Moreover, to check the quality of DNA extracted from colorectal cancer patients and the reliability of both amplification and hybridization steps, a positive control probe (PC) is added to the chip. The sequence of this probe is contained in the PCR-amplified sequence but outside codon 12 and 13. For all oligonucleotides, a 5' end decathymidine linker has been introduced to improve the oligonucleotide accessibility, which results in an increased hybridization signal.

4.3. Preliminary Studies on Oligonucleotide Hybridization

The ability of the silicon chip to detect known mutations is analyzed by using oligonucleotides as targets. The main steps of the process are described in **Fig. 3**. The assay is based on the allele-specific hybridization principle and

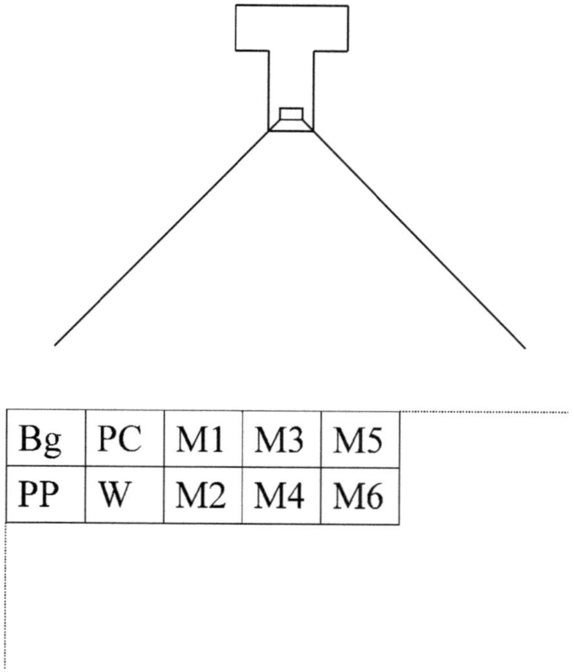

Fig. 2. Probe pattern of the K-ras DNA chip. PP: polypyrrole homopolymer; W: polypyrrole copolymer bearing the wild-type K-ras codon 12 sequence; M1–M6: polypyrrole copolymers with the six possible mutated sequences (M1–M3-first base, M4–M6-second base) on K-ras codon 12, PC: positive control, Bg: a nonpolymerized electrode used for background measurement.

Table 2
Sequence of the Probes Grafted onto the K-ras Silicon Chip

Probe name	Amino acid	Sequence
W	Gly	5' Py-$(T)_{10}$–GGA GCT **GGT** GGC GT 3'
M1	Ser	5' Py-$(T)_{10}$–GGA GCT **AGT** GGC GT 3'
M2	Arg	5' Py-$(T)_{10}$–GGA GCT **CGT** GGC GT 3'
M3	Cys	5' Py-$(T)_{10}$–GGA GCT **TGT** GGC GT 3'
M4	Asp	5' Py-$(T)_{10}$–GGA GCT **GAT** GGC GT 3'
M5	Ala	5' Py-$(T)_{10}$–TGG AGC T**GC** **T**GG CG 3'
M6	Val	5' Py-$(T)_{10}$–GGA GCT **GTT** GGC GT 3'
PC	Outside codon 12	5' Py-$(T)_{10}$–GCC TTG ACG ATA CAG CTA 3'

the aim is to find the hybridization/washing procedure allowing the detection of all seven possible sequences on codon 12 under the same operating conditions. Biotinylated oligonucleotides fully matched to those addressed to the

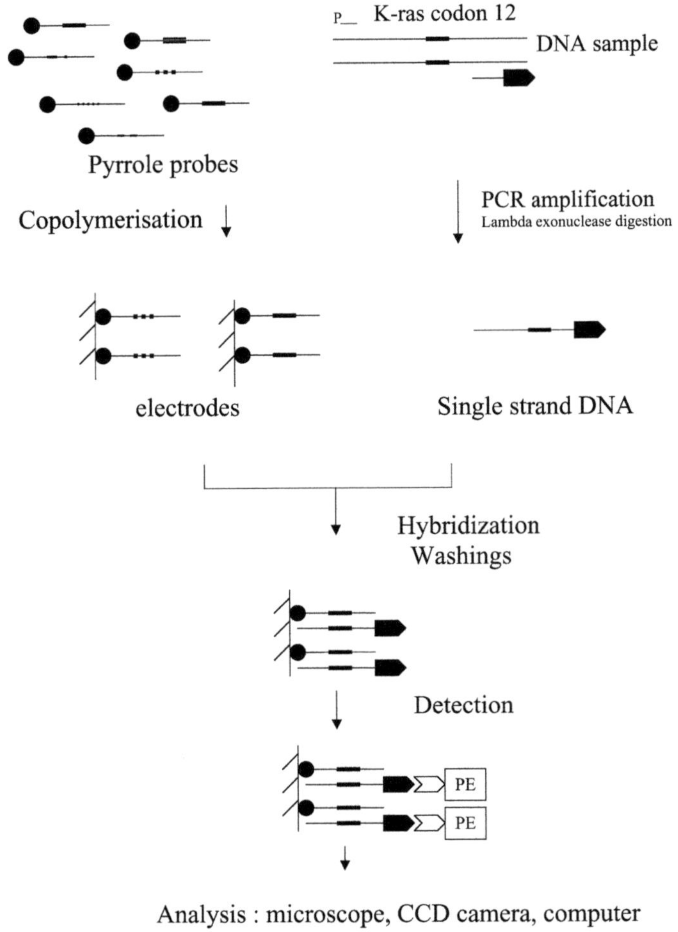

Fig. 3. Procedure for *K-ras* codon 12 mutation detection on the silicon chip. A portion of the *K-ras* gene encompassing the codon 12 sequence is amplified from the DNA sample by using two primers (one is biotin labeled ■▶, and the other is phosphate labeled [P]). Seven different oligonucleotide probes corresponding to the wild-type or mutated codon 12 sequence are addressed to individual gold microelectrodes by electrocopolymerization through their pyrrole extremity ●. The chip is then hybridized to a fraction of the single-strand DNA obtained by λ exonuclease digestion of the PCR product and washed. DNA duplexes are detected by streptavin-R-phycoerythrin [PE] labeling. The fluorescence emission is then analyzed through the use of a CCD camera connected to an image software (λ excitation: 500/550 nm; λ emission: 575 nm).

solid support are used in order to optimize the reaction parameters. First, 20-base-long oligonucleotides whose sequence had been previously optimized for the MUTA test ***(32)*** are copolymerized to the gold electrodes. Then, a reduc-

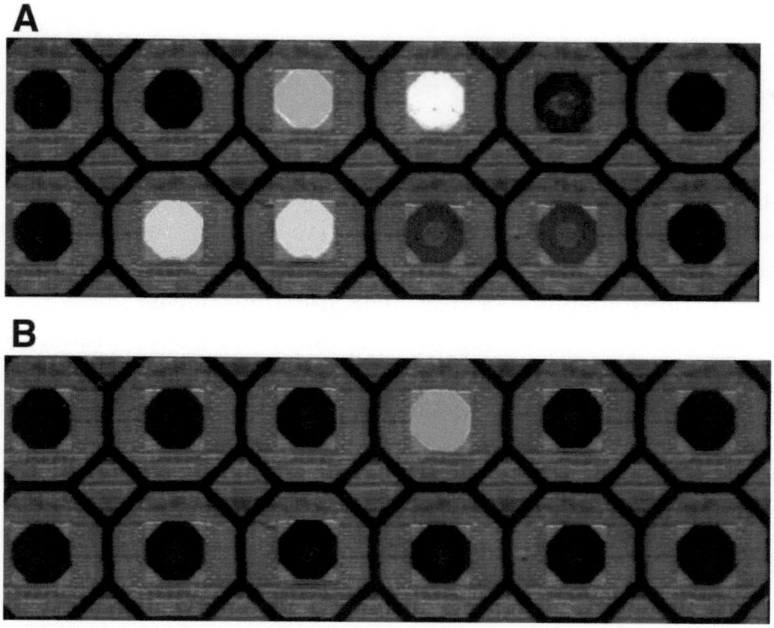

Fig. 4. Optimization of hybridization parameters on the K-ras silicon chip with biotinylated complementary oligonucleotides. The 14-base M3 biotionylated oligonucleotide probe was hybridized to the silicon chip and analyzed as described in **Subheadings 2.** and **3. (A)** Fluorescence signals under mild hybridization conditions; **(B)** fluorescence signal under optimal hybridization conditions.

tion of the length of the screening oligonucleotides (W_1, M1–M6) to 14 bases was made in order to increase the specificity. Hybridization of a particular oligonucleotide under mild conditions (low temperature: 37°C; high salt concentration: 0.5 mol/L Na^+) gives unspecific binding in addition to the annealing to the full-match sequence (*see* **Fig. 4A**). A correlation is found between the levels of fluorescence and the number of mismatches in the duplexes formed. The positive control (PC), whose sequence is outside the codon 12 region, produced no hybridization signal whatever the M1–M6 biotinylated probes was used. A 18-base-long sequence for the PC is kept in order to obtain a high-fluorescence signal that validated the entire process including PCR, hybridization, and detection. No nonspecific binding of the biotinylated oligonucleotide is observed on the nonaddressed gold microelectrode (Bg) or on the negative control electrode, which is composed of a homopolymer of pyrrole (PP). Better discrimination between codon 12 sequences is obtained when the hybridization temperature rose from 37 to 50°C, but an increase in temperature alone was not able to detect single-nucleotide mismatches. A specific hybridization is obtained with the introduction in the hybridization buffer of tetramethylammonium chloride at a final concentration of 1.8*M* (*see* **Fig. 4B**). Under these hybridization conditions, combining high temperature and an additive, a clear discrimination is made between a fully matched hybrid and a 1-bp-mismatched hybrid.

The detection limit is determined under mild hybridization conditions. We determined this value as the amount of biotinylated W probe allowing a mode fluorescence signal on the W electrode equal to twice the mode value on the PP electrode. Within the above-mentioned parameters, 0.1 fmol of W probe could be detected corresponding to a 10_{p}M detection limit range.

The characteristics of binding and accessibility of silicon-grafted ODN are similar to those observed using nylon membrane, because the optimal conditions allowing a perfect discrimination of mismatched duplexes are similar. The use of a product acting on the melting temperature ***(33)*** is especially efficient in equalizing duplex stabilities on both supports.

4.4. Characterization of the Assay With Cell Lines

In order to evaluate the ability of the methodology to analyze PCR products, amplicons are performed on genomic DNA from cell lines. A 117-bp-length DNA fragment was produced and its purity checked by agarose gel electrophoresis. Single-strand DNA was obtained by performing a symetric PCR with a 5'phosphorylated primer followed by a digestion with λ exonuclease. This approach results in the obtention of an intense fluorescent signal after hybridization. The operating conditions optimized on the basis of oligonucleotide hybridization are able to analyze homozygous (MiAPaCa-2 and SW620 cell lines) as well as heterozygous (LS 174T and SW 1116 cell lines) DNA.

The methodology described here does not require multiple steps subsequent to PCR (i.e., purification or postlabeling) to obtain reliable biological material. The amplicons to be analyzed are relatively short and are able to reassociate rapidly after heat denaturation, thus reducing hybridization efficiency. Several approaches have been described in order to generate single-strand DNA. Using asymmetric PCR ***(34)*** is not the best way because only relatively small amounts of single-strand DNA are produced under extensive optimization conditions. The use of T7 gene 6 exonuclease that digests 5' phosphorylated and 5' hydroxylated DNA, while blocked by phosphorothioate (*S*)-linkages, has been previously reported ***(35)***. Nevertheless, this method required modifications in the strand of interest by incorporation of sulfur bridges in one of the amplification primers. Lambda exonuclease ***(36)*** is able to convert double-strand amplified DNA to single strand and to enhance specific hybridization. This alternative is attractive because (1) the modification (5' phosphate residue) is

Table 3
Determination of Sensitivity on the Silicon DNA Chip

DNA sample ratio (MiaPaCa-2/LNCap)	Modal value of the fluorescent signal (UF)			
	M3 electrode	W electrode	PP electrode	Mx electrode[a]
100/0	136	28	24	22
50/50	85	79	25	24
25/75	70	90	23	23
15/85	58	120	27	25
10/90	42	129	24	25
5/95	27	141	25	23

[a]The values correspond to the mean of the signals from M1, M2, M4, M5, and M6 electrodes. Signal on the Bg electrode is 23 UF.

Table 4
***K-ras* codon 12/codon 13 Sequence of DNA From 75 Colorectal Cancer Patients Analyzed by Direct Sequencing**

Codon 12[a]							Codon 13[a]	
W[b]	**M1**	**M2**	**M3**	**M4**	**M5**	**M6**	**W**	**M4**
GGT	**A**GT	**C**GT	**T**GT	G**A**T	G**C**T	G**T**T	GGC	G**A**C
54	2	0	3	7	1	8	72	3

[a]Nucleotides in bold are the mutated nucleotides.
[b]W, wild type.

not in the hybridizable strand, (2) the production of single strand is very efficient, and (3) this approach can be applied to the multiplex PCR.

The sensitivity of the method is investigated by reconstructing samples with various dilutions of mutant DNA (MIA PaCa-2 cell line) in wild-type DNA (LnCap cell line). The first sensitivity was determined by mixing DNA in prior PCR. The generated symetric amplicons are then digested with λ exonuclease and hybridized to the chip. A K-ras mutated sequence is still unambiguously detected when the MiAPaCa-2 cell line represented only 10% of the initial material: a mode value of 42 UF on the M3 electrode (*see* **Table 3**). The background value was 23 UF.

4.5. Genotyping Human Colorectal DNA Samples

To demonstrate the reliability of the procedure, a study is conducted blind on DNA from 75 different patients with colorectal cancer. **Table 4** shows the

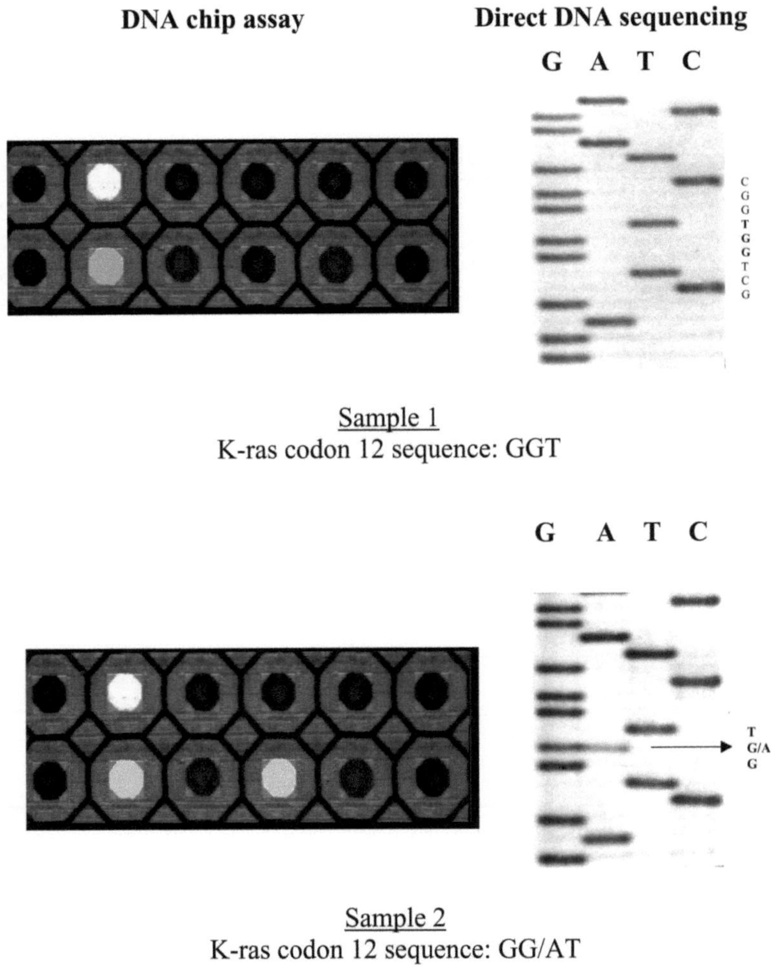

Fig. 5. Diagnosis of *K-ras* codon 12 mutations on human colorectal samples by both DNA chip assay and direct sequencing.

characteristics of human tumoral samples in term of exon 1 (codon 12, codon 13) K-ras sequence obtained by direct PCR product sequencing. Thirty-two percent of patients have an exon 1 K-ras mutation and 87.5% of the mutations are codon 12 alterations. The only K-ras codon 13-mutated allele found corresponded to GGC (Gly) → GAC (Asp). The genotypes scored by the polypyrrole DNA chip assay were 100% in agreement with conventional DNA sequencing results. All of the *K-ras* codon 12 mutations detected by direct sequencing were positive by polypyrrole DNA chip analysis and no false-positive result was obtained with the developed methodology. Moreover, three patients displayed a *K-ras* codon 13 mutation detected by direct sequencing and no nonspecific hybridization signal was observed on the electrodes corresponding to *K-ras* codon 12-mutated sequences. **Figure 5** shows an example of the data obtained from direct sequencing and DNA chip analysis for a wild-type (GGT) and a mutated (GG/AT) DNA.

5. Conclusion

The process of pyrrole copolymerization with biomolecules leads to the synthesis of polymer films bearing biological molecules such as oligonucleotides that can be addressed on the surface of a given electrode belonging to an array of microelectrodes. The easy electrosynthesis of polypyrrole films and their high chemical stability makes these materials very attractive candidates for biological arrays. Especially, their use allowed the detection of *K-ras* oncogene mutations on DNA samples providing from patients with colorectal cancer.

The hybridization allele-specific mutation detection method on the chip using the same process steps over the entire array is rapid. The cinetic reactions are fast, as the volume of reactions performed in the microchamber is low: 10 μL. Starting from genomic DNA, the detection of point mutations can be acccomplished within less than 4 h. Studies are performed in order to develop an automatic station for the hybridization and analysis steps.

The developed DNA chip based on electrocopolymerization on gold electrodes gives a support with a low autofluorescence, this allows the detection of less than 10% of mutated sequences within a mixed population of mutant/wild type sequences. This criterion is particularly important for studies in the oncology field. The direct sequencing performed with radioactive incorporation allows a sensitivity of around 15%, whereas this value is in the 5% range for our previously reported MUTA test ***(37)*** using tubes as solid support and serial hybridizations.

In order to cover the detection of the totality of *K-ras* mutations, it is possible to add screening probes for codons 13 and 61. Moreover, because 128 electrodes are available, we can expect to analyze other genes of interest whose mutations are implicated in cancer. The unambiguous discrimination among the seven potential alleles in the same region suggests that this technology may be useful in multiallelic gene analysis.

Moreover, the 3' end of the grafted ODN is free and extension by polymerases of the fixed ODN could be envisaged.

Finally, a quantitative application of the silicon device we have developed is conceivable because the amount of the grafted ODN is perfectly controlled.

6. Notes

1. Probes to be grafted are labeled at the 5' end with a pyrrole residue using previously described pyrrole–phosphoramidite building blocks and tailed with a $(T)_{10}$

spacer arm *(23)*. The chips are made using microelectronic technologies on a silicon support *(38)*. Electrosynthesis of polypyrrole films are carried out by potential sweeping between 0.35 and 0.85 V/SCE (saturated calomel electrode) in a solution containing both monomers of pyrrole and pyrrole-labeled oligonucleotides as previously described *(23)*. After reception and until use, store the MICAM® biochip under argon at +4°C.

2. The *K-ras* codon 12 sequence for each cell line was checked by standard direct automatic fluorescent sequencing.
3. Samples *(32)* from normal mucosa or tumor regions were selected macroscopically by the anathomopathologist and then immediately frozen in liquid nitrogen before nucleic acid extraction.
4. DNA extraction is performed as previously described *(37)*.
5. Amplification conditions: 32 cycles at 94°C for 30 s, 55°C for 30 s, and 72°C for 30 s.

References

1. Fujiyama, S., Tanaka, M., Maeda, S., et al. (2002) Tumor markers in early diagnosis, follow-up and management of patients with hepatocellular carcinoma. *Oncology* **62,** 57–63.
2. Numa, F., Umayahara, K., Suehiro, Y., et al. (2001) New molecular tumor markers for endometrial cancer. *Hum. Cell.* **14,** 272–274.
3. Fearon, E. R. (1993) K-ras gene mutation as a pathogenetic and diagnostic marker in human cancer. *J. Natl. Cancer Inst.* **15,** 1978–1980.
4. Kondo, H., Sugano, K., Fukayama, N., et al. (1994) Detection of point mutations in the K-ras oncogene at codon 12 in pure pancreatic juice for diagnosis of pancreatic carcinoma. *Cancer* **73,** 1589–1594.
5. Smith, G., Carey, F. A., Beattie, J., et al. (2002) Mutations in APC, Kirsten-ras, and p53 alternative genetic pathways to colorectal cancer. *Proc. Natl. Acad. Sci. USA* **99,** 9433–9438.
6. Bazan, V., Migliavacca, M., Zanna, I., et al. (2002) Specific codon 13 K-ras mutations are predictive of clinical outcome in colorectal cancer patients, whereas codon 12 K-ras mutations are associated with mucinous histotype. *Ann. Oncol.* **13,** 1438–1446.
7. Schimanski, C. C., Linnemann, U., and Berger, M. R. (1999) Sensitive detection of K-ras mutations augments diagnosis of colorectal cancer metastases in the liver. *Cancer Res.* **59,** 5169–5175.
8. Sidransky, D., Tokino, T., Hamilton, S. R., et al. (1992) Identification of ras oncogene mutations in the stool of patients with curable colorectal tumors. *Science* **256,** 102–105.
9. Hashimoto, T., Kobayashi, Y., Ishikawa, Y., et al. (2000) Prognostic value of genetically diagnosed lymph node micrometastasis in non-small cell lung carcinoma cases. *Cancer Res.* **60,** 6472–6478.
10. Hibi, K., Robinson, C. R., Booker, S., et al. (1998) Molecular detection of genetic alterations in the serum of colorectal cancer patients. *Cancer Res.* **58,** 1405–1407.

11. Bugawan, T. L., Begovich, A. B., and Erlich, H. A. (1990) Rapid HLA-DPB typing using enzymatically amplified DNA and nonradioactive sequence-specific oligonucleotide probes. *Immunogenetics* **32,** 231–241.
12. Hacia, J. G. (1999) Resequencing and mutational analysis using oligonucleotide microarrays. *Nature Genet.* **21,** 42–47.
13. Southern, E. M. (1996) High-density gridding: techniques and applications. *Curr. Opin. Biotechnol.* **7,** 85–88.
14. Guo, Z., Guilfoyle, R. A., Thiel, A. J., et al.(1994) Direct fluorescence analysis of genetic polymorphisms by hybridization with oligonucleotide arrays on glass supports. *Nucleic Acids Res.* **22,** 5456–5465.
15. Fodor, S. P. A., Read, J. L., Pirrung, M. C., et al. (1991) Light-directed, spatially addressable parallel chemical synthesis. *Science* **251,** 767–773.
16. Matson, R. S., Rampal, J., Pentoney, S. L., et al. (1995) Biopolymer synthesis on polypropylene support: oligonucleotide arrays. *Anal. Biochem.* **224,** 110–116.
17. Khrapko, K. A., Lysos, Y., Khorlin, A., et al. (1989) Hybridization of oligonucleotides as a method of DNA sequencing. *FEBS Lett.* **256,** 118–122.
18. Livache, T., Fouque, B., Roget, A., et al. (1998) Polypyrrole DNA chip on a silicon device: example of hepatitis C virus genotyping. *Anal. Biochem.* **15,** 188–194.
19. Pease, A. C., Solas, D., Sullivan, E. J., et al. (1994) Light-generated oligonucleotide arrays for rapid DNA sequence analysis. *Proc. Natl. Acad. Sci. USA* **24,** 5022–5026.
20. Yershov, G., Barsky, V., Belgovskiy, A., et al. (1996) DNA analysis and diagnostics on oligonucleotide microchips. *Proc. Natl. Acad. Sci. USA* **14,** 4913–4918.
21. Livache, T., Bazin, H., and Mathis, G. (1998) Conducting polymers on microelectronic devices as tools for biological analyses. *Clin. Chim. Acta* **278,** 171–176.
22. Livache, T., Bazin, H., Caillat, P., et al. (1998) Electroconducting polymers for the construction of DNA or peptide arrays on silicon chips. *Biosens. Bioelectron.* **15,** 629–634.
23. Livache, T., Roget, A., Dejean, E., et al. (1994) Preparation of a DNA matrix via an electrochemically directed copolymerization of pyrrole and oligonucleotides bearing a pyrrole group. *Nucleic Acids Res.* **11,** 2915–2921.
24. Wu, D. Y., Ugozzoli, L., Pal, B. K., et al. (1989) Allele-specific enzymatic amplification of β-globin genomic DNA for diagnosis of sickle cell anemia. *Proc. Natl. Acad. Sci. USA* **86,** 2757–2760.
25. Deng, G. A. (1988) Sensitive non-radioactive PCR-RFLP analysis for detecting point mutations at the 12th codon of oncogene c-Ha-ras in DNAs of gastric cancer. *Nucleic Acids Res.* **16,** 6231.
26. Holland, P. M., Abramson, R. D., Watson, R., et al. (1991) Detection of specific polymerase chain reaction product by utilizing the 5'–3' exonuclease activity of *Thermus aquaticus* DNA polymerase. *Proc. Natl. Acad. Sci. USA* **88,** 7276–7280.
27. Syvanen, A. C., Aalto-Setala, K., Harju, L., et al. (1990) A primer-guided nucleotide incorporation assay in the genotyping of apolipoprotein E. *Genomics* **8,** 684–692.

28. Bos, J. L., Verlaan de Vries, M., Jansen, A. M., et al. (1984) Three different mutations in the codon 61 of the human N-ras gene detected by synthetic oligonucleotide hybridization. *Nucleic Acids Res.* **12,** 9155–9163.
29. Landegren, U. (1993) Ligation-based DNA diagnostics. *Bioessays* **15,** 761–765.
30. Conner, B. J., Reyes, A. A., Morin, C., et al. (1983) Detection of sickle cell beta S-globin allele by hybridization with synthetic oligonucleotides. *Proc. Natl. Acad. Sci. USA* **80,** 278–282.
31. Iitia, A., Mikola, M., Gregersen, N., et al. (1994) Detection of a point mutation using short oligonucleotide probes in allele-specific hybridization. *Biotechniques* **17,** 566–573.
32. Lopez-Crapez, E., Chypre, C., Saavedra, J., et al. (1997) Rapid and large-scale method to detect K-ras gene mutations in tumor samples. *Clin. Chem.* **43,** 936–942.
33. Nguyen, H. K., Fournier, O., Asseline, U., et al. (1999) Smoothing of the thermal stability of DNA duplexes by using modified nucleosides and chaotropic agents. *Nucleic Acids Res.* **27,** 1492–1498.
34. Tombline, G., Bellizzi, D., and Sgaramella, V. (1996) Heterogeneity of primer extension products in asymmetric PCR is due both to cleavage by a structure-specific exo/endonuclease activity of DNA polymerases and to premature stops. *Proc. Natl. Acad. Sci. USA* **93,** 2724–2728.
35. Nikiforov, T. T., Rendle, R. B., Kotewicz, M. L., et al. (1994) The use of phosphorothioate primers and exonuclease hydrolysis for the preparation of single-stranded PCR products and their detection by solid-phase hybridization. *PCR Methods Appl.* **3,** 285–291.
36. Mitsis, P. G. and Kwagh, J. G. (1999) Characterization of the interaction of lambda exonuclease with the ends of DNA. *Nucleic Acids Res.* **27,** 3057–3063.
37. Sambrook, J., Fritsch, E. F., and Maniatis, T. (1989) In: *Molecular Cloning: A Laboratory Manual,* Analysis and cloning of eukaryotic genomic DNA. (Nolan, C., ed.), Cold Spring Harbor Laboratory Press, Cold Spring Harbor, New York, pp. 9–16.
38. Caillat, P., David, D., Belleville, M., et al. (1999) Biochips on CMOS: an active matrix address array for DNA analysis. *Sensors Actuators B* **61,** 154–162.

25

Microarray-Based CGH in Cancer

Ekaterina Pestova, Kim Wilber, and Walter King

1. Introduction

The detection of chromosome imbalances in malignancies has been a popular and useful approach in understanding key genetic loci and the molecular pathways of carcinogenesis. Alterations in gene dosage constitutes a major mechanism that leads to an imbalance in the gene products of oncogenes or tumor suppressor genes, resulting in the loss of normal cell division. One of the more robust technologies employed for determining alterations in gene dosage has been termed "comparative genomic hybridization" (CGH). CGH is a method that measures relative DNA copy differences between hybridized test DNA labeled with one fluorophore and reference DNA labeled in a spectrally distinct fluorophore. It was developed over a decade ago by Kallioniemi et al., who applied it to the study of copy number changes, in cancer cell lines and bladder tumors *(1)*. Two limitations of CGH technology are the inability to detect balanced changes, such as translocations and inversions, and the necessity for tumor purity (≥ 80%). Collectively, CGH studies done over the past decade have demonstrated that certain regions are more frequently altered. Moreover, the patterns of alterations seen in different cancers are not the same. As tumors progress, the frequency of copy number changes increase so that as much as 50% of the genome of solid tumors can be aberrant. Most of these changes are secondary effects because of the cell's inability to replicate and segregate its chromosomes in a normal fashion. The goal of CGH and other molecular techniques is to identify those genes that are key initiators of these events. Achieving this goal would not only aid in the understanding of the mechanism of specific cancers but would also provide valuable information for early diagnosis and, perhaps, effective treatment. In this regard, a major limitation of conventional CGH is that resolution is limited to about 5–10 Mb.

From: *Methods in Molecular Medicine, vol. 97: Molecular Diagnosis of Cancer*
Edited by: J. E. Roulston and J. M. S. Bartlett © Humana Press Inc., Totowa, NJ

The application of CGH technology to genomic microarrays (array CGH or matrix CGH) containing hundreds to thousands of large-insert DNA clones contained in artificial chromosomes, such as BACs, PACs, or P1s has improved both the resolution and speed of analysis. A recent publication by Beheshti et al. provides an overview of published methods used in CGH microarrays *(2)*. This key technology improvement was introduced by Pinkel et al. in their study of breast tumors *(3)*. In this seminal study, the investigators performed fine mapping of regions of gain or loss in the 20q region utilizing genomic microarrays. This region was reported to be amplified in both breast and ovarian tumors and breast cancer cell lines and was associated with a poor prognosis *(4,5)*. The improved resolution of microarrays identified several distinct regions of gains and losses not detected by conventional CGH. A more complex pattern of changes emerged from this study, demonstrating not only the boundaries and structure of regions but that multiple regions may be involved in breast cancer. There are other "hot spots" of copy number aberrations such as the q arm of chromosome 17, where copy number abnormalities are frequently associated with a number of solid tumors. The extent of copy number changes in gene-rich regions could provide a mechanistic explanation for tumor behavior and predict response to therapy. Similar approaches using CGH on cDNA arrays have been utilized in head and neck, breast, and nasopharyngeal carcinomas *(6–9)*. In each of these reports, the investigators examined the relationship between structural and functional changes by performing parallel microarray measurements of genomic copy alterations and expression levels. The consensus conclusion was that DNA copy number changes showed a highly correlative pattern with expression levels and that widespread DNA copy number alterations can lead directly to deregulation of gene expression.

Although microarray CGH technology can be applied in establishing a pattern of amplifications associated with cancer, a similar study examined the loss of a tumor suppressor gene, NF2, on 22q12, in Schwannomas. Specifically, investigators employed a tiling strategy to map the region of deletion and also establish a correlation between the extent of deletion and phenotype in 116 patients with different disease phenotypes *(10)*. The severe form of the disease has an early onset and patients contract other neurological tumors such as meningiomas, ependymomas, and astrocytomas. Studies employing other technologies seem to suggest a correlation between genotype and disease phenotype. However, the results of this study did not support this conclusion.

Profiling copy number changes with labeled genomic DNA from formalin fixed tissue or cell samples makes array CGH particularly well suited for this most widely accessible of clinical materials, permitting rapid correlations of observed changes with outcome data, such as survival, metastatic disease, and response to therapy. Additionally, changes can be correlated with disease stage and tumor grade, providing a molecular pathology fingerprint or classification of cancer types ***(11)***. Efforts are currently directed at determining whether these new classification modalities can translate into better disease treatments and outcomes.

Although most of the interest in multiplex analysis of solid tumors has centered on expression arrays and, more recently, protein expression, it is a fundamental tenet that copy number changes in specific chromosome regions is a frequent event and a major driver of carcinogenesis. Gaining an understanding of those changes will be an effort that is likely to broaden our understanding of the differences in cancers of the same or different type. With DNA being far more stable and accessible in archived tissue specimens than RNA, microarray CGH technology provides significant advantages in the identification of important targets for therapeutic development and disease management. To that end, it is the purpose of this chapter to detail the fundamental methodologies behind microarray-based CGH and to highlight important aspects for its implementation.

1.1. Print Stock Production

Consistent quality of isolated clone DNA is critical for reproducible experimental results. Genomic DNA clones are propagated in single-copy vectors, such as BACs, PACs, or P1s, that yield relatively small amounts of DNA from liquid culture. The DNA isolation method should minimize bacterial host DNA contamination and remove the majority of RNA. Manual alkaline-based procedures and column methods can be used; however, robotic DNA isolation, using an Autogen™, generates the most consistent DNA quality, especially when working with large numbers of clones. Spectrophotometry can be used for quantitation; however, fluorometry, which is not as sensitive to the presence of RNA or impurities in the DNA, is a more reliable means of quantitation. The isolated clone DNA itself can be printed; however, print stocks consisting of polymerase chain reaction (PCR) products representing the individual clones perform much more reproducibly.

1.2. Array Printing

There are numerous factors that affect the reproducibility of microarray printing, many of which need to be optimized for the individual arraying system. These include the type of arrayer, print pins, slide surface, spotting solution, temperature, and humidity. For genomic clone arrays, it is preferable to print the clones as close as possible to minimize the amount of required Cot-1 blocking DNA. Most arrayers use split pins that draw the solution up by capillary action and deposit nanoliter amounts of DNA per spot. Cleanliness and calibration of the pins are critical for the consistent spotting and robust hybridization results. Spotting solutions typically are 3X SSC, and 20–50% dimethyl sulfoxide (DMSO). DMSO denatures the DNA, resulting in improved surface binding, and the single-stranded nature can make the DNA more available for hybridization. In order to maximize signal-to-noise ratios, the degree of background fluorescence contributed by the slide itself should be minimal. Printing can be done on poly-L-lysine, amino-silane, or reflective-surface glass slides (listed in order of decreasing background fluorescence). Temperature and humidity have a significant impact on spot morphology, spot size, and DNA binding. Optimal conditions commonly are approx 22°C and 45% relative humidity. Typically, spot diameters range from 100 to 200 μm with 120- to 250-μm center-to-center spacing.

1.3. Genomic DNA Extraction

The size and purity of the extracted genomic DNA are essential for obtaining reproducible results with high sensitivity and specificity. The protocols in this chapter are optimized for genomic DNA extraction from blood and cultured cells, and they produce relatively intact, high-molecular-weight DNA. DNA that is heavily contaminated with other cellular components, or significantly degraded, will not label uniformly in random priming reactions, resulting in poor microarray hybridizations. For example, formaldehyde-fixed tissues may require experimentation to find the best extraction method prior to labeling the DNA. Several protocols optimized for DNA extraction from formalin-embedded tissues have been reported in the literature. Although most of the protocols have been optimized for PCR-based applications ***(12)***, several protocols have been applied to conventional CGH ***(13)*** and microarray CGH analysis ***(14)***. Conventional protocols for isolation of DNA from paraffin sections include removal of paraffin with xylene extraction at elevated temperatures (55°C), followed by proteinase K digestion, protein precipitation and/or phenol–chlorophorm extraction, and DNA precipitation. DNA yields from paraffin-embedded tissues depend both on the size and the age of the sample processed, as well as on the tissue-fixation conditions, digestion time, and storage ***(15)***. Reduced yields compared to fresh or frozen tissues are to be expected.

For fresh and frozen tissue specimens, blood, and cultured cells, Gentra Puregene™ DNA isolation kits are recommended for genomic DNA extraction. Depending on the tissue source, different kits and/or protocols may have to be used to prepare DNA adequate for microarray analysis. It is important to remember that the tissue sample should contain 80% or more tumor cells for CGH technology to detect single copy gains or losses. Therefore, microdissection may be necessary. For frozen tumors, use of stains such as Histogene™, which permits the identification of tumor cells while preserving the integrity of nucleic acids, have been used to aid in dissection ***(16)***. For isolation of DNA from small amounts of cultured cells, Gentra PureGene D-5500A (2×10^8 cells/g tissue) or D-5000A (8×10^8 cells/4 g tissue) kits are recommended. Protocol 2.5 for the extraction of chromosomal DNA from blood utilizes Gentra PureGene™ DNA Isolation KitD5000.

Upon the completion of the genomic DNA extraction protocol, quality and amount of the purified DNA should be assessed by measuring the absorbance ($A_{260/280}$) or by taking a fluorometry reading using Hoechst H33258 dye according to the manufacturer's protocol. Once the DNA concentration is calculated, a working solution at 25 ng/μL is made in 10 m*M* Tris-HCl and 1 m*M* EDTA, pH 7.4–8.0. The quality of the genomic DNA preparation is also assessed on a 0.8% agarose gel. For optimal results, isolated genomic DNA should be of a high molecular weight (>10 kb) and free of protein and RNA.

1.4. Labeling of Genomic DNA

For microarray CGH analysis, equal amounts of test DNA and normal reference DNA are labeled with Cy3- and Cy5-tagged nucleotides, respectively, by direct incorporation methods. By convention, target (sample) DNA is labeled with Cy3, whereas the reference DNA is labeled with Cy5. Several methods have been described in the literature for the preparation of labeled probe for microarray CGH analysis, including nick translation ***(3)***, random priming ***(17–19)***, and polymerase chain reaction (PCR)-based methods such as ligation-mediated PCR ***(20)*** and DOP-PCR ***(14)***. Random primer labeling is the preferred procedure for probe preparation samples when sample DNA amounts are not limiting. A random priming protocol for 100-μL reaction volumes with 100 ng input DNA is described below in **Subheading 3.6.** The GenoSensor Random Priming DNA labeling kit (Vysis, Inc) or BioPrime® DNA Labeling Kit (Invitrogen Life Technologies) is recommended for this procedure as a source of random octamer primers and Klenow enzyme. Labeled nucleotides (Cy3™ dCTP and Cy5™ dCTP) from Perkin-Elmer or Amersham could be used and have shown equivalent performance on microarrays. Random priming methods utilized by different laboratories may vary in the techniques used to reduce the size of genomic fragments prior to labeling. For example, restriction digest of the genomic DNA can be performed prior to random priming ***(21)***. In the protocol given in this chapter, labeled chromosomal DNA is digested by DNase I after labeling to reduce the size of the fragments to approx 200–800 bp. To remove unincorporated nucleotides and concentrate samples after labeling, reactions are precipitated twice with ethanol. To improve the recovery of the labeled DNA, a precipitation agent such as linear acrylamide, glycogen, RNA, or DNA is added. Alternatively, MicroSpin™ S-200 HR Columns

(Amersham Biosciences, cat. no. 27-5120-01) may be utilized instead of the first ethanol–salt precipitation.

1.5. Microarray Hybridization

The process of hybridization involves denaturation of probe DNA and hybridization of labeled probe in the presence of unlabeled Cot-1 DNA, which suppresses probe hybridization to highly repetitive sequences. Equal amounts of labeled target and reference DNA are mixed with a hybridization solution (50% formamide/2X SSC/10% dextran sulfate/Cot-1 DNA). Formamide, a chaotrope that lowers the melting point of duplexed nucleic acids *(22)*, is used to denature the labeled probe. The amount of each labeled probe used in hybridization is 2–4 μg in a 30-μL volume. The protocol herein is optimized for CGH microarrays with approx 1000 features arrayed over an area of approx 42 mm^2. The amount of probe and the final hybridization volume could be scaled up when using higher-density microarrays covering a larger spotting area. Because of the high complexity of both the probe and target, hybridization is carried out for 2–3 d. Mixing by gentle rocking was demonstrated to facilitate hybridization and is used in research laboratories *(3)*. After hybridization, microarrays are washed to remove unhybridized and nonspecifically bound probes. Washes can be performed in formamide-based buffers or aqueous washes could be applied to reduce time of the procedure. For an aqueous wash, slides are incubated for 4 min at 58°C in 1X SSC/0.1% NP-40, which is followed by a 4-min incubation in the 0.1X SSC/0.1% NP-40 jar at 58°C, a 1-min incubation at the room temperature in the 1X SSC, followed by a water rinse.

1.6. Microarray Analysis

Image acquisition for microarray analysis involves capturing or scanning the Cy3 and Cy5 signals on the microarray features (spots). To capture the slide image, either laser-based scanning systems or charge-coupled device (CCD)-based imagers are used. Scanning systems use narrow-band illumination (lasers) to excite the fluorophores and detect the resulting fluorescence with photomultiplier tube (PMT) detectors. To analyze dual-fluorophore samples, a scanning system can either excite and detect one color at a time (sequential scanning) or acquire both at once (simultaneous scanning) *(23)*. For example, one of the widely used commercial scanners, GenePix™ 4000 B Array Scanner (Axon Instruments Inc.), simultaneously reads at two excitation wavelengths (532 and 635 nm), and another popular scanning system, Packard BioScience's ScanArray™ Express, utilizes sequential scanning for up to five lasers. Microarray readers (e.g., GenoSensor™ Reader [Vysis, Inc.]) generally use wide-band illumination, such as a xenon lamp, and two or more excitation filters to give monochromatic illumination to the sample. A CCD is utilized to capture the resulting fluorescence *(24)*. The desired features of the reader system for CGH microarray imaging and analysis are maximal signal-to-noise ratio and linear dynamic range of the signal, minimal emission crosstalk between channels, and optimal image acquisition speed depending on the microarray spot density and desired throughput *(25)*. In addition to the properties of the reader hardware, the capacities of image analysis software supplied with a reader should be considered when choosing an image analysis platform.

Microarray image analysis requires correct identification of spots, subtraction of the background, calculation of ratios of target and reference signal intensities for individual spots, normalization to establish a fluorescence ratio baseline (the most representative ratio of the modal copy number of the sample DNA), and calculation of normalized ratios of target and reference signal intensities for each spot relative to the modal DNA copy number. Usually, microarray image data extraction software is supplied with a scanner, such as GenePix™ software (Axon Instruments Inc.), or QuantArray™ (Packard Biosciences). Several software packages integrate data acquisition, preprocessing, and analysis (GenoSensor™ analysis software [Vysis]). For the latest review of general microarray analysis tools, see the review by Holloway et al. *(26)*. In addition to these tools, image analysis and data processing packages are available from academic institutions, which are either specifically designed for array CGH analysis *(27)* or could be applied to array CGH analysis *(28)*.

1.7. Commercial Sources of Genomic DNA Microarrays

For those who would prefer to purchase ready-made microarray CGH components, kits, or microarray readers complete with analysis software, the GenoSensor System is available from Vysis (http://www.vysis.com). The GenoSensor Array 300 is a genomic array with 287 targets, spotted in triplicate, that include subtelomeric regions, microdeletions, oncogenes, and tumor suppressor genes. Next-generation, higher-density microarrays are under current development. A kit consisting of five microarrays together with preformulated hybridization buffer (cat. no. 32-801040) have been optimized for use with a labeling kit (cat. no. 32-801410). Together with the GenoSensor Reader, this system provides an alternative to custom array development. Spectral Genomics (http://www.spectralgenomics.com) is another vendor of whole-genome human BAC arrays. Arrays of 2- to 4-Mb resolution, spotted in duplicate, are available together as a complete hybridization system. The kit includes 2 arrays with 1003 nonoverlapping BAC clones from the RPCI BAC library spotted in duplicate, along with the necessary reagents and solutions for labeling and hybridization.

2. Materials

2.1. Clone DNA Isolation

1. Colony-purified stabs or glycerol stocks for clones of interest such as BAC, PAC, or P1s that contain large DNA inserts.
2. Luria broth (LB): 10 g tryptone, 5 g yeast extract, 10 g NaCl per liter (*see* **Note 1**).
3. 125-mL Baffled flasks.
4. Appropriate antibiotics (e.g., kanamycin or chloramphenicol).
5. 37°C Orbital shaker.
6. Autogen DNA isolation robot.
7. Autogen tube units.
8. Autogen reagent 1.
9. Autogen reagent 2.
10. Autogen reagent 3.
11. 70% and 100% Ethanol (EtOH).
12. Isopropyl alcohol.
13. TE: 10 m*M* Tris-HCl, pH 7.5, 1 m*M* EDTA.
14. 3*M* Sodium acetate (NaAc).
15. 2-mL capped tubes.
16. Centrifuge.
17. Speed-vac lyophilizer.
18. Fluorometer, such as Hoefer® DyNA Quant 200.
19. 10X TNE: 100 m*M* Tris-HCl, pH 7.4, 10 m*M* EDTA, 2*M* NaCl.
20. Hoechst H33258 dye (1 mg/mL in distilled water).
21. Pipettors.
22. Pipet tips.
23. 37°C Water bath.
24. 0.5-mL Snap-Cap tubes.
25. 10X React 2 buffer (Invitrogen).
26. *Hin*dIII restriction enzyme (10 U/mL) (Invitrogen).
27. 1% Agarose gel in 1X TAE containing EtBr at 0.5 mg/mL.
28. 50X TAE: 242 g Tris base, 57.1 mL glacial acetic acid, 100 mL of 0.5*M* EDTA (pH 8.0) per liter.
29. 6X Gel-loading buffer: 0.25% bromophenol blue, 0.25% xylene cyanol, 30% glycerol in H_2O.
30. 1-kb Ladder, ready-load (Gibco, cat. no. 10381-010).
31. Electrophoresis units, casting trays, combs, and power supplies.
32. Ultraviolet (UV) transilluminator.
33. Camera and film.

2.2. PCR Amplification of Clones

1. Gloves.
2. Pipettors.

3. Sterile, aerosol-resistant pipet tips.
4. 0.2-mL Polypropylene PCR 8-tube strips with separate 8-cap strips. Strips and caps should be free of RNase, DNase, DNA, pyrogens, and PCR inhibitors (Applied Biosystems, cat. nos. N801-0838 [tubes] and N801-0835 [caps]).
5. 0.5-mL Snap-Cap microcentrifuge tubes.
6. DNA Zap solutions 1 and 2 (Ambion, cat. no. 9890).
7. Multichannel calibrated pipettors (e.g., Matrix Technologies, 12.5 μL and 250 μL) (*see* **Note 2**).
8. *Mse*I restriction enzyme (10 U/μL) (New England BioLabs, cat. no. R0525S).
9. 10X One-Phor-All Buffer-Plus: 100 m*M* Tris-acetate (pH 7.5), 100 m*M* magnesium acetate, and 500 m*M* potassium acetate (Pharmacia, cat. no. 27-0901-02).
10. Primer 1: 5'TAACTAGCATGC resuspended to 100 μ*M* in TE.
11. Primer 2: 5' aminolinker AGTGGGATTCCGCATGCTAGT resuspended to 100 μ*M* in TE.
12. Sterile water (e.g., Milli-Q filtered and autoclaved).
13. 37°C Incubator.
14. PCR machine with a ramp rate that can reach 1.3°C/min. (e.g., Perkin-Elmer Gene Amp PCR System 9700).
15. T4-DNA ligase (5 U/μL) (Roche, cat. no. 799009).
16. 10X PCR buffer expanded long template 1 (Roche).
17. 3.5 U/μL expand long template PCR system (Roche).
18. 100 m*M* dNTP kits (Invitrogen, cat. no. 10297-018).
19. 100 m*M* ATP.
20. *Taq*/Pwo expanded long template polymerase (3.5 U/μL) (Roche).
21. 10X PE buffer II (without $MgCl_2$) (Perkin-Elmer).
22. 50 m*M* $MgCl_2$ (Perkin-Elmer).
23. AmpliTaq® (*Taq* polymerase, recombinant; 5 U/μL) (Invitrogen).

2.3. Preparation of Print Stocks

1. 45°C Oven.
2. Chilled 100% ethanol (EtOH).
3. 3*M* Sodium acetate (NaAc).
4. 70% Ethanol.
5. 20% Dimethyl sulfoxide (DMSO).

2.4. Array Printing

1. PCR print stocks representing desired clones.
2. 96-well or 384-well microtiter plates.
3. Arrayer.
4. Slides, such as Corning's CMT-GAP™ II or Nanofilm chrome-coated.
5. Stratalinker® UV crosslinker (Stratagene).

2.5. Genomic DNA Isolation From Blood

1. Vacutainer™ Sodium heparin blood collection tubes (Becton-Dickinson).
2. Gentra PURGENE DNA purification kit (cat. no. D5000).
3. Eppendorf phase lock gel tubes (cat. no. 0032007.961).
4. Pasteur pipet, glass.
5. Phenol equilibrated with buffer, pH 7.0.
6., Chloroform:Isoamyl alcohol (24:1).
7. Chilled 100% ethanol (EtOH).
8. 3*M* Sodium acetate (NaAc).
9. 70% Ethanol.
10. Isopropanol.
11. 15-mL Conical centrifuge tubes.
12. 10 m*M* Tris-HCl, pH 8.0.
13. 65°C Water bath.
14. Benchtop centrifuge (Beckman TJ-6 or equivalent).
15. Microcentrifuge.
16. 50 m*M* Sodium hydroxide.
17. Spectrophotometer.

2.6. Labeling of Genomic DNA

1. 2.5X Random primers (Vysis, cat. no. 32-801410).
2. dNTP mix (1.2 m*M* of each of dGTP, dATP, and dTTP and 0.8 m*M* of dCTP (Vysis cat. no. 32-801410).
3. 1 m*M* Cy3 dCTP, Cy5 dCTP (Amersham or PE Biosciences).
4. DNase I amp grade (Roche, Vysis, cat. no. 32-801410).
5. DNase dilution buffer (Vysis, cat. no. 32-801410).
6. Klenow enzyme (Vysis, cat. no. 32-801410).
7. DNase reaction buffer (Vysis, cat. no. 32-801410).
8. Male reference DNA (25 ng/μL) (Vysis, cat. no. 32-801410).
9. Female reference DNA (25 ng/μL) (Vysis, cat. no. 32-801410).
10. Stop buffer (0.5 *M* EDTA, pH 8.0) (Vysis. cat. no. 32-801410).
11. TE buffer, pH 7.4 (Vysis, cat. no. 32-801410).
12. 3*M* sodium acetate (Vysis, cat. no. 32-801410).
13. Precipitation reagent (Vysis, cat. no. 32-801410).
14. 100% EtOH.
15. 4°C Microcentrifuge.
16. 2-μL, 20-μL, 200-μL, and 1000-μL pipettors.
17. Vortex mixer.
18. 37°C Incubator.
19. 15°C, 37°C, and 100°C water baths.
20. DNase-free snap-lock 1.5-mL microcentrifuge tubes.
21. DNase-free aerosol-resistant pipet tips.
22. Powder-free gloves.

23. 2% Agarose gel in 1X TAE running buffer.
24. 6X Gel-loading buffer: 0.25% bromophenol blue, 0.25% xylene cyanol, 30% glycerol in H_2O.
25. 50-bp DNA ladder (Invitrogen, cat. no. 10416-014).

2.7. Hybridization of Labeled Probe to CGH Microarrays and Posthybridization Wash

1. Microarrays (Vysis, cat. no. 32-801040).
2. Hybridization coverslips (LifterSlip™; Erie Scientific Company, Vysis, cat. no. 32-801040).
3. Microarray hybridization buffer (Vysis, cat. no. 32-801040).
4. Coverslips, 18 mm (Corning, Vysis, cat. no. 32-801040).
5. Vortex mixer.
6. 37°C Incubator or heating block.
7. 45°C Slide warmer.
8. 80°C Water bath.
9. 0.5- or 1.5-mL Microcentrifuge tubes.
10. Fine-tip forceps.
11. 2-μL, 20-μL, and 200-μL pipettors.
12. Formamide.
13. Compressed filtered air.
14. Powder-free gloves.
15. 20X SSC.
16. 2X SSC/50% formamide wash. Mix thoroughly 105 mL formamide, 21 mL of 20X SSC, and 84 mL purified H_2O.
17. 1X SSC: Add 50 mL of 20X SSC to 950 mL purified H_2O.
18. 40°C Water bath.
19. Array DAPI solution (Vysis, cat. no. 32-801040).
20. Coplin jars with lids (Wheaton, cat. no. 900570).

3. Methods

3.1. Clone DNA Isolation

1. Inoculate 25 mL LB media in a 125-mL baffled flask containing kanamycin (25 mg/mL) or chloramphenicol (30 mg/mL) with cells from a single clone, using an inoculating loop to scrap cells from a colony-purified stab or glycerol stock.
2. Incubate flasks at 37°C for 16–18 h at 225 rpm in an orbital shaker.
3. Transfer 0.5–3 mL culture per each of six sections of an Autogen tube unit.
4. Fill the six reagent bottles according to manufacturer's instructions.
5. Clean reagent delivery tubes and prime pumps according to manufacturer's instructions.
6. Run program 4 for isolation of plasmid, cosmid, BAC, or PAC DNAs.
7. Upon completion of a run, pool six DNA suspensions (per clone) from a tube unit and transfer to a 2-mL centrifuge tube (approx 600 μL final volume).

8. Add 0.6 mL of 3 *M* NaAc, 1.5 mL of 100% EtOH; vortex and centrifuge at 12,000 rpm (approx 11,500*g*–13,000*g*) for 20–30 min at 4°C; carefully pour off supernatant.
9. Rinse pellet with 300 µL of 70% EtOH; centrifuge at 11,500*g*–13,000*g* for 5 min.
10. Carefully pour off supernatant or remove with a pipettor; briefly air-dry the pellet.
11. Thoroughly resuspend each clone in 100 µL TE.
12. For quantitation, prepare a sufficient amount of 1X TNE working solution with 1 µg/mL Hoechst dye, final concentration.
13. Calibrate the instrument against a 100-µg/mL standard according to the manufacturer's instructions.
14. For each clone, dilute 2 µL of isolated DNA into 2 mL of 1X TNE working solution and read concentration.
15. For each clone, remove 800 ng (or a maximum volume of 17 µL) of extracted DNA and transfer to a clean, 0.5-mL snap-cap tube. If necessary, add sterile water to a final volume of 17 µL. Add 2 µL of 10X reaction 2 buffer and 1 µL of *Hin*dIII enzyme. Digest DNA at least 2 h in a 37°C water bath.
16. Add 2 µL of 10X gel-loading buffer to entire digested DNA sample. Load entire volume into a single well of a 0.1% agarose gel and run overnight at 30 V against a 1-kb-ladder molecular-weight marker.
17. Do not continue with any DNA preparations that show significant contamination with host bacterial DNA, seen as a background smear of DNA in among the digested clone bands.

3.2. PCR Amplification of Clones

1. In order to reduce the opportunity for contamination events, all surfaces and pipettors should be cleaned with DNA Zap solutions according to manufacturer's instructions.
2. All reagents should be used exclusively for PCR. Use sterile, aerosol-resistant pipet tips and wear gloves at all times.
3. Dilute a sufficient amount of 10X One-Phor-All Buffer-Plus to a final concentration of 2X, store on ice.
4. Dilute a sufficient amount of *Mse*I enzyme to 0.4 U/mL with 10X One-Phor-All Buffer-Plus; store on ice.
5. To individual 0.5-mL tubes or 0.2-mL 8-strip PCR tubes, add 1.5 µL clone DNA (20–600 ng), 1 µL of 2X One-Phor-All Buffer-Plus, 1.5 µL sterile water, and 1 µL *Mse*I (0.4 U/µL). Incubate at 37°C overnight.
6. Based on the amount of input DNA, dilute *Mse*I-digested DNA to 1 ng/µL with sterile water.
7. Mix 1 ng (= 1 µL) of the digested DNA with 0.5 µL of 10X One-Phor-All-Buffer-Plus, 0.5 µL of 100 m*M* primer 1, 0.5 µL of 100 m*M* primer 2, and 5.5 µL sterile H_2O. Incubate the mixture at 65°C for 1 min in a PE9700 thermal cycler (or equivalent) and then ramp the temperature down to 15°C with a ramp speed of 1.3°C/min.

8. Make a sufficient quantity of 10 m*M* ATP by diluting 100 mM ATP 10-fold with sterile H_2O.
9. Keep ATP and T4 ligase on ice during addition to ligation reactions.
10. Once the temperature reaches 15°C (approx 45 min), pause the PCR program, place tubes on ice, and add 1 μL of 10 m*M* ATP and 1 μL T4-DNA ligase (5 U/μL). Return tubes to PCR machine and continue incubation at 15°C overnight.
11. Make a sufficient quantity of 10 m*M* dNTPs for both primary and secondary PCRs by diluting 100 m*M* stocks with sterile water (final of 2.5 m*M* each dNTP). Diluted dNTPs are stable at –20°C.
12. To each ligation reaction, add 3 μL of 10X PCR buffer expanded long template 1, 2 μL of 10 m*M* dNTPs, and 35 μL H_2O.
13. To melt off primer 2, incubate the reactions at 68°C for 4 min. Transfer the tubes to a clean area and add 1 μL expand long template PCR system (3.5 U/μL) to each tube. Change pipet tips after each addition. It is essential to swiftly add the polymerase mixture, recap, and place the tube immediately on ice to prevent significant reannealing of primer 2.
14. Return the tubes to the PCR machine and incubate under the following conditions: 68°C for 3 min, 94°C for 40 s, 57°C for 30 s, 68°C for 1 min, 15 s for 14 cycles, 94°C for 40 s, 57°C for 30 s, 68°C for 1 min, 45 s for 34 cycles, 94°C for 40 s, 57°C for 30 s, 68°C for 5 min, 4°C hold. The final 5-min incubation at 68°C will displace any reannealed primer 2 and extend the, now free, 3' ends.
15. Mix 3.5 μL each primary PCR reaction, 0.5 μL of 10X gel loading buffer, 1 μL sterile water. Run each mix on a 1% TAE gel containing 0.5 mg EtBr along with an appropriate molecular marker. Fragments should range in size from 70 to 1500 bp, with the majority of product between 200 and 800 bp.
16. For the secondary PCRs, mix, on ice, 1 μL of the primary PCR, 4 μL of primer 2, 10 μL of 10X PE buffer II (without $MgCl_2$), 2 μL of 10 m*M* dNTPs, 11 μL of 50 m*M* $MgCl_2$, 0.5 μL of AmpliTaq (2.5 U), and 71.5 μL of sterile water for each reaction.
17. Place tubes in the PCR machine and incubate under the following conditions: 95°C for 10 min, followed by 95°C for 30 s, 50°C for 30 s, and 72°C for 2 min for 45 cycles, 7 min at 72°C, followed by a 4°C hold. Yields range from 8 to 15 μg DNA/100 μL reaction, with each fragment containing a 5' aminolinker.

3.3. Preparation of Print Stocks

1. Reduce the volume of the secondary PCRs by about 50% to approx 50 μL by incubation at 45°C in an oven (such as a Techne Hybridizer HB-1D) for about 75 min.
2. Add 150 μL chilled 100% EtOH and 5 μL of 3 *M* NaAc to each tube. Chill at –20°C for 15 min. Centrifuge at 1700*g* for 90 min at 4°C.
3. Remove supernatant carefully with a pipettor. Add 150 μL of 70% EtOH to each tube and vortex until pellet comes loose. Centrifuge at 1700*g* for 45 min at 4°C.
4. Remove as much of the 70% EtOH as possible with a multichannel pipettor and air-dry pellets at room temperature for approx 90 min. Take care not to overdry the pellets or they will be difficult to resuspend.

5. Thoroughly resuspend each pellet in 15 μL of 20% DMSO. Store at –20°C.

3.4. Array Printing

1. Print stocks should be aliquoted into 96- or 384-well microtiter plates.
2. Duplicate or triplicate spotting of each clone increases confidence in hybridization results.
3. Slides must be handled with care and should be kept free of dust and fingerprints.
4. Load microtiter plate containing print stocks and print under previously established conditions.
5. Allow slides to dry in a dust-free area.
6. Bind DNA to slides by UV crosslinking at 65 mJ for 10–15 s using a Stratalinker (Stratagene, La Jolla, CA).
7. Printed slides should be stored in an airtight box at room temperature.

3.5. Genomic DNA Extraction From Blood

1. Collect whole blood in 10-mL green topped Vacutainer™ tubes.
2. Separate serum by centrifugation at 1000 rpm (approx 200*g*) for 10 min at room temperature in Beckman TJ-6 or equivalent centrifuge.
3. Using a glass Pasteur pipet, carefully withdraw the buffy coat cell layer. Measure the volume of the material collected and place in a fresh tube (1.5-mL microcentrifuge tube or 15-mL polypropylene conical tubes depending on the volume of the material).
4. Add three times the volume of RBC lysis solution, mix gently, and incubate 10 min at ambient temperature with intermittent gentle mixing.
5. Pellet white blood cells by centrifugation at 2000*g* for 10 min at room temperature, remove the supernatant.
6. Add 10 mL of the cell lysis buffer to the cell pellet. To facilitate cell lysis, mix the solution by pipetting up and down three to five times, or as necessary until the solution is homogenous. Samples are stable in the cell lysis solution for at least 18 mo at room temperature.
7. Add 50 mL of RNase A (4 mg/mL >80 U/mL) to the lysate and incubate at 37°C for 45 min; cool to room temperature.
8. Add 3.33 mL of protein precipitation solution, vortex vigorously for 20 s, cool on ice for 10 min, and pellet protein by centrifuging at 2000*g* for 10 min at room temperature.
9. Carefully pour the supernatant directly into a sterile conical tube containing 10 mL isopropanol and incubate for a few minutes to overnight prior to precipitation.
10. Precipitate DNA by centrifugation at 2000*g* for 5 min at room temperature, decant the supernatant, and invert the tube to drain residual isopropanol.
11. Wash the pellet with 10 mL of 70% ethanol at room temperature, precipitate at 2000*g* for 5 min at room temperature, invert the tube to dry the excess of ethanol, and allow to air-dry for 15–20 min, or until white DNA pellet becomes colorless (clear).

12. Resuspend the pellet in 0.833 mL of 10 m*M* Tris-HCl, pH 8.0 from 1 h to overnight at room temperature. To facilitate DNA resuspension, incubate at 65°C for 30 min to 1 h.
13. Determine the DNA concentration by spectophotometry (A_{260}) and/or by fluorometry, as described in **Subheading 3.1.** (*see* **Note 3**).
14. *Optional.* Extract DNA once with phenol and once with chloroform:isoamyl alcohol using the phase-lock gel tubes (Eppendorf), according to manufacturer's instructions. This step can be altered to the user's preference.
15. Add 0.1 vol of 3*M* NaAc and 2.5 vol of 100% ethanol. Incubate 1 h to overnight at –20°C.
16. Spin the tubes at 2000*g* for 5–10 min. Pour off the supernatant. Add 5–10 mL of 70% ethanol. Centrifuge for 5 min at 2000*g*. Pour off the ethanol and air-dry the pellet. Resuspend the pellet in 10 m*M* Tris-HCl, pH 8.0. Rehydrate DNA at 65°C for 1 h (it is very important to keep this incubation to a maximum of 1 h, because it may result in DNA degradation) or overnight at room temperature.

3.6. Random Primer Labeling of Genomic DNA

1. For each test and reference DNA, add 4 μL at a concentration of 25 ng/μL to 41.6 μL of TE buffer, pH 7.4, mix 40 μL with 2.5X random priming mix (random octamer primers) by gentle vortexing, and denature for 10 min at 100°C (*see* **Note 4**).
2. Chill tubes on ice for 10 min.
3. To each tube, add 10 μL of dNTPs, 2.4 μL of Cy3 or Cy5-dCTP (for labeling of test and reference, respectively), and 2 μL of Klenow enzyme (80 U).
4. Incubate at 37°C for 2 h in the dark; then, place tubes on ice.
5. For DNase I digestion, prepare DNase I dilutions and set up reactions strictly on ice. Dilute DNase amp grade 1:20 using DNase dilution buffer (make immediately before use and discard unused portion of the diluted DNase).
6. To each random priming reaction, on ice, add 17 μL of DNase reaction buffer and 3 μL of the 1:20 diluted Amp Grade DNase I. Mix gently by vortexing and quickly spin in a microcentrifuge.
7. Incubate at 15°C for 1 h in the dark; then immediately place tubes on ice and quench reactions with 6 μL of stop buffer; vortex.
8. To each reaction, add 0.1 vol of 3 *M* sodium acetate (12 μL), 1 μL of precipitation reagent, and 2.5 vol of cold (–20°C) 100% ethanol (350 μL); mix by vortexing after adding each reagent.
9. Incubate at –20°C for 1 h.
10. Centrifuge at 16,000*g*, 30 min at 4°C; remove supernatant and air-dry pellets.
11. Resuspend each pellet in 100 μL TE buffer with gentle vortexing.
12. Add 0.1 vol (10 μL) of 3*M* sodium acetate, and 2.5 vol (275 μL) of cold (–20°C) 100% ethanol; vortex briefly.
13. Incubate at –20°C. For best recovery, probes are incubated overnight.
14. Centrifuge at 16,000*g*, 30 min at 4°C; remove supernatant and then air-dry pellets until no visible liquid is present in tube.

15. Resuspend pellets in 4.0 μL of 10 m*M* Tris-HCl, pH 8.0. Be sure that the entire sample is resuspended by carefully washing the walls of the tube thoroughly. To facilitate resuspension, gently vortex and incubate at room temperature for 30 min.
16. Quickly spin the tubes to collect the sample at the bottom of the tube. Probes may be stored at –20°C if not used immediately for a gel analysis or hybridization reaction.
17. Test quality of the labeled DNA by agarose gel electrophoresis: Mix 0.5 μL of a sample with 1 μL of 6X gel-loading buffer and 8.5 μL of water and load on a 2% agarose gel. Use a 50-bp DNA ladder (Life Technologies) as a size marker. The gel may be stained with ethidium bromide before or after the run. If there is no DNA trailing above 200 bp, do not use the probe in array hybridization (*see* **Note 5**).

3.7. Hybridization of Labeled Probe to CGH Microarrays and Posthybridization Wash

1. Prewarm the hybridization buffer to 37°C for 30 min; vortex and spin prior to use to ensure that the solution is uniform. Quickly spin the tube to collect the solution at the bottom of the tube. Hold the hybridization buffer at 37°C until immediately before use (*see* **Note 6**).
2. In a 0.5-mL or 1.5-mL Eppendorf microcentrifuge tube, combine 25 μL of microarray hybridization buffer, 2.5 μL of test DNA probe, and 2.5 μL of reference DNA probe. Vortex and quickly spin the sample (*see* **Note 7**).
3. Place the microcentrifuge tube containing the hybridization mixture into an 80°C water bath and incubate for 10 min to denature the DNA.
4. Remove from the water bath, centrifuge at 12,000*g*–16,000*g* for 5 s and quickly transfer the microcentrifuge tubes containing the hybridization mixture to a 37°C incubator or covered heating block.
5. Incubate in the dark for 1 h.
6. Prewarm microarrays in a 37°C dry-air incubator for 30 min prior to use.
7. Place a paper towel folded in half on the bottom of a sealable (airtight) box. To the bottom of this box, add 16–18 mL of 50% formamide/2X SSC wash solution to saturate the paper towel (a 19 × 16 × 4-cm [7 1/2 × 6 × 1 1/2-inches] Nalgene utility box [cat no. 5700-0500] can be used). Place the box in 37°C dry-air incubator for 30 min to 1 h prior to use.
8. Place prewarmed microarrays on the slide warmer. Remove the tube containing the hybridization solution from the 37°C heating block. Mix gently and quickly spin. Draw the full amount of hybridization mixture into a pipet tip and slowly add the hybridization mixture onto the corner of the array. Be very careful not to touch the pipet tip to the DNA array area or introduce air bubbles (leave the microarray on the slide warmer).
9. Remove lint or dust from the hybridization cover slip (LifterSlip™) using filtered compressed air. Holding the hybridization cover slip at an angle, contact the hybridization solution on the microarray with the painted side of the hybrid-

ization cover slip touching the solution and slowly lower the hybridization cover slip to ensure that no air bubbles are introduced.

10. Place the microarray in prewarmed box in a 37°C incubator.
11. Repeat **steps 5–8** for the remaining microarrays (*see* **Note 8**).
12. Incubate for 60–72 h (*see* **Notes 9** and **10**).
13. Upon the completion of microarray incubation, prepare wash solutions. Label three glass Coplin jars with lids as 1, 2, and 3. Pour approx 50 mL of the 50% 2X SSC/formamide solution in each jar. Pour approx 50 mL of the 1X SSC wash solution into each of four glass Coplin jars with lids. Label the jars 4, 5, 6, and 7 (*see* **Notes 11–13**).
14. Remove microarrays from the 37°C incubator. Using fine-tip forceps, carefully remove the hybridization cover slip from each microarray by grabbing the overhanging edge and gently lifting up. Immediately immerse the microarray in the first 50% 2X SSC/formamide wash at 40°C (Coplin jar 1), agitate briefly, and incubate for 10 min.
15. Agitate each microarray and transfer to the second 50% 2X SSC/formamide wash (Coplin jar 2) at 40°C. Incubate for 10 min.
16. Agitate microarrays and transfer to the third 50% 2X SSC/formamide wash (Coplin jar 3) at 40°C. Incubate for 10 min.
17. Agitate as above and transfer to the first 1X SSC wash at room temperature (Coplin jar 4). Incubate microarrays in Coplin jar 4 for 5 min.
18. Repeat the above procedure for the second, third, and fourth 1X SSC washes at room temperature (Coplin jars 5, 6, and 7). Incubate in each wash for 5 min.
19. After removing array from last wash, rinse in purified H_2O for 1–2 s.
20. Briskly shake chip twice to get rid of the excess water, ensuring that the array area itself remains wet, and immediately apply coverslip containing DAPI mounting solution to the wet chip as described in **step 21** (*see* **Note 14**).
21. Pipet 20 μL of array DAPI solution onto the clean coverslip, turn it over, and carefully place it over the wet microarray. In order to avoid air bubbles, it is best to start at an angle at one side of the microarray and allow it to fall slowly onto the microarray. Store microarray in the dark, preferably in a box with an airtight lid prior to imaging.

4. Notes

1. Average DNA yield from 18 mL of culture is 5 μg when grown in Luria broth. Growing clones in a rich media, such as Terrific Broth, increases the DNA yield; however, the resulting DNA contains more impurities that negatively impact the quality of the print stocks.
2, If working with a large number of clones, multichannel pipettors and microtiter-style PCR plates are recommended for print stock production.
3. Before labeling, the quality of the DNA must be assessed. The DNA should be of high molecular weight and free of protein, RNA, and traces of phenol; the quantity determined by both spectrophotometry and fluorometry should not disagree more than twofold.

4. Because the labeling reaction produces additional copies of DNA, care should be taken to prevent sample contamination with foreign DNA.
5. The optimal probe length ranges from 100 to 2000 bp, with a majority of fragments around 200–800 bp, as assessed on a 2% agarose gel stained with ethidium bromide. Ideally, for best hybridization results, the size distribution of labeled DNA fragments should be comparable to the Cot-1 DNA. Although the random prime labeling protocol described is optimized to yield a specific size of fragments in a given time and temperature, there could be some variation depending on the source of DNA. Different methods of DNA extraction can have an effect on the labeling reaction as a result of variation in the size of fragments and purity of the DNA.
6. Because of the high content of the repetitive sequences present both in the probe and in the target clones on the microarray, hybridization of the labeled probe to microarrays is carried out in the presence of the excess of highly repetitive Cot-1 DNA. Because of the high concentration of Cot-1 DNA in hybridization buffer, the solution may appear cloudy or opalescent. It is extremely important that the hybridization buffer be homogeneous prior to the addition of the labeled probe (i.e., no visible clumps or precipitate). This can be accomplished by thoroughly mixing and prewarming the hybridization buffer to 37°C prior to combining with probes.
7. Labeled probes, dissolved in 4 μL of Tris buffer, could still contain some precipitate or undissolved material. Probes should therefore be microcentrifuged at 12,000*g*–16,000*g* for 1 min prior to combining with the microarray hybridization buffer. When removing the probe from microcentrifuge tubes, avoid any precipitate that may be collected at the bottom of the tube, as this material may produce clumps of probe on a microarray after hybridization.
8. Complete the loading of each individual microarray and place it in the humidified chamber before loading the next one. Do not store microarrays and tubes with hybridization solution at room temperature prior to loading. If multiple hybridizations are to be set up at one time, use a 37°C heating block to hold the tubes.
9. It is very important that the microarray does not dry during any hybridization step. Ensure that the hybridization chamber remains humidified to prevent evaporation of hybridization buffer. Drying of microarrays causes high background, decreased fluorescence, and poor or erroneous results will be obtained.
10. A high signal-to-noise ratio is essential for the detection of single-copy chromosomal gains and losses. In addition to drying, one of the possible causes of the nonspecific background is the use of colored pens (markers) to label microarrays. Certain types of pen or marker may leach off during the hybridization or wash steps, causing aberrant results by producing uneven autofluorescent background in either channel. Scribing of microarrays, or using black VWR markers (no. 52877-140), which do not cause significant background or auto-fluorescence, is recommended.
11. Adequate washing is vital to assay performance. Prior to transferring microarrays

from one bath to the next, agitate the microarray with a back and forth motion (approx 10 times). Do not wash more than five microarrays per Coplin jar. This allows for uniform access of the wash solution to each microarray. Optimally, washes should be done in reduced light if possible because Cy dyes, especially Cy5, are subject to photo bleaching ***(29)***.

12. Store formamide wash solutions covered at 2–8°C between uses and discard after washing 30 microarrays or after 2 wk of storage. If washes have been stored at 4°C, allow them to warm to 40°C in the water bath for approx 30 min. Prior to washing arrays, use a thermometer to check if washes are at 40±1°C. Prepare 1X SSC washes fresh and discard after use. Store stock wash solution (20X SSC) at ambient temperature for no longer than 6 mo.
13. Do not allow the microarrays to dry at any step upon completion of the hybridization, especially between washes (i.e., move chips quickly from one wash to the next). Avoid areas with high airflow when processing arrays. Do not allow chips to dry after the final rinse. As during hybridization, drying of microarrays could result in poor quality data ranging from lower hybridization signal and, consequently, significant loss of sensitivity and specificity, to a complete loss of signal. Mounting solution applied immediately to the chip prior to scanning reduces this quenching effect.
14. When applying the array DAPI solution, it is essential to prevent accumulation of dust particles on the microarray area. Remove any dust or lint from both sides of an 18 × 18-mm coverslip with a folded, lint-free paper tissue, being very careful not to touch the edges of coverslip with the wipes. It is best to use filtered compressed air to adequately remove all dust from the coverslip. Do not tap or squeeze the coverslip, as this may damage the target spots on the microarray surface. Store the array DAPI solution at –20°C in the dark. Allow solution to warm to room temperature prior to pipetting.

References

1. Kallioniemi, A., Kallioniemi, O. P., Sudar, D., et al. (1992) Comparative genomic hybridization for molecular cytogenetic analysis of solid tumors. *Science* **258(5083),** 818–821.
2. Beheshti, B., Park, P. C., Braude, I., et al. (2002) Microarray CGH. *Methods Mol. Biol.* **204,** 191–207.
3. Pinkel, D., Segraves, R., Sudar, D., et al. (1998) High resolution analysis of DNA copy number variation using comparative genomic hybridization to microarrays. *Nature Genet.* **20(2),** 207–211.
4. Courjal, F., Cuny, M., Rodriguez, C., et al. (1996) DNA amplifications at 20q13 and MDM2 define distinct subsets of evolved breast and ovarian tumours. *Br. J. Cancer* **74(12),** 1984–1989.
5. Tanner, M. M., Tirkkonen, M., Kallioniemi, A., et al. (1996) Independent amplification and frequent co-amplification of three nonsyntenic regions on the long arm of chromosome 20 in human breast cancer. *Cancer Res.* **56(15),** 3441–3445.
6. Redon, R., Hussenet, T., Bour, G., et al. (2002) Amplicon mapping and transcrip-

tional analysis pinpoint cyclin L as a candidate oncogene in head and neck cancer. *Cancer Res.* **62(21),** 6211–6217.
7. Kauraniemi, P., Barlund, M., Monni, O., et al. (2001) New amplified and highly expressed genes discovered in the ERBB2 amplicon in breast cancer by cDNA microarrays. *Cancer Res.* **61(22),** 8235–8240.
8. Pollack, J. R., Sorlie, T., Perou, C. M., et al. (2002) Microarray analysis reveals a major direct role of DNA copy number alteration in the transcriptional program of human breast tumors. *Proc. Natl. Acad. Sci. USA* **99(20),** 12,963–12,968.
9. Guo, X., Lui, W. O., Qian, C. N., et al. (2002) Identifying cancer-related genes in nasopharyngeal carcinoma cell lines using DNA and mRNA expression profiling analyses. *Int. J. Oncol.* **21(6),** 1197–1204.
10. Bruder, C. E., Hirvela, C., Tapia-Paez, I., et al. (2001) High resolution deletion analysis of constitutional DNA from neurofibromatosis type 2 (NF2) patients using microarray-CGH. *Hum. Mol. Genet.* **10(3),** 271–282.
11. Wilhelm, M., Veltman, J. A., Olshen, A. B., et al. (2002) Array-based comparative genomic hybridization for the differential diagnosis of renal cell cancer. *Cancer Res.* **62(4),** 957–960.
12. Bielawski, K., Zaczek, A., Lisowska, U., et al. (2001) The suitability of DNA extracted from formalin-fixed, paraffin-embedded tissues for double differential polymerase chain reaction analysis. *Int. J. Mol. Med.* **8(5),** 573–578.
13. Ghazvini, S., Char, D. H., Kroll, S., et al. (1996) Comparative genomic hybridization analysis of archival formalin-fixed paraffin-embedded uveal melanomas. *Cancer Genet. Cytogenet.* **90(2),** 95–101.
14. Daigo, Y., Chin, S. F., Gorringe, K. L., et al. (2001) Degenerate oligonucleotide primed-polymerase chain reaction-based array comparative genomic hybridization for extensive amplicon profiling of breast cancers : a new approach for the molecular analysis of paraffin-embedded cancer tissue. *Am. J. Pathol.* **158(5),** 1623–1631.
15. Srinivasan, M., Sedmak, D., and Jewell, S. (2002) Effect of fixatives and tissue processing on the content and integrity of nucleic acids. *Am. J. Pathol.* **161(6),** 1961–1971.
16. Mikulowska-Mennis, A., Taylor, T. B., Vishnu, P., et al. (2002) High-quality RNA from cells isolated by laser capture microdissection. Biotechniques **33(1)**, 176–179.
17. Cai, W.W., Mao, J. H., Chow, C. W., et al. (2002) Genome-wide detection of chromosomal imbalances in tumors using BAC microarrays. *Nature Biotechnol.* **20(4),** 393–396.
18. Snijders, A. M., Nowak, N., Segraves, R., et al. (2001) Assembly of microarrays for genome-wide measurement of DNA copy number. *Nature Genet.* **29(3),** 263–264.
19. Kraus, J., Pantel, K., Pinkel, D., et al. (2003) High-resolution genomic profiling of occult micrometastatic tumor cells. *Genes Chromosomes Cancer* **36(2),** 159–166.
20. Wessendorf, S., Fritz, B., Wrobel, G., et al. (2002) Automated screening for

genomic imbalances using matrix-based comparative genomic hybridization. *Lab. Invest.* **82(1),** 47–60.

21. Pollack, J. R., Perou, C. M., Alizadeh, A. A., et al. (1999) Genome-wide analysis of DNA copy-number changes using cDNA microarrays. *Nature Genet.* **23(1),** 41–46.
22. Trask, B. and Pinkel, D. (1990) Fluorescence in situ hybridization with DNA probes. *Methods Cell Biol.* **33,** 383–400.
23. Schermer, M. (1999) Confocal scanning microscopy in microarray detection, in *DNA Microarrays: A Practical Approach* (Schena, M., ed.), Oxford University Press, Oxford, pp. 17–42.
24. Che, D., Bao, Y., and Muller, U. R. (2001) Novel surface and multicolor charge coupled device-based fluorescent imaging system for DNA microarrays. *J. Biomed. Opt.* **6(4),** 450–456.
25. Mace, M. L., Rose, S. D., and McGuinness, G. (2000) Novel microarray printing and detection technology, in *Microarray Biochip Technology* (Schena, M., ed.), Eaton, Natick, MA, pp. 39–64.
26. Holloway, A. J., van Laar, R. K., Tothill, R. W., et al. (2002) Options available—from start to finish—for obtaining data from DNA microarrays II. *Nature Genet.* **32(Suppl.)** 481–489.
27. Jain, A. N., Tokuyasu, T. A., Snijders, A. M., et al. (2002) Fully automatic quantification of microarray image data. *Genome Res.* **12(2),** 325–332.
28. Saal, L. H., Troein, C., Vallon-Christersson, J., et al. (2002) BioArray Software Environment (BASE): a platform for comprehensive management and analysis of microarray data. *Genome Biol.* **3(8),** software0003.1–0003.6.p.
29. Buschmann, V., Weston, K. D., and Sauer, M. (2003) Spectroscopic study and evaluation of red-absorbing fluorescent dyes. *Bioconjug. Chem.* **14(1),** 195–204.

26

Tissue Microarrays

Ronald Simon, Martina Mirlacher, and Guido Sauter

1. Introduction

The rate of discovery of new genes involved in cancer and other diseases has increased heavily. The demand for analyses of these new genes in diseased tissues, especially human tumors, has grown at the same pace. To identify the most significant ones among all the emerging candidate cancer genes, it is often necessary to analyze a high number of genes in a high number of well-characterized tumors. Hundreds of tumors must be analyzed for each gene to generate statistically meaningful results. This leads to a massive workload in involved laboratories. Moreover, the analysis of multiple genes results in a critical loss of precious tissue material because of the number of conventional tissue sections that can be taken from a tumor block does usually not exceed 200–300. The tissue microarray (TMA) technology does significantly facilitate and accelerate tissue analyses by *in situ* technologies ***(1,2)***. In this method, minute tissue cylinders (diameter: 0.6 mm) are removed from hundreds of different primary tumor blocks and subsequently brought into one empty "recipient" paraffin block. Sections from such array blocks can then be used for simultaneous *in situ* analysis of hundreds to thousands of primary tumors on the DNA, RNA, and protein level. The TMA technique has a number of advantages as compared to the "sausage" block technique that was introduced more than 10 yr ago ***(3)***. The cylindrical shape and the small diameter of the specimen taken out of the donor block maximizes the number of samples that can be taken out of one donor block and minimizes tissue damage. The latter is important for pathologists because they can now give researchers access to their material and, at the same time, retain their tissue blocks. Punched tissue blocks remain fully interpretable for all morphological and molecular analyses that may subsequently become necessary, provided that the number of punches is reason-

From: *Methods in Molecular Medicine, vol. 97: Molecular Diagnosis of Cancer*
Edited by: J. E. Roulston and J. M. S. Bartlett © Humana Press Inc., Totowa, NJ

ably selected. Dozens of punches can be taken from one tumor without compromising interpretability.

Virtually all tissues are suitable to place into a TMA. Therefore, the range of TMA applications is very broad. One of the most distinct advantages of TMAs is that one set of tissues (which has been reviewed by one pathologist) with available clinical data can now be used for an almost unlimited number of studies. The TMA technique is not at all limited to cancer research, although this has been the predominant application to date. Typical TMAs used in cancer research include multitumor, progression, and prognostic arrays.

Multitumor TMAs are composed of samples from multiple tumor types. These arrays are utilized to screen different tumor types for molecular alterations of interest. For example, the largest multitumor TMA constructed by our group is distributed among 10 TMA blocks and contains 4788 tissue samples obtained from 129 different tumor types, 354 normal tissues, and 709 metastatic cancers. Sections from this TMA are now utilized in multiple studies to comprehensively analyze normal and neoplastic human tissues.

Progression TMAs have been used to study molecular alterations in different stages of one particular tumor type ***(1,4–6)***. For example, an ideal prostate cancer progression TMA would contain samples from either normal prostate or benign prostatic hyperplasia (BPH), prostatic intraepithelial neoplasia (PIN), incidental carcinomas (stage pT1), organ-confined carcinomas (pT2), carcinomas with extraprostatic growth (pT3–4), as well as metastases and recurrences after androgen-withdrawal treatment. TMAs are also suited to study progression within tumors. TMAs can easily include large numbers of pairs of primary tumors and their noninvasive precursor lesions, metastases, or recurrences after specific treatment. In our laboratory, we have constructed a TMA composed of tissues from 196 node-positive breast carcinomas. From each tumor, one sample was taken from the primary tumor and from each of three different metastases. Together with samples from 196 node-negative breast carcinomas, this "breast cancer metastasis TMA" contains almost 1000 tissue samples. In a recent study, we used this array to demonstrate a high concordance in the HER-2 amplification/overexpression between primary tumors and their nodal metastases ***(7)***.

Prognosis TMAs contain samples from tumors for which clinical follow-up data are available. As a proof of principle, these TMAs have been used to re-evaluate molecular alterations with known prognostic significance. Associations with prognosis were found on TMAs for ER, PR, and p53 positivity in breast cancer ***(8)***, cyclin E expression and Ki67 LI in urinary bladder cancer ***(4,9)***, and vimentin expression in kidney cancer ***(10)***. These data show that associations between molecular changes and clinical end points can be detected on TMAs containing just one single specimen per tumor, especially if the number of tumors included in a TMA is large.

Other TMA applications are obvious but have not been largely exploited yet. For example, the normal expression pattern of gene products can optimally be tested on TMAs containing all kinds of normal tissue. As for patient tissues, TMAs can be used for cell lines ***(11)*** and other experimental tissues such as xenograft tumors or tissues from animal models. TMAs are also ideal for organizing large tissue repositories or for studies investigating the impact of different fixations on staining procedures.

2. Materials

2.1. Sample Collection

1. Standard routine histology microscope for review of tissue sections.
2. Colored pens to mark representative areas on the slides (e.g., red for tumor, blue for normal, and black for premalignant lesions).
3. Sufficient working space; especially for large-scale projects that require extensive sorting of thousands of sections and blocks.

2.1.2. Preparing Recipient Blocks

1. Peel-A-Way Embedding Paraffin Pellets; melting point: 56–58°C (Polysciences Inc., PA, USA).
2. Slotted processing/embedding cassettes for routine histology (e.g., Electron Microscopy Sciences Inc., PA, USA; cat. no. 70070).
3. Stainless-steel base molds for processing/embedding systems (e.g., Electron Microscopy Sciences Inc.; cat. no. 62510-30).
4. Filter/filter papers.
5. Oven for melting paraffin (70°C).

2.1.3. TMA Making

1. Tissue arrayer (currently there are two commercial vendors for tissue arrayers (websites: http://www.beecherinstruments.com and http://www.chemicon.com) and supplies.
2. Premanufactured empty paraffin-recipient blocks.
3. Illuminated magnifying lenses and supplies (e.g., Luxo U wave II/70; Luxo Inc., Switzerland; cat. no. 27950) (optional).

2.1.4. TMA Sectioning

1. Standard routine histology microtome and supplies (e.g., Leica Microsystems Inc., IL, USA; Leica SM2400).
2. Slide label printer (e.g., DAKO Seymour glass slide labeling system; DAKO A/S, Denmark; product code S3416) or special slide marker (e.g., Securline Marker II, Precision Dynamics Corporation, CA, USA).

3. Boxes for slide storage.
4. Refrigerator for slide storage.
5. Paraffin Sectioning Aid-System (Instrumedics Inc., NJ, USA; cat. no. PSA) containing ultraviolet curing lamp, adhesive-coated PSA Slides, TPC solvent, TPC solvent can, hand roller, tape windows (optional).

2.1.5. TMAs From Frozen Tissues

1. Tissue arrayer and supplies (*see* **Subheading 3.1.3.**).
2. OCT Tissue-Tek compound embedding medium (Sakura BV, The Netherlands).
3. Dry ice to keep punching needles and recipient block in optimal cooled condition.
4. Freezer for frozen tissue storage (–70°C).

3. Methods

3.1. TMA Manufacturing

3.1.1. Sample Collection

Although a device is needed to manufacture TMAs, it must be understood that most of the work (approx 95%) is traditional pathology work that cannot be accelerated by improved (i.e., automated) tissue arrayers. This preparatory work is similar to what is needed for traditional studies involving "large" tissue sections. The major difference is the number of tissues involved, which can be an order of magnitude higher in TMA studies than in traditional projects. The different tasks related to sample collection are as follows:

1. Define exactly the TMA to be made (often TMA users realize that one critical control tissue has been forgotten only after completion of the TMA block). Include normal tissues of the organ of interest and—if possible—of a selection of other organs as well.
2. Generate a list of potentially suited tissues.
3. Collect all slides from these tumors from the archive.
4. One pathologist must review all sections from all candidate specimens to select the optimal slide. If possible, tumors should be reclassified at that stage according to current classification schemes and tissue areas suited for subsequent punching should be marked. Different colors are recommended for marking different areas on one section (e.g., red for tumor, black for carcinoma *in situ*, blue for normal tissue). It is advisable to have a freshly hematoxylin and eosin (H&E)-stained section if the actual block surface is not well reflected on the available stained section.
5. Collect the tissue blocks that correspond to the selected slides.
6. These blocks and their corresponding marked slides must be matched and sorted in the order of appearance on the TMA.
7. Define the structure (outline) of the TMA and compose a file that contains the identification numbers of the tissues together with their locations and real coor-

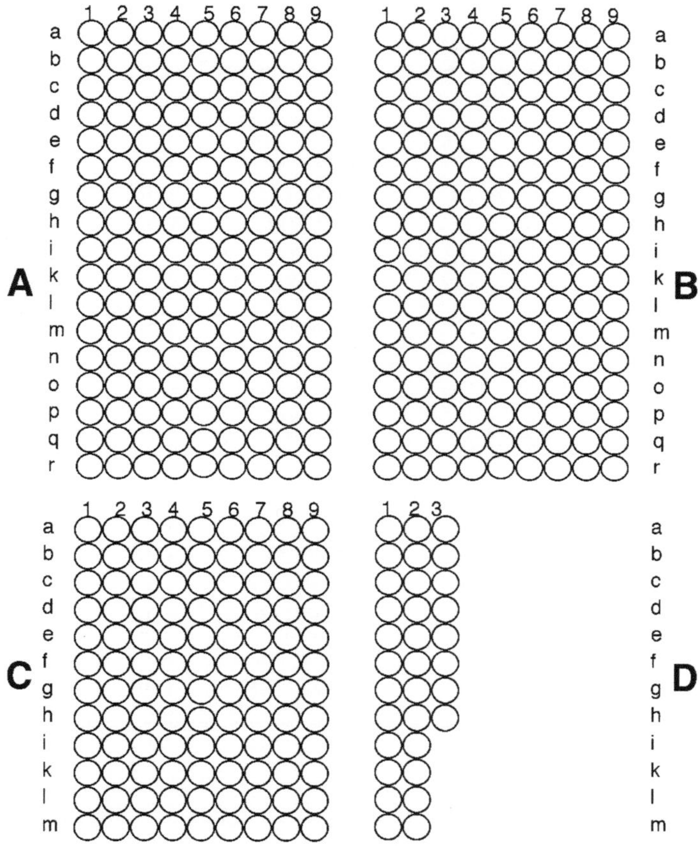

Fig. 1. A TMA outline example. The TMA has been divided into four subsections to facilitate navigation during microscopy.

dinates (as they need to be selected on the arraying device). A distance between the individual samples of 0.2 mm is recommended. To facilitate navigation on the TMA, we recommend arranging the tissues in multiple sections (e.g., quadrants). The distance between the quadrants may be 0.8 mm. For unequivocal identification of individual samples on TMA slides, it is important to avoid a fully symmetrical TMA structure. In most laboratories, capitalized letters define quadrants, whereas small letters and numbers define the coordinates within these quadrants. Examples of a TMA structure (outline) and data file containing the necessary information for making a TMA are given in **Fig. 1** and **Table 1**.

3.1.2. Preparing Recipient Blocks

In contrast to normal paraffin blocks, tissue microarray blocks are cut at room temperature. Therefore, a special type of paraffin is needed with a melting temperature between 55°C and 58°C (Peel-A-Way paraffin; *see* **Subheading 2.1.2.**).

Table 1
Example File for TMA Construction

loc	coord	loc	coord	loc	coord
A 1a	0/0	A 2a	0/800	A 3a	0/1600
A 1b	800/0	A 2b	800/800	A 3b	800/1600
A 1c	1,600/0	A 2c	1,600/800	A 3c	1,600/1600
A 1d	2,400/0	A 2d	2,400/800	A 3d	2,400/1600
A 1e	3,200/0	A 2e	3,200/800	A 3e	3,200/1600
A 1f	4,000/0	A 2f	4,000/800	A 3f	4,000/1600
A 1g	4,800/0	A 2g	4,800/800	A 3g	4,800/1600
A 1h	5,600/0	A 2h	5,600/800	A 3h	5,600/1600
A 1i	6,400/0	A 2i	6,400/800	A 3i	6,400/1600
A 1k	7,200/0	A 2k	7,200/800	A 3k	7,200/1600
A 1l	8,000/0	A 2l	8,000/800	A 3l	8,000/1600
A 1m	8,800/0	A 2m	8,800/800	A 3m	8,800/1600
A 1n	9,600/0	A 2n	9,600/800	A 3n	9,600/1600
A 1o	10,400/0	A 2o	10,400/800	A 3o	10,400/1600
A 1p	11,200/0	A 2p	11,200/800	A 3p	11,200/1600
A 1q	12,000/0	A 2q	12,000/800	A 3q	12,000/1600
A 1r	12,800/0	A 2r	12,800/800	A 3r	12,800/1600

1. The paraffin is melted at 60°C, filtered, and poured in a stainless-steel mold.
2. A slotted plastic embedding cassette (as used in every histology lab) is then placed on the top of the warm paraffin.
3. Recipient paraffin blocks are then cooled down for 2 h at room temperature and for an additional 2 h at 4°C. Blocks are then removed from the mold. It is important not to cool down the paraffin on a cooling plate because of the risk of block damage.
4. Quality check of the recipient blocks is important because they must not contain air bubbles.

Large recipient blocks (e.g., 30 × 45 × 10 mm) are easier to handle than the small blocks (e.g., 25–35 × 5 mm) that are typically used in routine histology labs.

3.1.3. TMA Making

Only if all of this preparatory work has been done can a tissue-arraying device be employed. Two different tissue-arraying systems are now commercially available (*see* **Subheading 3.1.3.**). Using these manually operated devices, excellent TMAs can be produced in the hands of a talented and experienced person. However, optimal arrays can be expected only after a significant training period, mostly including several hundred, if not a few thousand, punches. A patient and enduring personality as well as keen eyesight are important prerequisites for operators of the manual tissue arrayers. Early-generation automated tissue arrayers are available, but these devices are very expensive and do not accelerate the TMA manufacturing process.

The TMA manufacturing process consists of four steps that are repeated for each sample placed on the TMA:

1. Punching a hole in an empty (recipient) paraffin block.
2. Removing and discarding the wax cylinder from the needle used for recipient block punching.
3. Removing a cylindrical sample from a donor paraffin block.
4. Placing the cylindrical tissue sample in the premade hole in the recipient block.

Exact positioning of the tip of the tissue cylinder at the level of the recipient block surface is crucial for the quality and the yield of the TMA block. Placing the tissue too deeply into the recipient block results in empty spots in the first sections taken from the TMA block. Positioning the tissue cylinder not deep enough causes empty spots in the last sections taken from this TMA. However, a too superficial location of the tissue cylinder is less problematic than a too deep position because protruding tissue elements can, to some extent, be leveled out after finishing the punching process. The use of a magnifying lens facilitates precise deposition of samples, especially for beginners.

As soon as all tissue elements are filled into the recipient block, the block is heated at 40°C for 10 min. Protruding tissue cylinders are then gently pressed deeper into the warmed TMA block using a glass slide.

3.1.4. Array Sectioning

Regular microtome sections may be taken from TMA blocks using standard microtomes. However, the more samples a TMA block contains, the more difficult regular cutting becomes. As a consequence, the number of slides of inadequate quality increases with the size of the TMA, and, in turn, fewer sections from the TMA block can effectively be analyzed.

Using a tape-sectioning kit (Instrumedics) facilitates cutting and leads to highly regular nondistorted sections (ideal for automated analysis). In addition, the tape system may prevent arrayed samples from floating off the slide if very harsh pretreatment methods are used. However, the sticky, glued slides have the disadvantage of increased background signals between the tissue spots in immunohistochemistry (IHC) analyses. The tissue samples themselves do not show increased nonspecific background in IHC. The use of the tape-sectioning system is as follows:

1. Adhesive tape is placed on the TMA block in the microtome immediately before cutting.
2. A 3- to 5-µm section is cut. The tissue slice is now adhering to the tape.
3. The tissue slice is placed on a special "glued" slide (stretching of the tissue in a water bath or on a heating plate is not necessary).
4. The slide (tissue on the bottom) is then placed under ultraviolet (UV) light for 35 s. This leads to polymerization of the glue on the slide and on the tape.
5. Slides are placed into TPC solution (Instrumedics) at room temperature for 5–10 s. The tape can then be gently removed from the glass slide. The tissue remains on the slide.
6. Slides are dried at room temperature.

3.1.5. TMAs From Frozen Tissues

Recently, Fejzo and Slamon reported manufacturing of TMAs from frozen tissues using a commercially available tissue array device ***(12)***. Both commercially available arrayers can be utilized for frozen TMA making.

1. Recipient blocks are made from OCT that is frozen down in a Tissue-Tek standard cryomold. The resulting OCT block is mounted on top of a plastic biopsy cassette. As long as the recipient OCT block is sized exactly like a paraffin-recipient block (for which the arrayer had been constructed), no modifications of the arrayer were necessary to mount the block.
2. The recipient block must be surrounded with dry ice to prevent melting.
3. Tissue biopsies (diameter: 0.6 mm; height: 4–5 mm) are then punched from OCT-embedded tumor tissues and placed into the recipient OTC array block using a commercial tissue microarrayer. There are four main differences as compared to the procedure described for paraffin blocks.

   a. The same needle is utilized for making a hole in the recipient array block and for collecting the core biopsies. Switching to a larger needle is not necessary.
   b. It is important to keep the tissue in the needle frozen during the procedure. This can be done by precooling the needle with a piece of dry ice before punching and while dispensing the tissue core into the recipient block.
   c. Needles may easily bend or break. Therefore, punching and coring must be performed slowly with minimal pressure to prevent needle breakage.
   d. The frozen TMAs become more irregular and distorted than TMAs from formalin-fixed material. In fact, the commercially available arrayers have not been designed for making frozen arrays. Therefore, a larger space between samples is recommended (e.g., 1 mm).

4. Then 4- to 10-µm sections of the whole block are cut from the array block. A cryostat microtome (Microm GmbH, Germany) can be used with or without the Basic CryoJane Tape Transfer System and slides (Instrumedics).

3.2. TMA Analysis

3.2.1. General Considerations

TMAs are suited for all types of *in situ* analysis methods including IHC, fluorescence *in situ* hybridization (FISH), and RNA *in situ* hybridization (RNA-ISH). All protocols that can be used on large sections will also work on TMAs. Examples of stained TMA sections are shown in **Fig. 2**. The most significant difference as compared to traditional large-section studies is the high level of standardization that can be achieved in TMA experiments. All slides of one TMA study are usually incubated in one set of reagents, assuring absolutely identical concentrations, temperatures, and incubation times. Other minor variables that may have an impact on the outcome of *in situ* analyses, such as the age of a slide (time between sectioning and use) or section thickness, are also fully standardized, as long as all tissues of one study are located on the same TMA section. As a result of this unprecedented standardization within each experiment, surprising interassay variations can occur if experiments are repeated under slightly different conditions. Often, these variations alter the threshold for detection of positivity, thus affecting the overall frequency of positive cases. In contrast, associations between examined parameters and clinico-pathological data are usually retained unchanged, because all groups within one TMA (low and high stage, good and bad prognosis) are equally affected by experimental variations. Large numbers of samples on a TMA, however, markedly increase the likelihood of finding significant associations, especially in case of suboptimal IHC or RNA-ISH.

3.2.2. Immunohistochemistry

In general, the same rules apply for IHC analysis on TMA as on large sections. The small size of the arrayed tissues on a TMA facilitates the staining interpretation because predefined criteria can be applied to a well-defined tissue area. This reduces interobserver variation of IHC interpretation.

For many immunohistochemical tumor analyses, the following information can be recorded:

a. Percentage of positive cells
b. Staining intensity (0, 1+, 2+, 3+)
c. Subcellular localization of the staining (membraneous, cytoplasmatic, nuclear)
d. Tissue localization of the staining (tumor cells, stroma, vessels)

For statistical analyses, tumors can be classified into three or four groups based on the percentage of positive cells and the staining intensity:

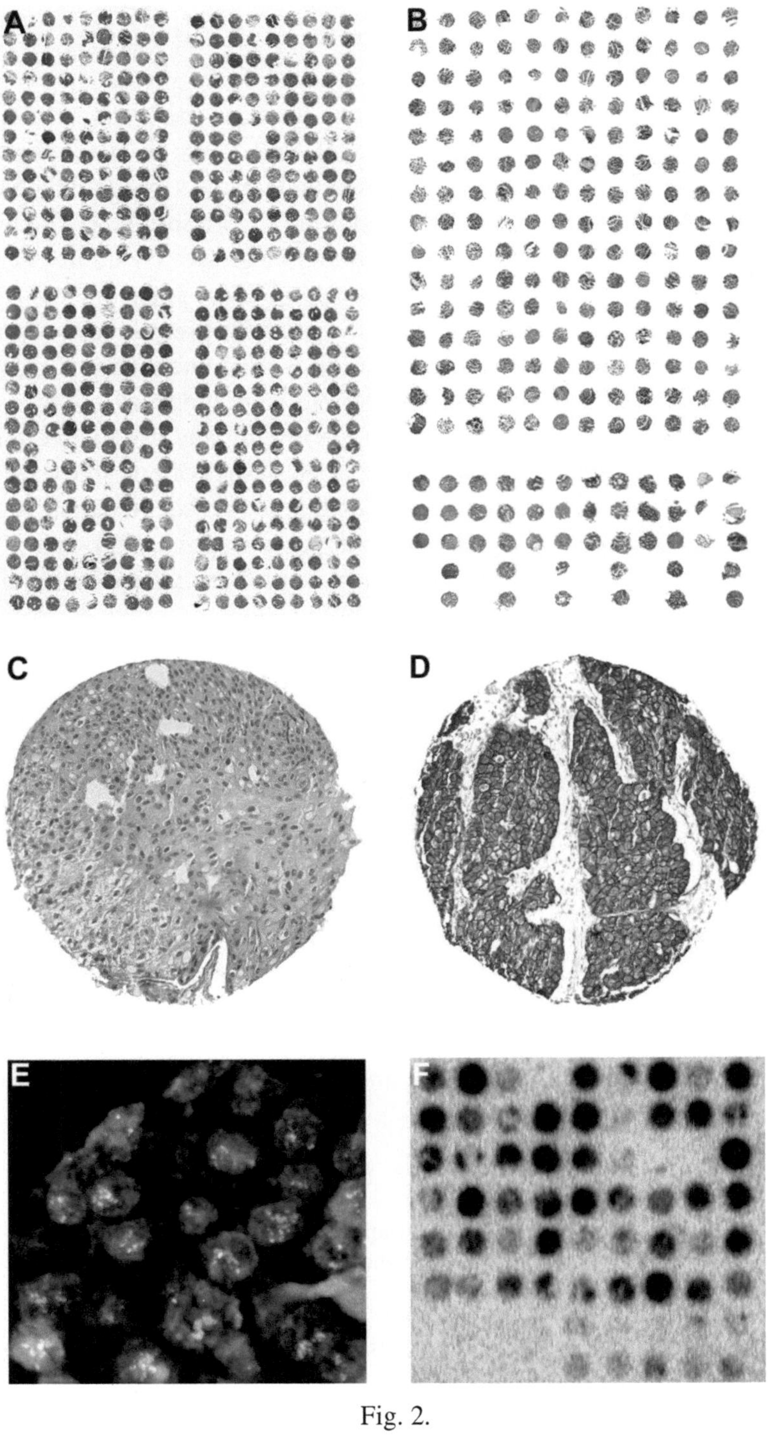

Fig. 2.

Negative:	No staining
Weak positivity:	1+ in 1–100% or 2+ in ≤20% of cells
Moderate positivity:	2+ in 21–79% or 3+ in ≤30% of cells
Strong positivity:	2+ in ≥80% or 3+ in >30 of cells

Some of the arrayed tissues may show false-negative or inappropriately weak IHC staining intensity as a result of variations in tissue processing (e.g., fixation medium and time). The large number of tissues included in a TMA will often compensate for this phenomenon, which is also encountered in large-section IHC analyses. At least a fraction of tissue spots yielding false-negative IHC staining results can be identified in control experiments assessing the antigen integrity of the samples (e.g., IHC detection of tissue-type-specific antigens like cytokeratins or vimentin). For tissues with a reasonable proliferative activity, Ki67 (MIB1) is an optimal quality control antibody. MIB1, which must lead to strong staining in all mitoses, is often falsely negative in suboptimally processed tissues.

It is highly recommended to use freshly cut sections for IHC analysis. The time-span between sectioning and immunostaining should be less than 2 wk. Studies have shown that staining intensity decreases significantly with time for many antibodies ***(13,14)***.

3.2.3. FISH

Because biopsies are all treated individually at the time when they are removed, fixed, and subsequently paraffin embedded, one must expect a certain degree of heterogeneity with respect to protein and nuclear acid preservation. The truth of this assumption is best illustrated in the outcome of FISH

Fig. 2. *(opposite page)* Examples of stained-tissue sections. H&E-stained sections of **(A)** a TMA from formalin-fixed, paraffin-embedded tissues containing 540 tissue spots and **(B)** a TMA from frozen tissue containing 228 tissue spots. Each tissue spot measures 0.6 mm in diameter. Missing samples result from the sectioning/staining process or indicate samples that are already exhausted. Note that the spot-to-spot distance is larger on the frozen TMA as compared to the paraffin TMA. **(C)** Magnification of a H&E-stained 0.6-mm tissue spot of a bladder carcinoma. **(D)** Immunohistochemistry against the Her2/neu protein in a breast cancer sample using the DAKO HercepTest. **(E)** FISH analysis of centromere 11 (green signals) and the cyclin D1 gene (red spots) in cell nuclei (blue staining) of a tissue spot (×630). The high number of cyclin D1 signals indicates a gene amplification. **(F)** RNA *in situ* hybridization on a frozen TMA made from normal and malignant kidney tissues. A radioactively labeled oligonucleotide was used as a probe against vimentin mRNA. The black staining intensity indicates the level of mRNA in each tissue spot.

analyses. As in large-section studies, TMA FISH analyses yield interpretable results in only about 60–90% of the analyzed tumors (depending on the quality and size of the FISH probe) at the first attempt.

Again, as in large-section studies, it is possible to achieve interpretability in a fraction of initially noninformative cases by changing experimental conditions. For example, an increased proteinase concentration for slide pretreatment will result in interpretable signals in some initially noninformative cases at the cost of overdigestion of some previously interpretable samples. In general, we do not attempt to improve the fraction of FISH-informative cases by changing experimental conditions. Because of the high number of tumors on our TMAs (usually >500), we tolerate a fraction of noninterpretable tumors rather than using too many precious TMA sections for additional experiments.

3.2.4. RNA-ISH

The question of whether RNA-ISH analysis can be reliably done on sections from archival tissue is disputed. Laboratories that feel confident in doing RNA-ISH analyses on formalin-fixed sections will also be able to execute such analyses on TMAs using the same protocols that are successful on large sections. As in IHC analysis, control experiments to detect expression of housekeeping genes (e.g., β-actin, GAPDH) may be performed to estimate the degree of RNA preservation in the different spots of a TMA, thus allowing exclusion of critical tissues from analysis. Alternatively, TMAs from frozen tissues may be utilized, especially for RNA quantification experiments. RNA-ISH yields reliable results because of the superior RNA preservation compared to formalin-fixed tissues.

4. Summary

The TMA methodology is now an established and frequently used tool for tissue analysis. The equipment is affordable and easy to use in places where basic skills in histology are available. Basically, all kinds of *in situ* analysis, like IHC, *in situ* hybridization, and *in situ* PCR assays may be adapted to TMAs with only slight (if any) modifications of the respective large-section protocols.

References

1. Kononen, J., Bubendorf, L., Kallioniemi, A., et al. (1998) Tissue microarrays for high-throughput molecular profiling of hundreds of specimens. *Nature Med.* **4,** 844–847.
2. Bubendorf, L., Kononen, J., Koivisto, P., et al. (1999) Survey of gene amplifications during prostate cancer progression by high-throughout fluorescence *in situ* hybridization on tissue microarrays. *Cancer Res.* **59,** 803–806.

3. Battifora, H. (1986) The multitumor (sausage) tissue block: novel method for immunohistochemical antibody testing. *Lab. Invest.* **55,** 244–248.
4. Richter, J., Wagner, U., Kononen, J., et al. High-throughput tissue microarray analysis of cyclin E gene amplification and overexpression in urinary bladder cancer. *Am. J. Pathol.*, **157,** 787–794.
5. Bubendorf, L., Kolmer, M., Kononen, J., et al. (1999) Molecular mechanisms of hormone therapy failure in human prostate cancer analyzed by a combination of cDNA and tissue microarrays. *J. Natl. Cancer Inst.* **91,** 1758–1764.
6. Bubendorf, L., Kononen, J., Koivisto, P., et al. (1999) Survey of gene amplifications during prostate cancer progression by high-throughput fluorescence *in situ* hybridization on tissue microarrays. *Cancer Res.* **59,** 803–806.
7. Simon, R., Nocito, A., Hübscher, et al. Patterns of HER-2/amplification in primary and metastatic breast cancer, *J. Natl. Cancer Inst.* **93,** 1141–1146.
8. Torhorst, J., Bucher, C., Kononen, J., et al. (2001) Tissue microarrays for rapid linking of molecular changes to clinical endpoints. *Am. J. Pathol.* **159,** 2249–2256.
9. Nocito, A., Bubendorf, L., Tinner, E. M., et al. High representativity of proliferation assessment and histologic grading on bladder cancer tissue microarrays. *J. Pathol.*, submitted.
10. Moch, H., Schraml, P., Bubendorf, L., et al. (1999) High-throughput tissue microarray analysis to evaluate the significance of genes uncovered by cDNA microarray screening in renal cell carcinoma. *Am. J. Pathol.* **154,** 981–986.
11. Simon, R., Struckmann, K., Schraml, P., et al. (2002) Amplification pattern of 12q13-q15 genes (MDM2, CDK4, GLI) in urinary bladder cancer. *Oncogene* **21,** 2476–2483.
12. Fejzo, M. S. and Slamon, D. J. (2001) Frozen tumor tissue microarray technology for analysis of tumor RNA, DNA, and proteins. *Am. J. Pathol.* **159,** 1645–1650.
13. Bertheau, P., Cazals-Hatem, D., Meignin, V., et al. (1998) Variability of immunohistochemical reactivity on stored paraffin slides. *J. Clin. Pathol.* **51,** 370–374.
14. Jacobs, T. W., Prioleau, J. E., Stillman, I. E., and Schnitt, S. J. (1996) Loss of tumor marker-immunostaining intensity on stored paraffin slides of breast cancer. *J. Natl. Cancer Inst.* ***88,*** 1054–1059.

Index

MIX
Papier aus verantwortungsvollen Quellen
Paper from responsible sources
FSC® C105338

If you have any concerns about our products,
you can contact us on
ProductSafety@springernature.com

In case Publisher is established outside the EU,
the EU authorized representative is:
Springer Nature Customer Service Center GmbH
Europaplatz 3, 69115 Heidelberg, Germany

Printed by Libri Plureos GmbH
in Hamburg, Germany